BIPOLAR DISORDER

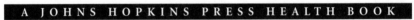
A JOHNS HOPKINS PRESS HEALTH BOOK

FRANCIS MARK MONDIMORE, M.D.

Bipolar Disorder

A Guide for Patients and Families

Second Edition

THE JOHNS HOPKINS UNIVERSITY PRESS   BALTIMORE

NOTE TO THE READER. This book is not meant to substitute for medical care of people with bipolar disorder or depression, and treatment should not be based solely on its contents. Nor is it meant to offer legal advice, which must be obtained from a practicing attorney.

The Johns Hopkins University Press
2715 North Charles Street
Baltimore, Maryland 21218-4363
www.press.jhu.edu

LIBRARY OF CONGRESS CATALOGING-IN-PUBLICATION DATA
Mondimore, Francis Mark, 1953–
    Bipolar disorder : a guide for patients and families / Francis Mark Mondimore. — 2nd ed.
    p. ; cm.
    Includes bibliographical references and index.
    ISBN 0-8018-8313-X (alk. paper) — ISBN 0-8018-8314-8 (pbk. : alk. paper).
    1. Manic-depressive illness—Popular works.   2. Affective disorders—
    Popular works.   I. Title.
       [DNLM: 1. Bipolar Disorder—Popular Works.   2. Bipolar Disorder—therapy—
    Popular Works.   WM 207 M741b 2006]
    RC516.M64   2006
    616.89′5—DC22   2005021215

A catalog record for this book is available from the British Library.

Figures 2-1, 2-4, 2-5, 5-1, 5-2, 6-1, 10-1, 16-3, and 16-4 by Jacqueline Schaffer

Contents

Preface

About 2 percent of the population suffers from some form of bipolar disorder. Winston Churchill, George Frederick Handel, Lord Byron, Virginia Woolf, Edgar Allan Poe, Napoleon Bonaparte, and Vincent van Gogh are only a few of the politicians, writers, artists, and musicians who, despite having bipolar disorder, left a mark of greatness upon the world.[1] Most persons who are affected by this illness, however, are ordinary people who want nothing more than to get back to their everyday lives after they or their family members have been diagnosed with it. This book is written for them.

We psychiatrists have at times become a little complacent about this disease. When lithium became widely available in the United States in the mid-1970s, many psychiatrists thought that the battle to control the illness had been won. Indeed, lithium was—and still is—a miracle drug for many of those who suffer from what was then known as "manic-depression." More recent studies, however, indicate that a substantial proportion of patients have a relapse of their illness despite taking lithium—according to some studies,[2] as many as half. But even as we become more aware of the sobering facts about the difficulty of successfully treating this illness, an explosion of developments in science and medicine is occurring that holds great promise for those affected by the disease. In this book I shall relate this good news.

Clinical research has shown again and again that many relapses of bipolar disorder occur not because of medication failure, but rather because patients stop taking medication and drop out of treatment. Perhaps patients don't understand that relapse and repetition of illness episodes are the hallmark of the illness, that *abruptly* stopping medication has been shown to be especially risky, that medication side effects can often be treated or controlled, and that new medications are becoming available all the time. I hope this book helps those who face difficult treatment decisions to make well-informed and intelligent choices.

A survey of patients with bipolar disorder and other mood disorders done by the National Depressive and Manic-Depressive Association in the early 1990s found that 36 percent of those who responded to the questionnaire did not seek professional treatment until more than *ten years* after their symptoms began.[3] Seventy-three percent of the bipolar patients in this study had received at least one incorrect diagnosis before being identified as having bipolar disorder—often many years after they had first sought help. The average respondent had seen 3.3 physicians before being correctly diagnosed. Why is this illness so difficult to identify correctly? One reason is that full-blown manic-depressive illness is only one of the several forms this chameleon disorder can take—and may in fact be less common than the milder forms (the so-called soft bipolar disorders). We are realizing that many patients with these milder forms of the disorder benefit from treatment with mood-stabilizing medications, too. But they can do so only if treatment is sought and the correct diagnosis is made. We shall see why many patients who have a bipolar disorder are labeled "neurotic" or receive a diagnosis of a "personality disorder." Another purpose of this book is to spread the word that symptoms of mild depression and subtle "mood swings" may be the only manifestations of a mild form of bipolar disorder that can be effectively treated.

Like any other serious illness, bipolar disorder affects not only the person who suffers from the disease but family, friends, and colleagues as well. Family support is crucial to the effective management of symptoms. The disrupted relationships and interpersonal conflicts that the symptoms of the illness can cause make bipolar disorder all the more difficult and complicated to treat. Information and understanding are part of the treatment for this disease too, and this book was written not only with the patient in mind but for his or her family and friends as well.

Bipolar disorder can be a fatal disease. Although the figures vary among studies, about 15 percent of persons with bipolar disorder commit suicide;[4] many more make suicide attempts. These are preventable deaths, because very effective treatments for this illness exist. I hope that the information this book provides about the treatment of bipolar disorder addresses some of the reasons why individuals are reluctant to enter treatment and dissuades some from stopping treatment against medical advice. Yes, it is my hope that this book will save lives.

Acknowledgments

I wish to thank those who have contributed to this project. Thanks to Robert Bright, M.D., Charles Casat, M.D., Rhonda Crow, Caroline Gretick, Sallie Mink of the Depression and Related Affective Disorders Association (DRADA) at Johns Hopkins, and Jenny Rosenthal of the Public Library of Charlotte and Mecklenburg County, who reviewed the manuscript and provided valuable feedback and much-needed encouragement.

Thanks to Jacqueline Schaffer for her handsome illustrations and to the staff of the Alan Mason Chesney Medical Archives at Johns Hopkins for the portrait of Dr. Adolf Meyer.

Special thanks to all the talented and dedicated staff of the Johns Hopkins University Press, who have been such a pleasure to work with on this as well as on my previous projects. *Thanks* is a flimsy word indeed to express my sincere and deep appreciation for the editorial skills and constant encouragement of my editor, Jacqueline Wehmueller.

Thanks, as well, to Jay Allen Rubin for countless cups of tea and for putting up with so many hours of a closed office door at home.

PART I

SYMPTOMS, SYNDROMES, AND DIAGNOSIS

A former professor of mine once told me, "When you can't figure out *what* the patient has, he or she probably has bipolar disorder." I remember thinking at the time that this was one of the most foolish things I had ever heard a Johns Hopkins faculty member say. But over the years I have come to realize that he was right (and also to realize that you don't get appointed to the faculty at Johns Hopkins by saying foolish things).

Bipolar disorder is the chameleon of psychiatric disorders, changing its symptom presentation from one patient to the next, and from one episode to the next even in the same patient. It is a phantom that can sneak up on its victim cloaked in the darkness of melancholy but then disappear for years at a time—only to return in the resplendent but fiery robes of mania. Although both depression and mania had been described over two millennia previously by Greek and Persian physicians—several of whom thought that the conditions were linked in some way—it wasn't until the early part of the twentieth century that a German psychiatrist, Emil Kraepelin, convincingly presented the idea that these opposite conditions were two sides of one pathological coin, the two profiles of a Janus-faced disease that he called manic-depressive insanity.

Why did it take over two thousand years for someone to solve a puzzle with only two pieces? Because, as my professor knew, there are so many more than two pieces to this mysterious disorder. The depressed phase can be merely gloomy or profoundly despairing; torpid and lethargic, or agitated and churning. The manic phase can be no more than an enthusiastic glow, or it can be an exultant, transcendental fervor, frenzied panic, or delirious, crashing, raving psychosis. Sometimes opposite moods seem to be combined, as inseparable as smoke and fire, mood states that have been given names like *depressive mania, manic stupor, agitated depression,* and more recently and more simply *mixed affective states.* The tendency of the illness to hibernate— for symptoms to spontaneously disappear for years, even decades at a time—adds to the confusion, perplexing the diagnostician and lulling the patient into dangerous complacency regarding the need for treatment.

In this first part, then, there are four chapters examining the symptoms, the syndromes, and the diagnosis of bipolar disorder. In chapter 1, "Normal and Abnormal Mood," we review the many symptoms of bipolar disorder, collected into three main clusters: *mania, depression,* and the *mixed mood states.* I have not minimized the severity of the symptoms in this chapter; I present all the possible symptoms of the illness, many of them frightening and terrible. But it is important to remember that not every person with bipolar disorder develops all the possible symptoms, and also that modern treatments usually prevent the development of the worst of them, many of which are now rarely seen even by psychiatrists.

In chapter 2, "The Diagnosis of Bipolar Disorder," I discuss the different forms the disorder can take. The diagnosis of bipolar disorder is complex, and there is still some disagreement about how the different symptom clusters are related to one another. Are there several different diseases of mood with different causes? Is there a group of disorders that share common features *and* common causes? Are these illness forms essentially the *same* disorder differing only in details of expression? Do these different forms remain the same over time in each patient, or can one form develop into another? The answers to many of these questions remain unknown. Nevertheless, there are several forms of the illness that can be reliably identified and separated from one another. Identifying one or another of these forms allows for predictions about the course of the illness over time and about the type of treatment that has the best chance of being effective.

In chapter 3, "A Summary of the Diagnostic Categories of Bipolar Disorder in *DSM IV,*" I review the official classification system of the illness that is currently used by the American Psychiatric Association (and by many psychiatrists in the rest of the world). This chapter might be considered optional reading and will probably be of more interest to students and professionals concerned with the details of illness classification and diagnostic categories.

In chapter 4, "The Mood Disease," I show how psychiatrists came to realize that bipolar disorder is indeed a disease. For decades, persons afflicted with mood disorders were often given the covert message by their physicians that they themselves were to blame for their symptoms. Depression and other mood symptoms were blamed on emotional immaturity or "maladjustment" rather than being recognized as expressions of disordered functioning of the brain. It was only with the discovery of effective pharmaceuticals that psychiatry realized that bipolar disorder is indeed a disease—as real as diabetes or hyperthyroidism.

Normal and Abnormal Mood

BIPOLAR DISORDER IS A *MOOD* DISORDER, ONE OF SEVERAL EMOTIONAL disorders whose main symptom is an abnormality of mood. The first step in understanding the illness, then, is to understand what we mean by the word *mood*. Perhaps more to the point, I want to talk about what *psychiatrists* mean by the word. The dictionary isn't much help here; it defines *mood* simply as "a conscious state of mind or predominant feeling."[1] The "predominant feeling" part of this definition begins to capture the psychiatric concept, but mood is much more than just a feeling.

Our mood includes our happiness or sadness, our state of optimism or pessimism, our feelings of contentedness or dissatisfaction with our situation, and even physical feelings such as how fatigued or robust we feel. Mood is like our emotional temperature, a set of feelings that expresses our sense of emotional comfort or discomfort.

When individuals are in a good mood, they are confident and optimistic, relaxed and friendly, patient, interested, content. The word *happy* captures part of it, but good mood includes a lot more. People in a good mood usually feel energetic and have a sense of physical well-being; they sleep soundly and eat heartily. It's easy for them to be sociable and affectionate. The future looks bright and the moment ripe for starting new projects. When we're in a good mood, the world seems a wonderful place to live in; it feels good to be alive.

When we're in a low mood, an opposite set of feelings takes over. We tend to turn inward and may seem preoccupied or distracted by our thoughts. The word *sad* captures some of the experience, but low mood is a bit more complicated. There may be a sense of emptiness and loss. It's difficult to think about the future very much, and when one does, it's hard not to be pessimistic or even intimidated by it. We may lose our temper more easily and then feel guilty about having done so. It's difficult to be affectionate or sociable, so we avoid others and prefer to be alone. Energy is low. Self-doubt takes over; we become preoccupied, worrying about how other people see us.

Abnormal Mood

Some of life's more common stresses and the normal human reactions to them are such common experiences that common terms have been coined for some mood changes—and most people recognize these mood changes as quite normal. Moving to a new community where we don't know anyone often leads to a sense of dislocation and loneliness that we know as homesickness, an unpleasant experience that may last for days or even weeks and that everyone has probably experienced at one time or another. When someone close to us dies, a profound sense of sadness and loss occurs that can become temporarily incapacitating—the deep sorrow that we call bereavement or mourning. At the time of various milestones of personal achievement, we experience changes of mood in the other direction. On the occasion of a graduation or wedding or the birth of a child, a person can be filled with joy and pride and a sense of limitless optimism that can be nearly overwhelming. We wouldn't call any of these moods "abnormal," even though they may be extreme.

Like many other things we can measure in human beings—body temperature, blood pressure, or hormone levels, for example—a person's mood state normally varies within a certain range. People are not in the same mood state all the time; it is quite normal for everyone to have ups and downs of mood. Do persons with bipolar disorder simply have higher ups and deeper downs? Well, it's certainly true that the bipolar patient's ups and downs are sometimes so far outside the range of normal that it doesn't take a psychiatrist to know that something is very wrong. But to say that persons with bipolar disorder simply have more extreme ups and downs of mood isn't quite right. Rather, the symptoms of bipolar disorder seem to be caused by a defect in the brain's *regulation* of mood.

Laura is a forty-year-old vice-president of one of the largest banks in the country.[2] When I walked out into the waiting room to call her for our first appointment, she was sitting with a lap-top computer balanced on her knees and a cellular telephone held up to her ear. "No,

Steve, that's not good enough," she was saying into the phone as she nodded to me. "No, that won't work either, we need the last quarter's *real* numbers, not an estimate. Listen, I'm . . . ah . . . in the doctor's office. I'll call you in an hour." I raised my eyebrows and shook my head. "Make that two hours. Bye." Click, click, snap, the LEDs went dark, phone and computer were shut, and in a moment we were sitting in an interviewing room.

"I made this appointment as soon as I could after I read this." Laura handed me a pamphlet called *A Guide to Depressive and Manic-Depressive Illness*. The local chapter of the National Depressive and Manic-Depressive Association had been handing them out at a local shopping mall during a health fair recently. "I've known for years that something was wrong, but I didn't know what. Reading this has made me think medication might help."

"What have you noticed that's 'wrong,' as you put it?" I asked.

"I go into these, these *things*," she started. "I get this wired, can't-slow-down feeling. I've always called it 'the crazies,' and I usually crash after it's over. Sometimes I can't get out of bed for days."

"You seem to have a very high stress job," I offered. "Maybe that's part of the problem."

"You sound like my mother. 'You don't have to take *every* promotion they offer you,' she says. But this isn't just stress, there's something else going on. The worst part is, I think these things are getting worse."

Laura's use of phrases like "the crazies" and "these things" seemed to indicate that she felt that these feelings were foreign, not like her normal feelings.

"Are you saying that sometimes your feelings and moods are controlling you rather than the other way around?" I asked.

Laura sat up straight in her chair. "That's the best way I could possibly describe it," she said decisively. "I can *feel* them coming on; it's almost physical. But I know they're . . . well, *mental*, I guess, is the best way to put it." Her face suddenly clouded over. "Does this mean I'm mentally ill?"

"Well," I said, "we know that there are illnesses that affect mood, and mood is certainly a mental state. But we have a lot more to talk about before I'll be able to say just what explains your 'crazies' the best."

Laura looked slightly relieved and said, "Well, that's why I'm here, for an explanation." She picked the brochure up from the edge of the desk. "This is the best explanation I've come across yet," she said thoughtfully. "And that means I can get rid of them, right? There's a treatment that will get rid of them?"

"There are many treatments for mood disorders. It may just take some time to find the one that works best."

"Then I came to the right place," she said as she sat back in her chair again. "'You're not crazy,' my mother said. 'You don't need to see a psychiatrist.'"

"Well, I think your mother was at least half right," I said.

Laura smiled for the first time. "OK, then let's—" Suddenly a beep-beep-beep sounded from her jacket pocket. She took out her cellular phone again. I started to get up. "If that's, um, confidential," I offered, "I can—"

Laura pushed a button, and the beeping stopped. She put the phone back in her pocket. "No, that can't possibly be as important as this. It can wait. I want to give you my undivided attention."

"Excellent!" I thought to myself. "This is a woman who understands priorities."

Imagine a person whose body temperature regulation system doesn't work correctly—a person who suddenly starts shivering on a warm sunny day or breaks out into a sweat in a room in which everyone else is chilly. This person's reactions to warm and cold are abnormal; his or her body "thinks" it is cold when it isn't, he or she feels hot when the temperature is cool. We can think of mood disorders as problems with *emotional* temperature regulation.

In mood disorders, the mood becomes disconnected from the individual's environment, and feelings of "happy" and "sad" take on rhythms and fluctuations of their own. Sometimes the fluctuations are mild, and the affected person only seems to have *more* ups and downs than other people have and to have mood fluctuations that are more difficult to understand. But because they don't get profoundly depressed or irrationally "high," their problems are dismissed as being due to a difficult personality or "immaturity." Sometimes, on the other hand, the mood states are so extremely abnormal that a person's ability to judge reality is shattered; behavior can be bizarre and frightening. (It is in some of these cases that a diagnosis of schizophrenia can be mistakenly made in an individual and proper treatment go wanting.) If the mood-disorder patient and his or her situation are examined with enough care, however, the basic underlying problem will be found: a problem with regulation of mood.

Since the basic problem in bipolar disorder is one of *regulation* of mood, the disorder can present different symptoms at different times. Persons afflicted with the classic form of the illness have periods of severe *depression* as well as periods of *mania* (a mood state that is in some ways the opposite of depression). The observation that these two mood states both occur at various times during the course of the illness gave rise to the older name for the disorder: manic-depressive illness. Both of these opposites of mood occur in affected persons because the brain mechanisms that normally regulate mood don't work properly. This observation—that the mood states of affected persons move to either of the two polar opposite extremes of mood—gives the disorder its modern name: bipolar disorder. In the following sections we'll take a closer look at these opposites, or poles, of bipolar disorder: the manic state and the depressed state, as well as an abnormal mood state in which the two opposites seem to be combined, a condition simply called a *mixed mood state*. After becoming familiar with these mood syndromes, we shall be able, in chapter 2, to see how their various combinations define the different forms of bipolar disorder.

A word you will frequently come across in discussions of mood disorders is *affect* (pronounced with the accent on the first syllable). To be precise, *affect* refers to the appearance of a person's mood state. *Mood* refers to the patient's inner experience, while *affect* refers to what others observe about a person's mood, the external signs of mood. (Psychiatrists talk of a patient's affect being depressed or irritable and so forth.) But for our purposes, *affect* can be considered a synonym for *mood*. (The mood disorders were at one time called *affective disorders.*)

The Manic Syndrome

The manic state, or more simply *mania,*[3] is the most extreme and dramatic of the symptom clusters of bipolar disorder. Many persons who have some of the forms of bipolar disorder never have a full-blown manic episode. But since mania is the most unmistakable and probably the most dangerous of the abnormal mood states associated with mood disorders, it is a good place to start.

In the manic state, the mood regulator switches into "high." Mania usually starts gradually and may take weeks to develop fully. Although the symptoms may be almost imperceptible at first, they gradually become more extreme, more unpleasant, and more unmistakably pathological (see table 1-1).

In the early stages of mania, the mood state of affected persons begins gradually to move "upward," and they find themselves filled with pleasant feelings of exuberance—what a physician writing almost a hundred years ago called "a welling up of a sense of well being and an overflowing of the spirits."[4] This heightened sense of well-being and confidence grows and expands and gradually evolves into euphoria. One bipolar patient described it this way:

> The world was filled with pleasure and promise; I felt great. Not just great, I felt *really* great. I felt I could do anything, that no task was too

TABLE 1-1 Symptoms of Mania

Mood Symptoms	Bodily Symptoms
Elated, euphoric mood	Increased energy level
Irritable mood	Decreased need for sleep
Grandiosity	Erratic appetite
	Increased libido
Cognitive (Thinking) Symptoms	
Feelings of heightened concentration	*Symptoms of Psychosis*
Accelerated thinking ("racing thoughts")	Grandiose delusions
	Hallucinations

difficult. My mind seemed clear, fabulously focused, and able to make intuitive mathematical leaps that had up to that point entirely eluded me . . . not only did everything make perfect sense, but it all began to fit into a marvelous kind of cosmic relatedness.[5]

And here we confront one of the many ironies of this illness: at the onset of an episode of the disorder, it is not uncommon to feel *better* than usual. As one manic patient said, "If I'm ill, this is the most wonderful illness I've ever had."[6]

Changes in thinking accompany the changes in mood. The feeling that one is thinking more clearly and more rationally than usual is especially common in the early stages of mania. This is an especially troublesome symptom, since such a mental state hardly makes a person suspect that something is wrong. Not only does thinking seem clearer than usual to the manic patient, but a feeling that mental processes are moving *faster* than usual also develops. As with the mood changes, there is often a very gradual onset to these alterations in thinking. At first there may be only a pleasant sense of nimbleness of thinking. Invariably, however, thinking processes accelerate: "quick" becomes "fast" and finally "racing." A vivid description of this acceleration of thinking—illustrating what psychiatrists call *flight of ideas*—comes from a collection of patient accounts written early in the twentieth century:

My thoughts ran with lightning-like rapidity from one subject to another. All the problems of the universe came crowding into my mind, demanding instant discussion and solution—mental telepathy, hypnotism, wireless, telegraphy, Christian science, women's rights, and all the problems of medical science, religion and politics.

Thoughts chased one another through my mind with lightning rapidity. I felt like a person driving a wild horse at a weak rein, who dares not use force but run[s] his course, following the line of least resistance, mad impulses rush through my brain carrying me first in one direction then in another.[7]

Racing thoughts are a symptom so typical of mania that the diagnosis becomes doubtful if this symptom is absent. This tumbling, jumbled jumping from one thought to another becomes progressively worse and more unpleasant as the episode develops.

As the manic individual's thinking speeds up, his or her speech does as well. Rapid or *pressured* speech (the term normally used by psychiatrists), like racing thoughts, is nearly always seen in mania. Manic individuals speak more and more quickly as the episode develops, attempting to express the ideas that are whirling through their consciousness at ever faster speeds. A psychiatric text from the beginning of the twentieth century mentions one early researcher who actually counted the number of syllables per minute spoken by manic patients. He found that manic patients spoke 180 to 200 syllables per minute, compared with 122 to 150 syllables per minute in nonmanic persons.[8]

Sometimes the racing thoughts and pressured speech lead to an outpouring of frenzied writing:

I made notes of everything that happened, day and night. I made symbolic scrapbooks whose meaning only I could decipher. I wrote a fairy tale . . . I noted down cryptically all that was said or done around me at the time, with special reference to relevant news bulletins and to jokes which were broadcast in radio programs. The time, correct to the nearest minute, was written in the margin. It was all vitally important. [I was convinced that] the major work [that] would be based on this material would be accurate, original, provocative and of profound significance.[9]

The feelings of exuberance and overconfidence that characterize mania can lead to several patterns of behavior typical of the manic state: spending sprees, sexual promiscuity, and overuse of alcohol and other intoxicating substances.

Spending sprees can be extravagant and financially catastrophic, because the manic person has no concern for where the money will come from when the bills come due. The increased sexual feelings of this stage of mania may lead to infatuations and even betrothals. One early psychiatric expert noted that "incomprehensible engagements, also pregnancies, are not rare in these states. I know cases in which the commencement of [mania] was repeatedly announced by a sudden engagement."[10] The lack of inhibitions typical in mania may also lead to promiscuity as well as to uncharacteristic bisexual or homosexual behaviors in some persons, perhaps by "releasing" suppressed feelings.

We shall explore the complex relationship between bipolar disorder and substance abuse in chapter 15. Suffice it to say here that increased and un-characteristic use of intoxicating substances is frequently seen in mania.

One way to understand this hedonistic triad of mania—spending sprees, sexual overactivity, and increased substance abuse—is to group these behaviors together as expressions of an increase in "motivated behaviors" seen in mania,[11] an exaggeration of the normal drives toward pleasurable goals.

There are almost always changes in sleeping and eating habits in mania. Decreased need for sleep is in fact one of the first symptoms to develop in mania—often a clue for individuals who have been manic before that an-other episode may be starting. Food intake is usually reduced because manic individuals simply don't have time to eat. Constantly distracted by new thoughts and ideas they feel pressed to act on, they just can't sit still long enough to finish a meal. The ensuing weight loss can be dramatic.

As the combination of euphoric mood and mental quickness develops, the manic individual begins to feel tremendously self-confident, even fear-less. This is the so-called *grandiosity* of the manic state. Fears of unpleasant consequences disappear altogether, and reckless enthusiasm takes over. The affected person may seek out new adventures and experiences with no regard for the possible adverse repercussions. This is one of the points at which the manic person can begin to lose touch with reality—when the grandiose thinking leads the individual to start *believing* the great things he or she feels capable of.

In a landmark work on bipolar disorder that we'll discuss in detail in chapter 4, the German psychiatrist Emil Kraepelin recorded the symptoms and course of the illness he called *manic-depressive insanity*. (I quote Krae-pelin extensively here and in the following chapter. Not only did Kraepelin write some of the most vivid and enduring descriptions of the symptoms of bipolar disorder ever written, but his insights into the different forms and the course of the illness have proven to be correct again and again.) Krae-pelin's description of the grandiose delusions of mania, written in 1896, is classic:

> The patient asserts that he is descended from a noble family. That he is a gentleman; he calls himself a genius, the Emperor William, the Em-peror of Russia, Christ, he can drive out the devil. A patient suddenly cried out on the street that he was the Lord God, the devil had left him. Female patients possess eighty genuine diamonds, are leading singers, leading violinists, Queen of Bavaria, Maid of Orleans, a fairy;

they are pregnant, are going to be engaged to St. Francis, are to give birth to the redeemer . . . the Messiah.[12]

Modern patients are more likely to become convinced that they are president or prime minister rather than king or queen, a rock star rather than a great violinist, but the feelings that lead to such beliefs are the same: a fantastic, indescribable feeling of mental power and significance. Feelings of religious inspiration are very common. Patients may feel that they are a modern prophet, the founder of a new religion, a reincarnation of Christ, even a new god.

The "feeling good" stage of mania is sometimes very short-lived, and the elated mood and grandiosity can be quickly replaced by angry, irritable mood. Quoting Kraepelin again:

> The patient is dissatisfied, intolerant, faultfinding . . . even rough. Trifling external occasions may bring about extremely violent outbursts of rage. In his fury, he thrashes his wife and children, threatens to smash everything to smithereens . . .
> . . . At the most trifling affront it may come to outbursts of rage of extraordinary violence . . . clamorous abuse and bellowing, to dangerous threats with shooting and stabbing, to blind destruction and actual attacks.[13]

Sometimes the manic individual alternates quickly between elation and irritability for a time, but usually an irritable, unpleasant mood becomes predominant. It is often this irritability that brings the patient to medical attention.

As the manic state continues to develop, pressured, racing thoughts, increased energy level, and loss of inhibitions lead to more grossly disorganized and disturbed thinking and behavior. A psychiatric textbook written in the 1950s described this stage as follows:

> Driven by greater pressure of activity, terror and excitement, [the manic person] becomes violent, attacks his neighbor, begins to shout all kinds of accusations against his alleged persecutors . . . Distortions [and] misinterpretations . . . are now elaborated into delusions of persecution accompanied by violence and panic, the patient runs down the street nude, sets fire to the house, starts an argument with the police, shoots a gun on the street or starts suddenly to preach the gospel in a frenzied manner . . . If crossed or interfered with in any way he becomes abusive, destructive, homicidal.[14]

Thinking patterns not only spin faster and faster but also become more bizarre. Hallucinations can develop, and beliefs called *delusions* can occur.

The very best modern written descriptions of the symptoms of severe mania are those of Kay Redfield Jamison. Dr. Jamison's nearly unique qualification to set them down is that she is an internationally recognized medical expert on bipolar disorder who suffers from it herself. This passage by Dr. Jamison is what I give medical students to read so that they can learn about the symptoms of severe mania:

> Although I had been building up to this for weeks and certainly knew something was seriously wrong, there was still a definite point when I knew I was insane. My thoughts were so fast that I couldn't remember the beginning of a sentence halfway through. Fragments of ideas, images, sentences, raced around and around in my mind like the tigers in a children's story. Finally, like those tigers, they became meaningless melted pools. Nothing familiar to me was familiar. I wanted desperately to slow down but could not. I felt my mind encased by black lines of light that were terrifying to me. My delusions centered on the slow painful deaths of all the green plants in the world—vine by vine, stem by stem, leaf by leaf they died, and I could do nothing to save them. Their screams were cacophonous. Increasingly, all my images were black and decaying.[15]

These passages vividly make the point that the manic state is not pleasant—even if it may sometimes start out that way. Those unfamiliar with the illness sometimes think that persons with bipolar disorder simply experience swings of mood between "happy" and "sad." As the foregoing illustrates, this is not usually true. The full-blown manic state is not only intensely unpleasant but also very dangerous. The danger arises not only from the increased risk of violence toward others (or toward self) but also from the physical stress the syndrome causes.

The combination of severe manic symptoms and the physical stress from such frenzied hyperactivity can lead to what Kraepelin called *delirious mania* in which there is "profound clouding of consciousness and extraordinary and confused hallucinations . . . The patients become stupefied, confused, bewildered and completely lose orientation for time and place."[16] Fortunately it is now rare for a psychiatrist to see patients suffering from this severest form of the manic state, but in Kraepelin's time and even more recently, mania had a significant mortality rate. Persons with mania died "in a state of progressive exhaustion,"[17] suffering dehydration and cardiovascular collapse.

In 1973, just as lithium, the first effective treatment for bipolar disorder, was becoming available, a study from the National Institutes of Health attempted to describe a typical manic episode from beginning to end.[18] Patients who had been admitted to a research unit that was trying to figure out how to use lithium safely and effectively for the treatment of bipolar disorder were carefully observed. The course of their symptoms was meticulously documented and described. The authors concluded that three stages could be described in a manic episode:

[Stage I]: Increased psychomotor activity which included increased . . . rate of speech and increased physical activity . . . Euphoria predominated, although irritability became obvious when the patients' many demands were not instantly satisfied . . . Expansiveness, grandiosity and overconfidence. Thoughts were coherent though sometimes [disconnected]. Also frequently observed during this stage were increased sexuality or sexual preoccupations, increased interest in religion, increased and inappropriate spending of money, increased smoking, telephone use and letter writing. Some of the patients were aware of the mood change on some level and described the feeling of "going high," having racing thoughts and feeling like they were in an airplane. At this stage the patients were not out of control.

[Stage II]: Pressure of speech and . . . activity increased still further. Mood, although euphoric at times, was now more prominently characterized by increasing [unpleasantness] and depression. The irritability observed initially had progressed to open hostility and anger, and the accompanying behavior was frequently assaultive. Racing thoughts progressed to . . . increasing disorganization. Preoccupations that were present earlier became more intense with earlier . . . grandiose trends now apparent as frank delusions.

[Stage III]: A desperate, panic stricken, hopeless state experienced by the patient as clearly [unpleasant], accompanied by frenzied and frequently even more bizarre . . . activity. Thought processes that earlier had been only difficult to follow now became incoherent . . . Delusions were bizarre . . . hallucinations were present [in about one-third of the patients].

More recently some researchers have questioned whether or not typical manic episodes include all of these stages. Specifically, some researchers believe that stage III mania (or *dysphoric mania,* as it has come to be called) occurs only in a subgroup of patients with bipolar disorder. There is some evidence that these patients have a variant of the disorder and may need medications different from what others with more typical bipolar disorder would need. (More on this in "Mixed States," later in this chapter.) Nevertheless, this study on the "stages of mania" was important because its investigators used modern clinical methods to document just how very sick patients with mania can get. Even more important, it made the researchers realize that it would be easy to misdiagnose a very disorganized patient in stage III mania as having schizophrenia, a psychiatric illness that requires a very different treatment approach and has a very different prognosis from bipolar disorder.

The Hypomanic Syndrome

In 1881 a German psychiatrist named Mendel published a book about the manic state called *Die Manie* and in it proposed that another term be used for states of mild euphoria and hyperactivity that did not progress to full-blown mania. He called this condition *hypomania,* "similar to the state of exultation in typical mania [but] with a certain lesser grade of development."[19] (The prefix *hypo-* comes from a Greek word meaning "under.") Hypomania can best be thought of as consisting of the symptoms that are present at the beginning of a manic episode (stage I in the study described above): the elated mood, the increased energy level, the rapid thinking and speaking, and sometimes a bit of the irritability. Norman Endler, another psychologist who himself suffered from a mood disorder and wrote of his experiences with the illness, described hypomania this way:

> Most of the time I was busy, busy, busy; taping records, playing tennis, skiing, writing manuscripts, talking . . . reading, going to movies, staying up at night, waking up early in the morning, always on the go—busy, busy, busy. Furthermore, I was boasting about all the energy I had that enabled me to keep up this fast pace . . . Instead of occasionally "idling" in neutral I was always in overdrive.[20]

Although persons in the hypomanic stage do not have the severe mental disorganization of mania and are by definition not agitated and frenzied to the point of violence toward themselves or others, hypomania can nevertheless have unpleasant consequences. Feelings of increased confidence can lead to foolish investments in real estate or the stock market, and patients can squander personal resources on grandiose and risky business ventures. Increased sexual feelings can lead to extramarital affairs or promiscuity—actions that can be life-threatening in the age of HIV disease. The irritability of hypomania can lead to arguments and disagreements with family, colleagues, or neighbors that can sour relationships, sometimes irreparably. Dr. Endler described it this way:

> As a hypomanic, I didn't stop to analyze my thoughts, feelings, or behavior. I was much too busy and didn't always stop to think about what I was doing . . . I was critical of others and occasionally told some people off publicly. I was not so concerned about . . . the effect my be-

havior had on [others]. I was aggressive, talked incessantly, and interrupted others while they were speaking. Whenever I had a thought I felt compelled to utter it, and I didn't always censor my thoughts and feelings. At times I seemed to have lost my sense of judgment. I was having a good time, I was narcissistically preoccupied with myself, but (without being aware of it) I was making my wife miserable.[21]

Persons with even mild hypomania can quit a good job in a burst of overconfidence or irritability, withdraw a life's savings for a get-rich-quick scheme, or simply begin to drive their car too fast—all behaviors with potentially devastating consequences.

Words like *seductive* and *addictive* are frequently applied to the hypomanic syndrome. Because individuals in a hypomanic state feel so good, they seldom seek treatment. Even for persons who have a history of previous manic or depressive episodes of bipolar disorder and perhaps should know that trouble is brewing, the giddy delight of being hypomanic often seems too delicious to interrupt. Persons whose abnormal mood states are successfully controlled with medication sometimes stop treatment to recapture the wonderful feelings that accompany hypomania.

Because hypomanic individuals are *not* psychotic, they often cannot be involuntarily treated for their illness because criteria for involuntary treatment insist upon "dangerous" behaviors. (We shall discuss involuntary treatment in chapter 22.) Hypomanic persons can avoid treatment for weeks, even months (see table 1-2), consequently ruining their financial status, credit rating, employment history, relationships, and health.

As we shall see in a later section, many patients go through episodes of

TABLE 1-2 Length of Time before Hospitalization for Mania in Ninety-four Manic Patients

Time	Percentage of Patients	
	Male	Female
14–30 days	69	62
3 months	11	11
6 months	11	10
1 year or more	6	15

Source: Data from George Winoker, *Mania and Depression: A Classification of Syndrome and Disease* (Baltimore: Johns Hopkins University Press, 1991), 13.

Note: Notice that some patients have symptoms for many months before receiving needed treatment. During this time, hypomanic symptoms can wreak havoc on their lives.

hypomania only and never become completely manic. Others have both hypomanic and manic episodes. Observations about the frequency and intensity of hypomanic versus manic episodes in different individuals are beginning to suggest that the classic "manic-depressive disorder" with episodes of full-blown mania and depression may be only one of many forms of the illness. (We shall discuss this new way of thinking about bipolar disorder in chapter 2, in the section "Bipolar Spectrum Disorders.")

The Syndrome of Depression

The depression of bipolar disorder is both easier and more difficult to describe and discuss than mania or hypomania. It is easier to discuss because depression is a more familiar set of feelings: everyone, whether suffering from bipolar disorder or not, has gone through periods of depressed mood. But the depressive syndrome of bipolar disorder is more difficult to discuss for that very reason: it is a very different experience from "normal" depression. In modern psychiatric terminology, this abnormal depressed mood state is called *major depression* (see table 1-3).

When persons who do not suffer from a mood disorder go through a period of low mood, such as after a romantic disappointment, the loss of a job, or a period of homesickness, not only is their depressed mood temporary,

TABLE 1-3 Symptoms of Depression

Mood Symptoms	*Bodily Symptoms*
Depressed mood	Sleep disturbance:
Dysphoric mood	insomnia
Diurnal variation of mood (early-morning depression, mood improving as day goes on)	hypersomnia
	Appetite disturbance:
	weight loss
Guilty feelings	weight gain
Loss of ability to feel pleasure (anhedonia)	Loss of interest in sex
Social withdrawal	Fatigue
Suicidal thoughts	Constipation
	Headaches
	Worsening of painful conditions
Cognitive (Thinking) Symptoms	
Poor concentration	
Poor memory	*Symptoms of Psychosis*
Indecision	Delusional thinking
Slowed thinking	Hallucinations
	Catatonic states

but they retain the normal *reactivity* of mood. Anyone who has attended a funeral and then returned to the home of the bereaved afterward has probably observed this normal reactivity of mood, perhaps even in themselves. Mourners who might have been grief-stricken during the funeral service or at the grave site can afterward often relax, reminisce about good times with the person who has died, and enjoy catching up with friends and relatives perhaps not seen for a long time. The reactivity of mood is also retained in the lonely or homesick person who goes to the movies and loses himself or herself in a good film. We are able to dispel the feelings of bereavement, isolation, or disappointment—even if it's only for a few hours—if the depressed mood is a "normal" one.

The most significant feature of the depressed mood of the syndrome of depression is that instead of being reactive, the mood is *constricted*. Years ago AM radio stations used to give away free radios, gifts that came with only one catch: they couldn't be tuned to any of the sponsoring station's competitors. These radios were built to receive only the signal of the station that gave them away. The mood state of the person suffering through a depressed episode of bipolar disorder is like one of those radios, "set" to receive only one mood signal: depression. The mood of the syndrome of depression is a relentless, pervasive gloom that continues from one day to the next and from which the afflicted person cannot rouse himself or herself. As Pulitzer Prize–winning novelist William Styron said of his own depression, "The weather of depression is unmodulated, its light a brownout."[22]

In these constricted mood states, depressed individuals can find their thinking dominated by thoughts of sadness and loss, regret and hopelessness. Guilty ruminations are especially characteristic of the syndrome of depression, and psychiatrists often make a special point to ask about guilty feelings when examining a person being evaluated for depression. Ruminations on themes of guilt, shame, and regret are common in the depressed states of the mood disorders, and they are uncommon in "normal" depression. Persons experiencing the normal depressed mood that comes after a personal loss usually attribute their bad feelings to the fact that a loss has occurred; only in unusual circumstances will they feel that they are to blame for their problem and be preoccupied by guilty feelings or feelings of shame. The individual with a depressive syndrome, on the other hand, frequently feels to blame for his or her troubles, and sometimes for other people's troubles as well. The presence of guilty preoccupations is very significant for making a diagnosis of the syndrome of depression.

Feelings of inadequacy and worthlessness are similarly significant and especially common in the syndrome of major depression. Psychologist Norman Endler described how depression caused him to be tormented by feelings of incompetence even at the height of a successful academic career:

[When I became depressed] I was positive I was a fraud and a phony and that I didn't deserve my Ph.D. I didn't deserve to have tenure; I didn't deserve to be a Full Professor; I didn't deserve to be a Fellow of the American Psychological Association and the Canadian Psychological Association; I didn't deserve the research grants I had been awarded; I couldn't understand how I had written the books and journal articles that I had and how they had been accepted for publication. I must have conned a lot of people.[23]

Another typical symptom of major depression is the loss of interest in usually pleasurable activities. This can be understood as another aspect of the loss of normal reactivity of mood. The depressed person is unable to derive any pleasure from listening to music, going to a movie, engaging in the sports or hobbies that usually provide enjoyment. This loss of the ability to feel pleasure has come to be called *anhedonia* (derived from the Greek word for "pleasure"). In his novel *The Sorrows of Young Werther,* Johann Wolfgang von Goethe has his main character express a loss of responsiveness to the joys and beauty of nature by saying, "Nature lies before me as immobile as in a little lacquered painting, and all this beauty cannot pump one drop of happiness from my heart to my brain."[24] Patients describe food losing its taste, colors draining away from sunrises and landscapes, flowers losing their textures and perfumes—everything becoming bland, dull, and lifeless. For some, the bright and beautiful things of the world become a source of anguish rather than pleasure. The nineteenth-century Austrian composer Hugo Wolf described a terrible sense of sorrowful isolation during his depressions, a feeling of separation from the world of ordinary pleasures—all the more painful when it occurred in springtime:

What I suffer from . . . I am quite unable to describe. This wonderful spring with its secret life and movement troubles me unspeakably. These eternal blue skies, lasting for weeks, this continuous sprouting and budding in nature, these coaxing breezes impregnated with spring sunlight and fragrance of flowers . . . make me frantic. Everywhere this bewildering urge for life, fruitfulness, creation—and only I . . . may not take part in this festival of resurrection, at any rate not except as a spectator with grief and envy.[25]

Just as the manic syndrome infuses the affected person with feelings of inexpressible joy, the syndrome of depression brings indescribable anguish. Many individuals who have suffered from depression have struggled to describe the feelings, and even great writers seem to falter in the attempt. Quoting William Styron again: "If the pain were readily describable most of the countless sufferers from this ancient affliction would have been able to confidently depict . . . their torment. Healthy people [cannot] imagine a form of torment so alien to everyday experience. For myself, the pain is most closely connected to drowning or suffocation—but even these images are off the mark."[26]

Sometimes the "indescribable" mental discomfort seen in major depression is a feeling that seems different from the sad, pessimistic mood people usually mean by the word *depression*. Instead, people with major depression may have a tense, irritable, miserable sort of mood called *dysphoria*. (Remember that the term *dysphoric mania* is used to describe a tense, unpleasant, irritable mood that can be seen along with the agitation and hyperactivity of the manic state.)

The changes in thinking and physical well-being caused by the syndrome of depression are perhaps easier to describe. Energy level and thinking as well as mood are affected—in an opposite direction of polarity from that seen in mania. The depressed person experiences slowing and inefficiency in thinking and a feebleness of memory and concentration. Information processing and reasoning falter, and simple decisions can become overwhelming dilemmas. Quoting Endler again: "My indecisiveness was the worst of all. I couldn't decide what to eat or what to wear. I couldn't decide whether to get out of bed or to stay. I couldn't decide whether to shower or not to shower. I could never decide what to do because I didn't know myself."[27]

These *cognitive* functions (from the Latin *cognoscere*, meaning "to know") become progressively debilitated as the depression deepens, but even in milder depressions, ordinary mental tasks seem to require extraordinary effort. Kraepelin described the severe cognitive slowing he observed in his severely depressed patients: "[The patient's] thoughts are as if paralysed . . . immobile. He is no longer able to perceive or to follow the train of thought of a book or conversation . . . he has no memory, he has no longer command of knowledge formerly familiar to him [and] must consider a long time about simple things."[28] In the elderly, these sorts of thinking problems can be so severe that depression is misdiagnosed as Alzheimer's disease.

Severe depression almost always causes a change in sleeping pattern. Depressed persons frequently suffer from insomnia—but also from its opposite, sleeping too much (*hypersomnia* is the technical term). In the depression associated with bipolar disorder, hypersomnia seems especially common, perhaps more common than in other types of depression, where insomnia predominates.

There is sometimes seen in depressed persons a peculiar rhythmic pattern of sleep disturbance and mood changes throughout the day, called *diurnal variation of mood* (*diurnal* is a word used in biology to refer to a twenty-four-hour cycle). Persons with this pattern fall asleep at the usual time and without much difficulty but wake up very early in the morning after only a few hours of sleep. Lying awake hours before sunrise, they experience their lowest mood of the day, and minor problems and regrets seem magnified and overwhelming during this early-morning period. I recall one patient who told me that during those early-morning hours, "I lie awake thinking about every stupid thing I've ever done in my life." American author F. Scott Fitzgerald, who described his struggles with depression in the 1936 autobiographical work *The Crackup,* gave a vivid account of this mood pattern. He experienced the worst of his moods during the predawn hours, recalling that "at three o'clock in the morning, a forgotten package has the same tragic importance as a death sentence." For Fitzgerald, these nocturnal agonies were the worst part of his depressions, which he called "the dark night of the soul."[29] Individuals notice a gradual lifting of their mood as sunrise approaches, and when the morning light comes they can often rouse themselves and start their daily activities. As the day goes on, their mood continues to improve little by little until by day's end they feel nearly back to normal. They go to bed and can often fall asleep normally, but several hours later, it's "three o'clock in the morning" again: they awaken depressed, and the cycle repeats itself.

Novelist William Styron experienced a very striking diurnal variation in his mood during his depression, but with a reversal of the usual pattern: "While I was able to rise and function almost normally during the earlier part of the day, I began to sense the onset of the symptoms at mid-afternoon or a little later—gloom crowding in on me, a sense of dread and alienation and . . . stifling anxiety."[30]

The disruptions of various bodily rhythms that occur in depression and mania have convinced many scientists that some persons with mood disorders have a disturbance of their *chronobiology* (from *chronos,* the Greek word for "time"). Persons with mood disorders have been observed to have disturbances in the normal rhythmic pulsing of various hormone levels, in body temperature fluctuations, the sleep-wake cycle, and other natural rhythms. Later in this book we shall examine connections between these natural rhythms and mood and shall look at other cycles: the monthly cycles of mood in women with premenstrual mood symptoms (chapter 14) and the twelve-month cycles of persons with seasonal affective disorder (chapter 16).

Appetite is usually disturbed in depressed individuals. As with sleep problems, changes occur in both directions, and patients may eat too much or too little. Individuals can lose or gain a significant amount of weight during periods of depression. As might be expected, the depressed person loses interest in sex, perhaps best understood as part of his or her inability to experience pleasurable activities of any kind, the "anhedonia" of depression.

Of the other bodily symptoms that occur in depression, a sense of fatigue with prominent low energy and listlessness is one of the most striking.

Here is Endler: "[My] fatigue [was] extreme to the point of exhaustion. I was too tired to make decisions and felt as if I had a huge weight on my back that wouldn't allow me to achieve anything . . . No matter how long I stayed in bed and slept I never felt rested and refreshed . . . When I did get out of bed I was lethargic. I was slow as molasses."[31] Headaches, constipation, and a feeling of heaviness in the chest are common, as are other more difficult-to-describe sensations of physical discomfort. Here is Styron: "I felt a kind of numbness, an enervation . . . an odd fragility—as if my body had actually become frail, hypersensitive and somehow disjointed and clumsy. Nothing felt quite right . . . there were twitches and pains, sometimes intermittent, often seemingly constant, that seemed to presage all sorts of dire infirmities."[32]

It is not clear whether these symptoms are caused by depression itself or arise from the lack of restful sleep, the lack of exercise, and the poor eating habits that depression brings on. Persons who have preexisting painful medical conditions such as arthritis or inflammatory bowel disease are usually more bothered by the physical symptoms of these illnesses when they are depressed. The connections between depression and problems with fatigue seen in chronic fatigue immunodeficiency syndrome (CFIDS) and the painful joint and muscle disease fibromyalgia are well known but poorly understood. Depression seems to lower the pain threshold: depressed individuals seem more sensitive to pain and are more distressed by it.

Some persons may be willing to seek treatment for these physical symptoms but reluctant to mention their mood problems. This can cause patients with depression to end up getting all kinds of tests and treatments for physical illnesses from their physicians when their real problem is depression.

Just as in the syndrome of mania, persons suffering through an episode of the depression of bipolar disorder can experience the distortions of thinking that psychiatrists call *delusions*. As their view of the world and of themselves is increasingly colored by their pervasive mood changes, depressed individuals can come to believe that terrible things are happening all around them: "I was positive that I was going to be fired from the university because of incompetence and that [my family] would become destitute—that we would go broke," wrote Endler. "I felt guilty at the prospect of not being able to support my family."[33] In addition to such *delusions of poverty*, delusions can arise from the uncomfortable physical sensations of depression. Patients believe they have cancer, AIDS, or some other terrible illness. Kraepelin described the increasingly bizarre *hypochondriacal delusions* he sometimes observed in his patients: "[The patient believes he is] incurably ill, half-dead, no longer a right human being, has lung disease, a tapeworm, cancer in his throat, cannot swallow, does not retain his food . . . Face and figure have changed; there is no longer blood in his brain, he does not see any longer, must become crazy, remain his whole lifetime in an institution, die, has already died." Patients with these sorts of beliefs may refuse to eat or drink, convinced that their body cannot absorb the food. *Paranoid delusions*, beliefs that one is in danger or the victim of evil people and forces, can also occur. Quoting Kraepelin again:

> Everywhere danger threatens the patient . . . strange people are in the house; a suspicious motorcar drives past. People mock him, are going to thrash him, to chase him from his post in a shameful way, incarcerate him, bring him to justice, expose him publicly, deport him, throw him into the fire, drown him. The people are already standing outside; the bill of indictment is already written; the scaffold is being put up; he must wander about naked and miserable . . . His relatives also are being tortured . . . his family is imprisoned, his wife has drowned herself; his parents are murdered; his daughter wanders about in the snow without any clothes on.[34]

It's easy to understand why suicidal thinking and behavior are so common in the syndrome of major depression: compared with the horrors of such delusional imaginings, death may seem a welcome alternative. It's also possible to understand why delusionally depressed persons can occasionally be dangerous to others as well as to themselves: delusionally depressed individuals can come to believe that those close to them are in similar danger of gruesome persecution and would be better off dead.

Hallucinations occur in severe depressions, but not as frequently as in mania (see table 1-4). The hallucinations are consistent with the mood and are frightening, even horrifying: "The patients see evil spirits, death, heads of animals . . . crowds of monsters . . . dead relatives . . . The patient hears his tortured relatives screaming and lamenting . . . his food tastes of soapy water or excrement, of corpses and mildew."[35]

TABLE 1-4 Delusions and Hallucinations in Bipolar Disorder:
Mania versus Depression

Category of Symptoms	Percentage of Patients
Delusions	
Mania	44
Depression	12
Hallucinations	
Mania	14
Depression	8

Source: Data from D. W. Black and A. Nasrallah, "Hallucinations and Delusions in 1,715 Patients with Unipolar and Bipolar Affective Disorders," *Psychopathology* 22 (1989): 28–34.

Some seriously ill patients sink into a state of lethargy and despair that is called *depressive stupor*. Styron's description of this horrible condition is the best I have ever read:

> I had now reached that phase of the disorder where all sense of hope had vanished, along with the idea of a futurity; my brain . . . had become less an organ of thought than an instrument registering, minute by minute, varying degrees of its own suffering . . . I'd feel the horror, like some poisonous fog bank, roll in upon my mind, forcing me to bed. There I would lie for as long as six hours, stuporous and virtually paralyzed, gazing at the ceiling.[36]

Just as few modern psychiatrists have ever seen the most extreme stage of mania, so-called *delirious mania*, it is also fortunately rare today to see a patient depressed to the point of unresponsiveness and immobility that psychiatrists call *catatonia*. Kraepelin, describing patients of an era when virtually no treatment was available for this terrible condition, starkly describes the deepest abyss of depression: "The patients lie in bed taking no interest in anything. They betray no pronounced emotion; they are mute, inaccessible; they pass their [bowel movements] under them; they stare straight in front of them with [a] vacant expression of countenance like a mask and with wide open eyes."[37]

Electroconvulsive therapy (ECT), which we shall discuss in more detail in chapter 10, is a very effective treatment for these extreme states of the depressive syndrome. Although there have been misguided attempts to ban this safe and effective treatment technique in the United States, and equally misguided activists still occasionally appear in the media to disparage ECT, it fortunately remains available to treat this most extreme stage of depression, rescuing these individuals from a kind of living hell.

Mixed States

Another type of abnormal mood can be seen in bipolar disorder, a strange combination of both the frenzied intensity of mania and the horrors of deep depression that has been called a *mixed state* (sometimes, *mixed affective state*). Kay Jamison described these states as the most terrible expression of the illness for her: "On occasion, these periods of total despair would be made even worse by terrible agitation. My mind would race from subject to subject, but instead of being filled with . . . exuberance and cosmic thoughts . . . it would be drenched in awful sounds and images of decay and dying; dead bodies on the beach, charred remains of animals, toe-tagged corpses in morgues."[38]

Although psychiatrists do not yet agree on the defining characteristics

TABLE 1-5 Symptoms in Ten Patients with Mixed Mania (Dysphoric Mania)

Symptoms	Percentage of Patients
Depressed mood	100
Irritable mood	100
Increased activity	100
Insomnia	93
Pressured speech	93
Hostility	79
Flight of ideas	43
Anxiety attacks	43
Delusions (depressive)	36
Delusions (nondepressive)	21

Source: Data from Frederick K. Goodwin and Kay Redfield Jamison, *Manic-Depressive Illness* (New York: Oxford University Press, 1990), 49.

for this mood state, they have long recognized that symptoms of depression and mania seem to exist almost simultaneously in some patients (see table 1-5). This state represents a distinct variety of abnormal mood that is separate from depression and typical mania yet combines features of both. The accelerated thinking and hyperactivity typical of the manic state remain its most striking features, but instead of a euphoric mood, these changes become combined with a depressed, despairing, desperate mood. Kraepelin described patients with "flight of ideas, excitement and anxiety" who were at the same time "anxiously despairing."[39] Other labels used for the mixed state are "mixed mania" or "dysphoric mania."[40] As we shall see in chapter 2, there is some evidence that this mood state does not occur in all patients with bipolar disorder and that, when it does occur, a different treatment approach is necessary.

Just as full-blown mania is unmistakable, so is a full-blown mixed state. But in the same way that a state of mild hypomania can be difficult to distinguish from elevated but normal mood, milder mixed states can be difficult to recognize. These milder mixed states sometimes last only a few hours. Whenever a patient tells me about being troubled by uncomfortable angry "rages," I suspect that he or she may be having mild mixed states.

Mixed states are very dangerous because the patient has negative, depressing thought patterns together with excess energy, restlessness, and an inner sense of pressure and tension. This negative energy puts patients in mixed states at high risk for hurting themselves with suicidal behaviors. And it is often while in a mixed state that an individual is propelled into a variety of self-destructive behaviors that are not immediately life-threatening. Persons in mixed states may cut or burn themselves. Patients have told me that these desperate behaviors help them shift a terrible inner pain and tension to "the outside" and that the physical pain is somehow easier to deal with than the painful agitation of a mixed state.

Another type of mood "mixture" occurs when, rather than a true mixture of both mania and depression simultaneously, there is very rapid alternation between the two states. Kraepelin described "transition periods from one state to another, which often [extended] over weeks" during which his patients seemed depressed one moment and manic nearly the next:

> Manic patients may transitorily appear not only sad and despairing, but also quiet and inhibited. A patient goes to bed moody and inhibited, suddenly wakes up with the feeling as if a veil had been drawn away from his brain, passes the day in manic delight in work, and the next morning, exhausted and with a heavy head, he again finds in himself the whole misery of his state. Or the hypomanic exultant patient quite unexpectedly makes a serious attempt at suicide.[41]

Recently the term *ultra-rapid cycling* has been proposed for these rapid alternations in mood seen in some bipolar patients.

Now that you have some familiarity with the symptoms of bipolar disorder, I can talk about diagnosis. As I have already said, most people with bipolar disorder never develop all the possible symptoms of the illness. It is the presence or absence of certain symptoms as well as the pattern of mood symptoms that allows a diagnosis of a particular type of bipolar disorder. And once a diagnosis has been made, a treatment plan can be developed. In the next chapter you'll see how the diagnostic process works.

Although the same morbid process lies at the foundation of all these forms [of manic-depressive illness], they are yet so different in clinical behavior, in course, and in prognosis, that one might perhaps speak of a morbid group springing from a common root.

EMIL KRAEPELIN

The Diagnosis of Bipolar Disorder

WHEN LITHIUM BECAME AVAILABLE IN THE 1970S AS A TREATMENT FOR bipolar disorder, psychiatrists started to realize that not all cases of bipolar disorder were the same. For some patients, lithium was indeed a miracle; their symptoms were completely controlled by it, and their illness seemed simply to end. But other patients—often those with more severe symptoms and more frequent episodes of abnormal mood—didn't respond as well to the medication. Did these people have bipolar disorder, or something else? Patients who had been thought to have "cyclothymic personality disorder"— a diagnostic category in an old edition of the diagnostic manual of the American Psychiatric Association—also saw their troublesome and unpredictable mood variations stop when they took lithium; did these people have bipolar disorder, and not a personality problem after all? Was this a milder form of "manic-depressive" illness, or a different disorder altogether? Did it matter? What difference does diagnosis make, anyway?

Diagnostic classification has two purposes in medicine: to make predictions about the course of an illness, and to aid the clinician in selecting the treatment most likely to be effective. In the practice of psychiatry, since the physical basis for most psychiatric illnesses has yet to be discovered, classification systems are largely derived from studying groups of patients with different combinations of symptoms and seeing if the different groups vary in the course of their illness or in their response to medications.

As lithium and other medications have become available to treat mood disorders, the classification system for bipolar mood disorders has continued to evolve. In the sections that follow, various subtypes of bipolar disorder are described. These are the subtypes that currently seem to make sense to clinicians because they serve one of the two purposes of diagnosis mentioned above: they allow for a better prediction of the course of the illness, and they allow for a rapid selection of effective therapy—saving the patient time that would be wasted on a trial of an ineffective medication.

Psychiatric Diagnosis

At least once a month, it seems, I see a patient who asks to be "tested for bipolar disorder." It's not an unreasonable request. Unfortunately, it's not a request that can be satisfied—not just yet. There's not a blood test or an x-ray or a biopsy that can make the diagnosis of bipolar disorder (or, for that matter, that can be used to confirm the diagnosis of most of the problems psychiatrists treat).

The reason for this sorry state of affairs is that the biological and chemical basis of bipolar disorder remains a nearly complete mystery; no one knows what to test for. Despite literally hundreds of years of examining the bodily fluids and brain tissues of individuals with mood disorders—first with the naked eye, then with microscopes, later with x-rays and scanning devices, and more recently with incredibly sophisticated biochemical probes—no one has been able to find in patients with this illness any abnormalities that can be accurately and reliably measured as an aid in diagnosing the disorder. Although work in the genetics of bipolar disorder holds the promise that genetic markers for the illness may be discovered in the not too distant future—suggesting that a blood test might be possible that will identify at least some cases of the illness—and although some individuals with bipolar disorder have been identified as having subtle brain-scan abnormalities (see "Picturing Bipolar Disorder in the Brain" in chapter 18), again suggesting a possible diagnostic tool, the clinical applications of these findings are still far off. Modern psychiatrists are left with the same diagnostic tools that Emil Kraepelin and other nineteenth-century psychiatrists had: their eyes and ears.

We psychiatrists listen to the patient and to his or her family members describe symptoms—their onset, course, fluctuation, and impact upon the patient. We observe the patient for the signs of bipolar disorder described in chapter 1 by performing a *mental status examination,* the psychiatrist's equivalent of the physical examination; this examination consists of observing speech patterns and behavior, asking questions about mood and thinking processes, and evaluating other aspects of mental functioning such as concentration and memory. After this process of history taking and examination, a picture of the person and of his or her symptoms and the course of the trouble emerges. A particular diagnostic category that seems to be a good fit with the clinical information is identified. Once the diagnostic category of the illness is determined, we can make predictions about the future course of the symptoms and, perhaps more important, can select a treatment that has a good chance of relieving them. In the sections that follow we shall learn about the different forms of bipolar disorder the same way young physicians training to be psychiatrists do: by hearing from patients.

Bipolar I

It had been several years since I had seen Richard in the mood-disorders clinic. He looked great. Although he was only in his late thirties, some silver tones in his hair made him look a bit older and quite distinguished. I remembered that he had always dressed well, but today, in an obviously finely tailored suit, a crisp white shirt, and beautiful silk tie, he looked—well, like a million. I knew that this could be a very good sign—or a very bad sign.

"That's a handsome suit you've got on, Richard. Is it new?" I asked.

"I got it about a month ago," he said proudly, "in London. A terrific shop on Savile Row, the same one Prince Charles goes to." He smiled a little mischievously. "And I know what you're thinking: no, I wasn't manic when I bought it!"

Rich certainly knew what mania was, as did several members of his family. His wealthy parents had taken control of his financial affairs in a legal-guardianship proceeding; for years he hadn't even been able to write a check at the supermarket. Rich had first developed manic symptoms during law school, making down payments on not just one Porsche but three before a check bounced. He had angrily stormed into the bank's branch office to protest, created quite a scene, and ended up in jail, where an astute nurse fortunately arranged an immediate psychiatric evaluation. Richard was in a local psychiatric hospital and had taken his first dose of lithium before his parents even knew what had happened.

He stopped taking his lithium within a month of leaving the hospital and started having manic symptoms almost immediately. This time his manic enthusiasm turned to travel rather than cars, and he used a credit card to buy an airline ticket to Fiji. He made it as far as Los Angeles before his mania turned dysphoric and irritable again. He had started yelling at and shoving a security guard who wanted to examine his luggage and wound up in jail again—this time with federal charges. After a talk with a good lawyer, another hospitalization, more lithium, a leave from law school, and a move back home, he had come for treatment at the university outpatient clinic where I was training.

Richard's father also suffered from bipolar disorder and knew, from his own turbulent experiences with the illness, just how to handle the situation. A pair of scissors to the credit cards, a power of attorney, and going along with Richard to the psychiatrist's appointments made the difference—as did the fact that Richard was an intelligent fellow who (eventually) learned from experience as well. Moreover, he learned from his father that a paternal uncle who had been killed in a car accident when Rich was a child had also actually probably died from the disease; the single-passenger accident had most likely been a suicide. Rich made the decision to take control of the illness rather than let it control him. And as with most things, once he decided to do so, Rich applied himself to staying well with energy and determination.

There was a time after he broke up with a girlfriend when severe depressive symptoms almost necessitated another hospitalization for Rich; he spent fourteen to sixteen hours in bed every day for nearly three weeks and put on almost fifty pounds. Fortunately, family support, an excellent psychologist in the clinic who saw him for therapy, and a higher lithium dose for several months got him through. After about a year of stable mood, he got into a local law school to finish his studies and eventually graduated at the top of his class. He had taken a job in New York but now had returned home. "I couldn't pass up the opportunity to open my firm's new branch office in my hometown, could I?" he beamed.

Rich brought me up to date. A little hypomania had occasionally emerged during the summers while he was working in New York, especially if he was working too hard and didn't watch his sleep habits. But Rich had obviously remained serious about his mental health; he monitored his moods and saw his psychiatrist regularly. Most important, he was making career decisions that reflected his knowledge of his illness. "I think the pace will be slower here than in New York. I may not become a millionaire as quickly," he said a little sadly, "but there will also be less risk of getting sick, blowing it all, and having to start over again. So . . . I had my last lithium level done three months ago, and it was 0.8. When do you want me to get another?"

It looked as if the suit had been a very *good* sign.

———————————————————————————————

Bipolar I is the designation for the classic variety of bipolar disorder, characterized by full-blown manic attacks and deep, paralysing depressions. A schematic representation of the moods of bipolar I appears in figure 2-1.

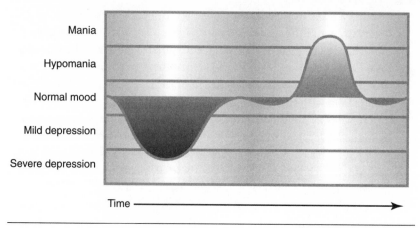

FIGURE 2-1 Mood changes in bipolar I

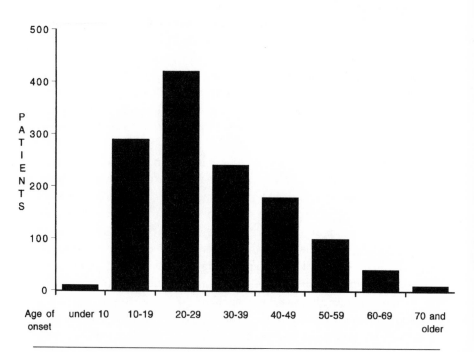

FIGURE 2-2 Age of onset of bipolar disorder in 1,304 patients. These data were compiled from ten different studies carried out between 1969 and 1984. Notice that early adulthood is the peak time for the onset of the disorder.

Source: Frederick K. Goodwin and Kay Redfield Jamison, *Manic-Depressive Illness* (New York: Oxford University Press, 1990), 132. Copyright © 1990 by Oxford University Press, Inc. Used by permission of Oxford University Press, Inc.

The pattern of abnormal mood episodes seems to vary widely, and the rhythm of the illness is almost as individual as the patient who has it. Symptoms of bipolar I usually begin in the late teens or early twenties (see figure 2-2), although onset at later ages is not uncommon.[1]

Bipolar I is what physicians refer to as a relapsing and remitting illness; during the course of the illness, its symptoms come and go. This feature of bipolar I—it is actually a feature of *all* mood disorders—makes it difficult to diagnose, difficult to treat, and fiendishly difficult to study. This deserves a closer look.

THE DISEASE THAT SLEEPS

When we think about illnesses of the body, we usually think of diseases that have a beginning, a middle, and an end. Take, for example, pneumonia, an infection of the lungs caused by bacteria. The disease begins when fever, cough, chest pains, and breathing problems appear. These symptoms build and worsen over a period of hours or sometimes days. Before the antibiotic era, patients reached what was called a *crisis* point, when their bodies' natural defenses had mounted their best effort against the bacterial invaders, and the patient either started getting better or died. Either the patient killed off the bacteria or vice-versa, but in any case the disease process came to an end. (Fortunately we can now administer antibiotics that usually give the patient's defenses the crucial edge against the bacterial invader.)

How about a disease not caused by a foreign invader like bacteria but instead one in which the body seems to turn on itself, a disease like cancer— say, leukemia? In this case a white blood cell in the body develops an abnormality that causes it to start reproducing uncontrollably. Most of the cells in the body reproduce from time to time, in order to replenish those that wear out. It is thought that most cancers are caused by an error during cell duplication that results in an abnormality in the control center of one of the new cells, probably involving DNA. This abnormality causes the cell to start reproducing continuously. More and more abnormal cells are produced, and in the case of leukemia they fill the bloodstream and lymph nodes such that the normal cells cannot do their job properly, the immune system fails, and the patient dies. Many types of leukemia are now curable. The cures basically involve using ingenious methods to eradicate every single cancer cell, eliminating the abnormally reproducing cells altogether; when the abnormality is eliminated from the body, things return to normal. Again, the illness begins when something goes wrong in the body, and it ends (is cured) when the abnormality is corrected and eliminated. The illness is finished for good.

Bipolar disorder is very different from these diseases because it does not simply have a beginning, a middle, and an end. Or perhaps it is more accurate to say that the illness seems to have many beginnings and endings: the symptoms of bipolar disorder can develop in an individual, and then *without any treatment at all* the symptoms may go away for years at a time—a pattern that is nearly unique among the diseases that afflict humankind.

Since most people are more familiar with diseases that end when their symptoms go away, it is often very difficult for patients and their families to understand that although the symptoms of bipolar disorder can go into *remission* after treatment (or even spontaneously), they almost inevitably will come back if treatment to prevent their return is not in place. The hallmark of bipolar illness—especially bipolar I—is the tendency of the illness to *relapse*. No matter how well the symptoms of any one episode are treated, the illness does not end but instead seems merely to hibernate—and *symptoms can come back at any time.*

THE NATURAL HISTORY OF BIPOLAR I

Now, back to a description of the characteristics of bipolar I. Fortunately many excellent clinical studies about the course of bipolar disorder were done in the years before effective treatments for it were available; these studies document and illustrate the pattern of bipolar-disorder symptoms that exists if the illness is not treated—what physicians call the *natural history* of the illness.[2]

How many episodes of illness did patients have in the days before treatment was available? How long did episodes last? What was the length of time between episodes?

In a 1942 study, the records of sixty-six patients with "manic-depressive psychosis" were studied; some of these individuals had been followed for up to twenty-six years. Although a few patients seemed to have had only one episode of illness in the period of study, about one-third had two to three episodes, about one-third had four to six episodes, and about one-third had more than seven (see table 2-1). A few had twenty or more episodes.[3] Unfor-

TABLE 2-1 Number of Episodes of Illness in Sixty-six Patients with Bipolar Disorder

Number of Episodes	Percentage of Patients
1	8
2–3	29
4–6	26
More than 7	37

Source: Data from Thomas A. C. Rennie, "Prognosis in Manic-Depressive Psychosis," *American Journal of Psychiatry* 98 (1942): 801–14.

Note: This study was done before the availability of any treatments for bipolar disorder.

tunately, when a diagnosis of bipolar I is made, there is no way to know whether the individual will have another two or three episodes during his or her lifetime or more than twenty.

How long did episodes of mania or major depression last before effective treatments were available? In the 1942 study, the average duration was about six and a half months. But we also know that depressions and manias were sometimes shorter and sometimes lasted much longer. Kraepelin, writing at a time when there were essentially no effective treatments, noted that

the duration of individual attacks is extremely varied. There are some which last only eight to fourteen days, indeed we sometimes see that states of moodiness or excitement . . . do not continue in these patients longer than one or two days or even only a few hours. For the most part, however, a simple attack usually lasts six to eight months. On the other hand, the cases are not at all rare, in which an attack continues for two, three or four years, and a double attack [can] double that time. I have seen manias, which even after seven years, indeed after more than ten years, recovered, and a state of depression which after fourteen years recovered.[4]

Modern psychiatrists no longer see patients who are manic for years at a time. Effective modern treatments abort these episodes, and the patient is usually better in a few days—weeks at the most. Modern psychiatrists do, however, see patients who seem to become manic again and again, month after month, year after year—often every time they stop taking medication. Do these patients have many episodes, or do they have many relapses of a single episode of several years' duration? I tend to think it's the latter, but the rhythm of the illness makes research very difficult.

How about the time between attacks? For many persons with bipolar disorder, modern treatments are quite effective at keeping the episodes from recurring. But how long did remissions last in the days before these treatments were available? Kraepelin noted that the time between episodes could be years, even decades. Among 703 "intervals" that he studied in his patients, Kraepelin found one case in which forty-four years separated one episode of illness from the next.[5] However, many subsequent studies have shown that, if untreated, episodes of bipolar disorder occur more and more frequently in individual patients (see figure 2-3). The illness seems to accelerate if untreated, and in the days before treatment was available, mood episodes tended to recur more and more frequently as patients aged. This acceleration has profound implications for treatment and prognosis, as we shall see in chapter 20.

Another finding in these older studies is that some patients tend to "switch" from a depression to a manic episode without an interval of normal

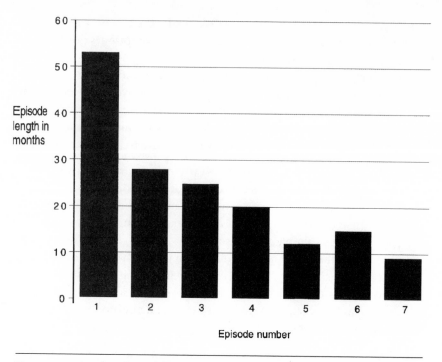

FIGURE 2-3 Acceleration of illness in one hundred patients. This graph shows that the cycle length of episodes of bipolar disorder (the time from the onset of one episode to the onset of the next) becomes shorter and shorter in patients whose symptoms are not well controlled and who continue to have episodes of the illness.

Source: Data from P. P. Roy-Burne, R. M. Post, T. W. Uhde, T. Porcu, and D. Davis, "The Longitudinal Course of Recurrent Affective Illness: Life Chart Data from Patients at the NIMH," *Acta Psychiatrica Scandinavia* 71, suppl. 317 (1985): 1–34.

TABLE 2-2 Features of Bipolar I

Mood
Fully developed manic episodes
Fully developed depressive episodes

Other Features
Untreated episodes average six months
Hallucinations and delusions frequently seen
Triphasic episodes
Relapses more frequent as patient ages

mood. In a 1969 study, the course of one hundred manic episodes was described.[6] Many individuals were noted to have a period of depression of several weeks' or months' duration that switched into a manic episode, again of
several months' duration. In a few of these patients, there followed another
switch and the beginning of a third phase of the episode: a long period of depression. In this study, about half of the patients' manic episodes showed at
least one switch—a depression either before or after their manic episode.
There have been several studies that suggest that patients who "switch" from
depression to mania have a more difficult-to-treat form of illness than those
who switch from mania to depression.[7]

Bipolar I is the classic manic-depressive illness, with fully developed
manic episodes and episodes of severe depression, and it is also characterized by long periods of "hibernation" in which the symptoms temporarily
disappear (see table 2-2). The number of episodes varies enormously, but patients who have only one or two episodes seem to be the exception rather
than the rule. Before effective treatments became available, the average
length of each episode if untreated was about six months—but episodes that
lasted years were not at all uncommon.

Bipolar II

Robert was a thirty-nine-year-old accountant who had been seeing a
psychologist for treatment of depression for about three months. Both
he and his therapist were frustrated because despite the best efforts of
both, Robert's depression seemed to be getting worse.

"I can usually pull myself out of these things—or at least I can usually slog through them until they finish," he told me at our first appointment. Right away, his description of his depressions as "these
things" made me feel pretty certain that this fellow had a mood disorder. Robert's moods had an alien, external quality to him; they came
upon him like a fog bank rolling in, lasted for a few weeks, and then
slowly dissipated. Where they came from and where they went was a
complete mystery to Robert. He would sleep away the weekends, put
on weight, fall behind in his work. "This has been happening to me
since college," he said, "and I really want it to stop." In fact, this was not
the worst his depressions had ever gotten. Shortly after graduation,
Robert had had such a severe depression that he had spent most of the
summer at home in his room. At one point he had seriously contem-
plated suicide. The only reason he hadn't gotten into treatment then
was because he had felt he was no worse off than his mother.

Robert's mother was a closet alcoholic. "There was always one of those huge bottles of wine in the refrigerator," he told me. "It always seemed either full or half full, and when I was in high school I realized that this was because she drank about a half a gallon every day." Robert's mother had never had any treatment for either her drinking problem or for depression, but his description of the long "naps" she took most afternoons and the "sick headaches" that put her in bed for weeks sounded like more than alcoholism—more like a smoldering depression *complicated* by alcohol addiction. Another red flag for a mood-disorder diagnosis: a positive family history.

Robert had always blamed his melancholic moods on his childhood. The memories of his shame and worry about his mother seeped back into his consciousness during these times, as did guilty feelings that he had put hundreds of miles between himself and his mother now, hadn't seen her in over two years, and could bring himself to call her only on holidays. Here was more evidence pointing to a mood disorder: guilty feelings and painful preoccupations with the past that seemed really to bother him only when his mood changed. Though I wasn't quite through taking his history, I was already thinking about which antidepressant to recommend to him when Robert gave me another piece of information that changed everything.

"I even feel like my *thinking* is slower than usual. I'll never get through tax season unless I do something to get some help—or unless one of my highs kicks in."

"One of your . . . ?"

"I call it a high. But it's not like I'm manic-depressive or anything. It's just that sometimes when things get back to normal I'm so relieved and happy that—oh, I don't know, it just feels so good not to be depressed."

"Do you find that you're especially productive during these times?" I asked.

"Oh, definitely. One year I came out of a depression just in time for tax season. I didn't feel overwhelmed like I usually do. It was spring, and I wasn't depressed for a change, and I had just met the girl I was going to marry—in fact we got married that summer, and so of course things settled back down. But that was a great year."

"Do other people notice?"

"Um, yes, especially at the office. 'Slow down, Rob.' 'Take it easy, Rob.' Sometimes I get irritated by that."

I had a few more questions to ask, but I was beginning to think about how to tell this fellow that he probably had "manic-depression" after all.

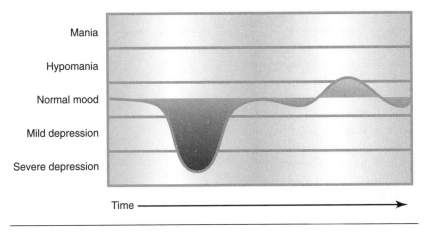

FIGURE 2-4 Mood changes in bipolar II

Bipolar II is characterized by fully developed depressive episodes and episodes of *hypo*mania. A schematic representation of the moods of bipolar II appears in figure 2-4.

When lithium became available in the United States in the 1970s and researchers were trying to find better diagnostic criteria for bipolar disorder, several of them noticed that there was a large group of patients who didn't have a history of fully developed manic episodes but who seemed to be bipolar nonetheless. They had severe depressions, but their "highs" never developed into mania. Were these patients "manic-depressives" who were still early in the course of their illness and simply hadn't had time to have a fully developed manic episode? Several studies attempting to answer this question concluded that these patients did *not* usually go on to fully developed mania. In one study, fewer than 5 percent of the patients with recurrent depressions and hypomania ever became manic.[8] Several studies showed as well that these patients often had relatives who also had a bipolar mood disorder characterized by major depressions and hypomanias.[9] Although patients with bipolar II sometimes have family members who have bipolar I or depressive disorders (without either mania or hypomania), the disorder frequently seems to "breed true": family members of persons with bipolar II who have mood disorders also tend to have bipolar II symptom patterns.[10]

Since bipolar II is a rather new way of classifying bipolar disorders, we can't go back into the research literature of the days before lithium and look for statistics on the course of untreated bipolar II. So we don't know for sure if bipolar II patients have longer or shorter or more frequent or less frequent episodes of illness. Nevertheless, modern studies indicate that there are a few typical features of bipolar II (see table 2-3).

TABLE 2-3 Features of Bipolar II

Mood
Fully developed depressive episodes
Hypomanic episodes

Other Features
Increased sleep and appetite during depressions
Depressions sometimes more chronic
Bipolar II history in family members
Later age at first hospitalization
Fewer hospitalizations
Possible increased risk for alcoholism

Bipolar II patients seem to have more problems with depression—in fact the depression is sometimes so prominent that many receive a diagnosis of depressive disorder and don't get treatment for bipolar disorder at all. In a study from the National Institutes of Health published in 1995, 559 patients diagnosed with a depressive disorder were followed over time, some for up to eleven years. It was reported that almost 9 percent of them developed symptoms of bipolar II.[11] The first hypomanic episode could usually be documented within several months of the onset of severe depression, but sometimes it took up to nine years for the correct diagnosis to become clear. Some of these 559 "depression" patients also developed a manic episode— that is, they turned out to have bipolar I—but this was far less common (only 3.9 percent). This study also found that bipolar II patients had longer depressive episodes (52.2 weeks) than bipolar I patients (24.3 weeks). Bipolar II patients have also been found to be at higher risk for alcoholism.[12]

What is the relationship between bipolar I and bipolar II? At present, there are only interesting speculations. As noted above, it is fairly clear that bipolar II is not merely a prelude to "full-blown" manic-depressive illness— that is, bipolar II patients are not in the early stages of bipolar I. These two conditions really seem to be separate illnesses, and bipolar II can perhaps best be thought of as a milder form of bipolar I.

There is some evidence to suggest that bipolar II is actually more common than bipolar I. Researchers from Johns Hopkins University published a study in 1993 showing that when the family members of individuals with bipolar disorder (I or II) are evaluated for mood disorders, bipolar II shows up most often.[13] Even when family members of individuals with bipolar I were studied, bipolar II was more frequent (see table 2-4).

TABLE 2-4 Family Histories of Bipolar I and Bipolar II Patients

	Family Members of Bipolar I Patients	Family Members of Bipolar II Patients
Percentage diagnosed with bipolar I	15.5	2.1
Percentage diagnosed with bipolar II	22.4	40.4

Source: Data from Sylvia Simpson, Susan Folstein, Deborah Meyers, Francis McMahon, Diane Brusco, and J. Raymond DePaulo, "Bipolar II: The Most Common Bipolar Phenotype?" *American Journal of Psychiatry* 150 (1993): 901–3.

These researchers suggested that instead of thinking of bipolar II as a less severe form of bipolar I, it might be more accurate to think of the relationship the other way round. Bipolar II might be the more common and "simpler" disorder, and bipolar I its more complicated and more severe form. Perhaps individuals with bipolar II, the simpler disorder, have only one mood-disorder gene. Bipolar I might be the result of multiple "hits," either when multiple genes are affected or because of some other combination of abnormal genes and environmental events.

Cyclothymic Disorder

Phil was a thirty-one-year-old recently married man whose wife had insisted that he come to the local community mental-health clinic because of his "mood swings." He had never had any psychiatric treatment before and wasn't sure he really needed any now. "I'm doing this for her, Doc. I'm not crazy," he said as he sat down. "If you really want to know, I think *she's* the one with the problem."

"What do you mean?"

"Well, don't get me wrong. She's a great girl, and I really love her, but . . ." He seemed to be having a hard time admitting something. "She's an only child, and she's—well, I admit it, she's more mature than I am, and she can't, oh, I don't know . . . just go with the flow."

I smiled a little and shook my head. "Sorry, Phil, I'm not getting it."

"Well, I don't think my mood swings are *that* bad. I think she's overreacting to them. Everyone has good days and bad, don't they?"

"Well, yes, that's true, of course, but some people seem to have runs of extremely good days and of extremely bad days that they can't quite account for. Have you ever experienced anything like that?"

In fact Phil never knew when he went to bed at night just what his mood might be when he got up. He sold expensive sailboats for a living and was usually good at it—in fact sometimes he was great at it, but he needed those "great" times to offset the down times. During the down times, which lasted up to a week, Phil would miss work, sleep ten to twelve hours a day, lose interest in everything—including sex with his wife—and be just miserable. Then he would suddenly awake one morning with boundless energy, confidence, and enthusiasm and sell more boats in two days than he had the previous week. But there was a down side to the "up" times too—sometimes Phil would get impatient with customers, pressure them too much, and lose a sale he might otherwise have made. He also drank too much during these times and had even been arrested once for "driving under the influence."

School had been similar: uneven and unpredictable performance. Sometimes he got A's and B's and other times D's and F's. His high school teachers thought him bright but "not mature enough for college" and suggested that he work for a few years before attempting it, perhaps thinking a dose of life in the "real world" would teach Phil better self-control.

"But I *can't* control how I feel; that's just the way I am. I've just learned how to live with it."

And this was, of course, exactly the point. Phil thought that everyone lived at the mercy of their moods and learned how to "go with the flow," as he put it—learned how to adjust his or her schedule and activities according to unpredictable fluctuations of mood. It was only when he got married that he got an objective observer—his wife— who noticed that Phil's moods had a life and rhythm of their own. "She keeps telling me that everyone *doesn't* have mood swings like I do, but I think she's wrong. What do you think?"

"Well, I think you married a very astute young woman. I think she might be right."

Cyclothymic disorder (-*thymia*, from the Greek word for "mind," is used in psychiatry to refer to mood) is characterized by frequent short periods (days to weeks) of depressive symptoms and of hypomania separated by periods (which also tend to be short, on the order of days to weeks) of fairly normal mood. By definition, the patient does not have either fully developed major depressive episodes or manic episodes. A schematic representation of the moods of cyclothymia appears in figure 2-5.

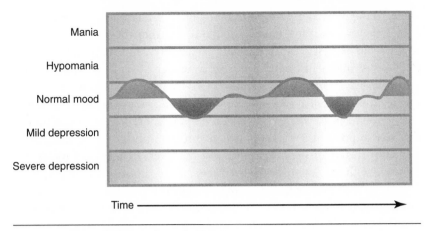

FIGURE 2-5 Mood changes in cyclothymia

Emil Kraepelin believed that "there are certain temperaments which may be regarded as rudiments of manic-depressive insanity. They may [exist] throughout the whole of life as peculiar forms of psychic personality without further development." Kraepelin described "cyclothymic temperament" as "characterized by frequent, more or less regular fluctuations of the psychic state to the manic or to the depressive side."[14] He reported that 3 to 4 percent of his patients had the cyclothymic temperament but speculated that many more persons might have similar illnesses that "run their course outside of institutions." Modern research on community populations has proven Kraepelin (as usual) quite correct. Several studies have shown that cyclothymic disorder probably affects 3 to 6 percent of the population.[15] Clearly most of these individuals are neither diagnosed nor treated for these mood problems (fewer than 6 percent of the general population ever receive treatment for any psychiatric problem).

Kraepelin's descriptions of the symptoms of cyclothymia are lively and vivid:

> These are the people who constantly oscillate hither and thither between the two opposite poles of mood, sometimes "rejoicing to the skies," sometimes "sad as death." Today lively, sparkling, beaming, full of the joy of life, the pleasure of enterprise, and the pressure of activity, after some time they meet us depressed, enervated, ill-humored, in need of rest, and again a few months later they display the old freshness and elasticity.[16]

For many years American psychiatric classification systems regarded cyclothymia as a personality problem. The concept of "temperament," which can be thought of as a person's usual manner of thinking, behaving, or reacting, captures the same idea. Cyclothymia was thought to be better understood as an expression of a person's personality than as an illness caused by an abnormality of brain chemistry. In earlier editions of the *Diagnostic and Statistical Manual* of the American Psychiatric Association (the *DSM*), the disorder was called *cyclothymic personality disorder*. This changed rather recently (in 1980), when *cyclothymic disorder* moved over to the mood-disorder section of the manual—where it remains today.

Individuals with cyclothymic disorder have very frequent ups and downs of mood with only comparatively few periods of "normal" mood (see table 2-5). As Kraepelin noted, they seem to "constantly oscillate . . . between the two opposite poles of mood." (This almost constant instability perhaps explains why psychiatrists thought of this as a "personality" characteristic for so long.) As might be expected, constant mood instability causes instability in many areas of the patient's life. In a 1977 study of forty-six patients with cyclothymia, the patients demonstrated a whole variety of oscillations of emotions and behavior—from sleep patterns to work habits to group affiliations (see table 2-6).[17]

Cyclothymic disorder begins early in life—in the late teens or early twenties.[18] Although many persons with cyclothymic disorder never develop more severe mood symptoms, a significant number of them eventually have a fully developed depression or manic episode—that is, they develop bipolar disorder. In one study, about 6 percent of patients with cyclothymic disorder eventually had a manic episode, putting them in the bipolar I category, but a higher number (25 percent) developed severe depression—that is, they turned out to have bipolar II.[19] However, perhaps half of patients with the cyclothymic pattern never develop symptoms of full-blown bipolar disor-

TABLE 2-5 Features of Cyclothymic Disorder

Mood
Frequent alteration between mild depression and mild hypomania
Short irregular cycles (days)
Only short periods of normal mood

Other Features
Patients often wake up with mood changes
Pattern appears in late teens, early twenties
Frequently mistaken for problem with "personality"
Sometimes develops into bipolar I or II

TABLE 2-6 Mood, Thinking, and Behavior Patterns in Forty-six
Cyclothymic Patients

Mood	Percentage of Patients
Irritable periods lasting a few days	50
Explosive, aggressive outbursts	50
Thinking	
Shaky self-esteem alternating between lack of self-confidence and overconfidence	75
Periods of mental confusion alternating with periods of sharpened creative thinking	50
Activity and Behavior	
Increased sleep alternating with decreased need for sleep	75
Unevenness in quantity and quality of work	75
Buying sprees, extravagance, or financial disasters	75
Repeated shifts in work, study, interest, or future plans	50
Drug or alcohol abuse	50
Extroversion alternating with introversion	50
Unexplained promiscuity or extramarital affairs	40
Joining new movement with enthusiasm, rapidly changing to disillusionment	25

Source: Data from H. Akiskal, M. K. Khani, and A. Scott-Strauss, "Cyclothymic Temperamental Disorders," *Psychiatric Clinics of North America* 2 (1979): 527–54, quoted in Frederick K. Goodwin and Kay Redfield Jamison, *Manic-Depressive Illness* (New York: Oxford University Press, 1990), 54.

der—a finding that makes cyclothymic disorder a true diagnosis in its own right.

Family-history studies indicate that there is some relationship between cyclothymia and other bipolar disorders. Patients with cyclothymia often have relatives with bipolar disorder but rarely have relatives suffering from depressions only.[20] As we shall see in chapter 6, treatment experiences seem to confirm this relationship: the mood swings of cyclothymic disorder often respond to many of the same treatment approaches as the bipolar disorders. This finding also confirms that cyclothymia is just as much a "chemical" problem as the other bipolar disorders, and that thinking of the mood swings of cyclothymia as arising from personality problems is not helpful in making treatment decisions.

Bipolar Spectrum Disorders

If you look at the end of the section on bipolar disorders in the fourth edition of the *Diagnostic and Statistical Manual* of the American Psychiatric Association, you will see the category "bipolar disorder not otherwise specified" (also, simply, "bipolar NOS"). This odd category exists because the developers of the *DSM* recognized that there are patients who seem to have *some* kind of bipolar disorder but who don't meet the diagnostic criteria for bipolar I or II or cyclothymia.

Maria is a violinist in the local symphony orchestra. She is nearly sixty but looks much younger. Born in what is now the Czech Republic, she defected to the United States during a tour of a chamber music group in the 1960s. Maria found herself in New York with only a small suitcase of clothes, her violin, and a charming European accent. She credits the latter two with her success in finding good work with several American orchestras over the years.

"I must tell you, Doctor, that my son has started taking lithium and Wellbutrin, just like me. His psychiatrist asked him about my medications and put my son on the same ones. It's so good to know he's being treated by a psychiatrist as brilliant as you."

"Now, now, it was hardly brilliant of me to—"

"Oh, yes, so humble, so modest you are, just like all geniuses."

This was a little game we had played for years, ever since we had come up with a combination of medications that controlled her mood symptoms—for the first time in many years.

Because she had moved to a new city every five years or so, Maria had seen many different professionals for her mood problems— mostly depression. For many of those years she had gotten no treatment at all but simply slogged through her periods of depression on her own. During the 1970s, a physician had given her a prescription for the tranquilizer Valium, and although it hadn't treated her depression very well, it numbed Maria's feelings enough to keep her going. When she moved to a new community, she would be able to get more prescriptions for Valium by reporting to her new doctor that it helped her—which, after a fashion, it did. During the really bad times, Maria used alcohol to augment the Valium's effect. By the time she was in her mid-forties she was well on her way to chemical dependency. One terrible year she lost a job because of missing several rehearsals and an important concert while in a week-long alcohol- and Valium-induced fog during a period of depression. Her husband left her, and a month later she got word that her son, also a talented musician, had dropped out of the prestigious conservatory he had been attending and had disappeared.

Maria's depression worsened to the point that she took a nearly fatal overdose of Valium and alcohol. It was only because the manager of the apartment building where she was living happened to go into her apartment that particular day that she ended up in a hospital rather than in the city morgue. She was eventually admitted to the psychiatric unit for treatment of her depression.

It was in the psychiatric hospital that she started taking an antidepressant for the first time, but the imipramine she was started on made things even worse. Within three days of starting on the antidepressant, Maria started to have manic symptoms. She started staying up all night furiously writing music, convinced that she had discovered new musical forms and new harmonies that would make her fabulously famous and even more fabulously wealthy. Her antidepressant medication was immediately stopped, and she was started on lithium. Within about ten days her mood was back to normal.

On lithium, her depressions were less frequent and less severe, but she continued to have several weeks of low mood every year, and it was during one of these that she had come to see me for the first time. "You were the first doctor to understand that I needed lithium *and* an antidepressant, and that makes you truly brilliant," Maria continued, a raised eyebrow emphasizing her slightly teasing tone.

I was the lucky recipient of a lot of gratitude—gratitude she sometimes archly exaggerated to keep me from taking myself too seriously—because her moods were stable for the first time in years on this combination of pharmaceuticals.

Starting a patient with a history of manic symptoms on an antidepressant is something psychiatric textbooks warn against—but Maria had had manic symptoms only once in her life, at age fifty-three, while taking an antidepressant. Did this really make her bipolar? She didn't have the history of manic or even hypomanic episodes that would make her fit the bipolar I or II diagnosis—yet she clearly had *some* type of bipolar disorder.

Psychiatrists have long recognized that there are many forms of bipolar disorder. Kraepelin noted that "it is fundamentally and practically impossible to keep apart in any way" the various forms of bipolar disorder, and that "everywhere there are transitions."[21] For many years various clinicians have described various types of "soft" bipolar disorder (see table 2-7), mostly in

TABLE 2-7 Indicators of "Soft" Bipolar Disorders

Family history of bipolar disorder
History of mania or hypomania caused by treatment with antidepressants
History of "mixed" mood states
Depressive, "hyper," or cycling temperament
Recurrent depressions

patients who came to be treated for depression and whose illness seemed related to bipolar disorder.[22] Terms like *pseudo-unipolar depression* and *bipolar III* have been coined to describe various types of severe depressions that have some features of bipolar disorder but do not fall into traditional categories for bipolar diagnoses. Often these patients have had a long history of depressive-like or manic-like features in their usual mood state, or "temperament," which are punctuated by the more severe mood symptoms that bring them to treatment.

As more treatments for bipolar disorder become available and as more research on the mood disorders is done, it is becoming clear that many patients who suffer from mostly depressive symptoms can benefit from treatment with medications for bipolar disorders and may in fact have a type of bipolar disorder.

Nathan is the fifty-five-year-old executive director of a philanthropic foundation. He describes himself as a "workaholic" who for years has worked sixteen- to eighteen-hour days and with only four to six hours of sleep a night. Nathan is famous around town for his buoyant optimism and the boundless energy that he says comes from "making a living giving away other people's money," but his staff knows that he can be impatient and driven when deadlines approach or personnel problems distract him from devoting himself 110 percent to his mission. He came to me for treatment of miserable, irritable, restless feelings that had bothered him for several years but had gotten much worse in the previous few months.

Nathan had had problems with depression before but had never received any treatment with medication. When he was twenty-five he had been depressed after a friend died in a freak accident while both of them were skiing. Nathan had been a graduate student at the time and nearly dropped out of school. When he was in his forties he went through several months of depressed mood, trouble concentrating on his work, and appetite and weight loss that he and his psychiatrist at the time labeled a "midlife crisis" exacerbated by some unpleasant changes in his job. He was in therapy for about three months, and he started feeling better after he embarked on the job search that eventually led to his current position with a prestigious foundation.

"Or maybe it was the other way around," he mused.

"What do you mean?" I asked.

"Maybe I was able to look for a new job because I was feeling better."

"Do you know if other people in your family have had trouble with depression?"

"My father left us when I was three, and they say he was in and out of psychiatric hospitals his whole life. Both his sisters were alcoholics; one committed suicide."

Nathan was proud that despite his childhood in a broken, impoverished home, he now headed a foundation, signed checks for millions of dollars every year, and was courted by presidents of hospitals and universities every day of the week. "So why do I feel this way?" he asked. "It can't just be stress; I thrive on stress. These hopeless feelings come over me, these 'what's the point?' feelings. Why now?"

Nathan suffers from one of the "soft" bipolar disorders that some researchers call *bipolar III*.[23] These patients have a baseline mood that is a bit "higher" than that of most people, a personality characteristic that has been called *hyperthymic temperament* (see table 2-8). Their usual energy level is high; they are cheerful, talkative, confident, and sociable. The down side of their personality style is that they tend to become irritated easily and can be impulsive, even reckless at times. They usually have a family history of bipolar disorder and are bothered by recurrent depressions. Antidepressant medication alone can make them more irritable and miserable or provoke a manic or hypomanic episode, but mood stabilizers can be very helpful.

TABLE 2-8 Features of Bipolar III

Family history of bipolar disorder
Hyperthymic temperament:
   Habitual short sleeper—less than six hours per day
   Cheerful, optimistic personality style
   Tendency to become irritable easily
   Extroverted and sociable
Recurrent depressions

For about half a century, psychiatry divided mood disorders into cases of unipolar depression, an illness characterized by only depressive symptoms, and bipolar disorders, in which patients suffer depressive episodes but also manic, hypomanic, or mixed states as well. Bipolar spectrum disorders seem to challenge this way of thinking; many of these patients have an illness that is dominated by depressive symptoms and shows only the slightest colorings of mania. They may have periods of elevated mood that they don't feel are particularly abnormal but that, when examined more closely, bear the hallmarks of hypomania: decreased need for sleep, increased energy, uncharacteristic overconfidence, and loss of inhibitions. As mentioned previously, periods of agitation and irritability that last only a few hours may represent mild mixed states. I have seen many patients who have been unsuccessfully treated with one antidepressant after another for what they have been told is "unipolar depression." Many of these patients have bipolar features to their illness that haven't been recognized as such. When one of the medications more typically used to treat bipolar disorder is prescribed for these patients, they frequently have a significant improvement in their depressive symptoms.

Some patients with this kind of problem become upset when I try to explain that a better treatment approach for their depression might be to treat it as a form of bipolar disorder; they worry that a diagnosis of bipolar disorder means they have a more serious problem than "just depression" or are "really crazy." This overlooks a couple of facts: first, depression is always a serious illness, and second, many people with bipolar disorder never develop full-blown mania or psychotic symptoms (which is what most people are thinking of when they use the pejorative term *crazy*). I sometimes use the term *complicated depression* to talk about these illnesses.

The important point to remember is that, despite what you might gather from reading short newspaper or magazine articles about depression and bipolar disorder, we haven't yet figured out how to classify these illnesses. It is becoming clear that many cases that seem to be "just depression" are related in some way to bipolar disorder. Many depressed patients who don't seem to have classic "manic-depressive illness" will nevertheless benefit from medications used to treat bipolar disorder.

Rapid-Cycling Bipolar Disorder

Soon after lithium became available for the treatment of bipolar disorder, psychiatrists noticed that some of the sickest bipolar patients didn't seem to derive much benefit from it. These patients clearly suffered from a bipolar mood disorder—they had severe manias and depressions—but they were set apart from other bipolar patients by the frequency of their episodes. Currently, rapid-cycling bipolar disorder is diagnosed if the patient has four or more episodes (mania, hypomania, depression, or mixed state) in one year.[24]

Early impressions and case reports seemed to indicate that there were features other than frequency of episodes that set rapid-cycling bipolar disorder apart from other bipolar disorders. It seemed to occur more often in females, usually began with a depressive episode, and was less responsive to lithium therapy. There also seemed to be some indication that patients with this pattern of illness were more likely to have a history of thyroid gland problems and to have been treated with antidepressant medications.[25] There were suggestions from some researchers that these last two factors—thyroid disease and treatment with antidepressants—might cause "normal" bipolar illness to switch into rapid-cycling illness.[26]

Of these two factors, the most interest has been focused on the possibility that treatment with antidepressant medications can cause the switch from "normal" bipolar disorder into a rapid-cycling form. One study examined the case records of 118 patients who were rapid cyclers (had had four or more episodes of abnormal mood in one year).[27] The researchers found that eighty-six of these patients seemed to have had a change of the course of their illness—that is, they had "switched" into a rapid-cycling pattern. The authors stated that "the majority" of these switched after they were treated with an antidepressant medication.

A more recent study casts some doubt on these findings and on the usefulness of talking about rapid cycling as a specific type of bipolar disorder.[28] In this study, 919 patients were followed over a five-year period, and any who met the criteria for rapid cycling (having had at least one episode of mania or hypomania and three additional episodes of any type during one year) were studied closely for the next five years. Forty-five patients turned out to meet the rapid-cycling criteria, and their family history, treatment course, and course of illness were compared with those of the "normal" bipolar patients.

The picture that emerged from these patients suggested that rapid cycling is a temporary phase of bipolar illness that some patients are prone to—not a particular type of bipolar illness. The rapid cycling stopped after a period of several months in forty-four out of the forty-five patients who were studied. These patients did not have rapid cyclers in their family, although they did have family members with "normal" bipolar illness. The link with thyroid disease and antidepressant treatment seemed weak, and these patients didn't seem any less treatable with lithium than other bipolar patients. As time went on, their rapid cycling gradually stopped. The only finding from the earlier reports that was confirmed was that more women than men had rapid cycling; nearly three-quarters of the patients with rapid cycling were women (bipolar disorder usually affects both sexes about equally).

Some bipolar patients (18.5 percent in this study) seem to go through a period of rapid cycling for some months during which their symptoms are more difficult to control—more women than men (I discuss this in more depth in chapter 14). Although there continues to be suspicion among many clinicians that antidepressant medications can cause some patients to start rapid cycling, the exact causes of rapid cycling remain a mystery, as does, unfortunately, the treatment steps that will prevent it.

Schizoaffective Disorder

Some patients have an illness that has features both of mood disorders and of a very different psychiatric illness: schizophrenia. In addition to mood-disorder symptoms such as depression, hypomania, or mania, these patients have the hallucinations, delusions, and other bizarre mental experiences typical of schizophrenia; they often receive the diagnosis of schizoaffective disorder.

As we have seen in chapter 1, many patients with bipolar disorder develop delusional beliefs or hallucinations. But in the mood disorders, these symptoms can be understood as arising out of the mood state. For example, in a severe depression a patient might have the delusional belief that he or she has a terrible illness like AIDS or has lost all of his or her money, or that family members are being tortured by kidnappers, all beliefs that are—well, depressing. Manic patients may hear the singing of angels or the voice of God—again, hallucinations that can be understood as coming out of the expansive, grandiose mood of mania. Delusions (false beliefs and ideas) and hallucinations (false sensory perceptions such as the hearing of voices) are said to be *mood congruent* when they can be understood as being part of the abnormal mood.

Persons with schizophrenia have bizarre delusions and hallucinations too, but they don't usually seem to bear any relation to a change in mood. Examples of schizophrenic delusions would be the belief that one's next-door neighbors are pumping poisonous gas into one's house, or that one's real spouse and children have been replaced by exact replicas, or that the FBI has implanted a transmitter in one's brain. Patients with schizophrenia sometimes believe that other people are reading their minds or putting into their heads thoughts that are not theirs. They might hear their own thoughts repeated to them aloud or hear the voices of unseen commentators describing their actions to other unseen persons. None of these symptoms has much relationship to mood changes.

When a person has bizarre delusions or hallucinations like those described above or has these kinds of symptoms during times when they do not seem to be in an episode of abnormal mood, the diagnosis of schizoaffective disorder is often made.

What is this disorder, and where does it belong in the classification of psychiatric disease? These are questions that have plagued psychiatry for many years; we still don't have very good answers to them.

Is schizoaffective disorder truly a separate disorder, an illness that shares symptoms with mood disorders and schizophrenia but is neither? If it is, it has been very difficult for researchers to agree on its defining symptoms. In an earlier version of *DSM*, the American Psychiatric Association's classification manual for mental illnesses, the diagnostic category of schizoaffective disorder was included without *any* listing of the symptoms that defined it.

I have seen patients who have been diagnosed with schizoaffective disorder who seem to me instead to have a severe case of a mood disorder that has been difficult to treat. Patients can be delusional and have hallucinations when they are very depressed or very manic, and if they are in a phase of ultra–rapid cycling, these symptoms can change rapidly and do not seem to make much sense in relation to their moods. I have seen patients diagnosed with schizoaffective disorder because they have prominent paranoid symptoms—that is, they believe that they are being watched or followed or talked about. Although paranoid symptoms are very common in some types of schizophrenia and not as common in the mood disorders, close questioning often reveals the mood component in these patients. In a book written during the last century called *A Mind That Found Itself*, Clifford Beers described his battle with a mental illness that was almost certainly bipolar disorder. In one scene he describes a train ride to the psychiatric hospital. As the train passed through the stations along the way, Beers noticed people standing on the station platforms reading the newspaper. He became convinced that they were reading about him. At first glance, this symptom doesn't seem to have any mood component, and in fact it is a rather typical symptom of schizophrenia called an *idea of reference*. Fortunately, however, Beers describes this symptom in great detail in his book and writes that he thought the people on the train platforms were reading about his long history of mental illness and about what a failure he had been. With this added detail—the themes of shame and failure in the symptom—the mood component becomes obvious and the real diagnosis clear: a mood disorder.

Another possible explanation for the mingling of symptoms of a mood disorder and of schizophrenia in one patient is that the patient may suffer from *both* illnesses. If one considers that bipolar I affects about 1 percent of the population and that about 1 percent of the population suffers from schizophrenia, then obviously, if there are no other factors operating to prevent the illnesses from occurring together, as many as 0.01 percent of the population will suffer from both disorders—that is, one in ten thousand. If one adds in other mood disorders such as bipolar II, cyclothymia, and the "soft" bipolar disorders, the numbers of persons with schizophrenia who also have a mood disorder will be even greater. Treatment experience would seem to support this idea: patients with a diagnosis of schizoaffective disorder seem to be most effectively treated with medications for mood disorders used in combination with medications for schizophrenia.

This said, there are some patients whose illness definitely seems to combine two disorders: patients who have the kind of bizarre delusions common in schizophrenia, which seem to have nothing to do with an abnormal mood, but who also have clear-cut episodes of depression and mania. This seems to be a rare disorder, but it is important not to miss it. I have occasionally seen patients whose psychiatrist seemed reluctant to make the diagnosis of schizoaffective disorder, perhaps not wanting to frighten patients and families with the diagnosis of an illness that is usually more impairing and difficult to treat than a bipolar disorder. This reluctance to diagnose, however, can result in the illness not being treated aggressively enough.

I once saw a patient whose psychiatrist had referred him for consultation because of what had been diagnosed as severe bipolar depression with psychotic symptoms that had responded poorly to many different treatments for mood disorders. This patient was certainly depressed, but his illness—which had required multiple hospitalizations and had become so disabling that he could no longer work or even live in his own apartment—had other features consistent with schizophrenia. For this patient, treatment for depression was only helpful up to a point. Only when he was also prescribed clozapine (Clozaril), a medication usually reserved for patients with severe schizophrenia who have failed to benefit from other medications, did he have a substantial recovery. Making a change in diagnosis and recommending a very different treatment approach was upsetting for this patient and his family at first—for just the reasons mentioned above. But the patient's parents also admitted that they had long suspected that their son had "more than just bipolar disorder," and with more careful explanations of my reasoning and further discussions with the patient and his family, we shifted the course of the treatment plan, ultimately with positive results. This is a lesson in the importance of making the correct diagnosis in mood disorders.

A diagnosis of schizoaffective disorder is in many ways more serious than that of bipolar disorder, as this illness shares some of the features of schizophrenia and some of the treatment challenges of that illness. Delusions and hallucinations may respond only incompletely to medication treatment, and more severe (and sometimes progressive) social and occupational impairment is not uncommon. For this very reason, however, it is even more important, if a diagnosis of schizoaffective disorder is being considered, to be extra careful in reviewing the symptoms and course of illness and to use information from as many sources as possible.

CHAPTER 3

A Summary of the Diagnostic Categories of Bipolar Disorder in *DSM IV*

INDIVIDUALS BEING TREATED BY A MENTAL-HEALTH PROFESSIONAL who read their diagnosis in their medical records or insurance statements often have questions about the diagnostic categories and terms that are used. Psychiatry is one of the few medical specialties that has a more or less official list of disorders and diagnoses, and in this chapter we'll take a closer look at the latest version of this list, the fourth edition of the *Diagnostic and Statistical Manual of Mental Disorders* (the *DSM IV*), developed and published by the American Psychiatric Association. I'll present a brief overview of the *DSM* and explain some of the diagnostic terminology for bipolar disorder.

What Is the *DSM*?

The roots of the *DSM IV* go back at least as far as the United States Census of 1840, which included the category of "idiocy/insanity" in its system for classifying American citizens. By 1880 there were seven categories into which persons with mental illness could be placed: mania, melancholia, monomania, paresis, dementia, dipsomania, and epilepsy.[1] In 1917 the American Medico-Psychological Association—the forerunner of the American Psychiatric Association—developed a statistical manual for use in mental hospitals that included various categories of diagnoses. As time went on other organizations interested in the statistics of mental illness, such as the Veterans Administration and the United States Army, developed their own statistical manuals. After World War II the World Health Association included a long section on mental disorders in the sixth edition of its *International Classification of Disease* (the *ICD 6*).

In 1952 the American Psychiatric Association published the *Diagnostic and Statistical Manual: Mental Disorders* (the *DSM I*), which differed from previous statistical manuals in that it contained a glossary that described the symptoms of the different disorders. Thus, in addition to containing an official list of categories of mental illness, the *DSM I* provided guidance to the clinician in making psychiatric diagnoses. By the time the third edition of the manual appeared in 1980, each category of psychiatric disorders had a list of *diagnostic criteria*—a list of the symptoms and other characteristics of each disorder that were thought to define it and to set it apart from other psychiatric disorders.

As its name now indicates, the *DSM* has become much more than a list of official diagnoses to be used to collect statistics on mental illness; it has developed into a valuable clinical tool, one that has proven immensely useful to clinicians and also to those who do research on psychiatric illnesses. Now, when a patient goes to a new doctor and his or her medical records indicate a diagnosis of, say, "panic disorder" or "anorexia nervosa," the new doctor knows—if the last psychiatrist did his or her job well, of course—that the patient has had certain symptoms and not others, and that the symptoms have troubled the patient for a certain period of time. Use of the *DSM* in research means that when you read a study of some particular psychiatric disorder in a professional journal and read that "the patients met the *DSM IV* diagnostic criteria" for that disorder, you can be sure that the patients all had a certain well-defined collection of symptoms and other characteristics in common, and that the researchers were not mixing, as it were, psychiatric apples and oranges in their study.

Because the *DSM* contains a list of psychiatric diagnoses followed by succinct and clearly written criteria for making those diagnoses, it has the unfortunate effect of making psychiatric diagnosis look easy. It is tempting for individuals who do not have any psychiatric training to regard it as series of symptom checklists that can be easily applied to make the diagnosis of mental illness. Well, why not?

First of all, it is only with an enormous amount of training and experience that one can gain an appreciation for the very wide range of *normal* emotions and behaviors and have a sense of what falls outside this normal range. Significant clinical experience and judgment are needed to decide what constitutes an "expansive mood" or an "increase in energy" that is clinically significant. I have been called to see "manic" patients referred by their counselors or their family members who turn out to be persons simply a bit more intense in manner than most people but whose mood state is perfectly within the normal range. The *DSM* is full of diagnostic criteria that use qualifiers like "clinically significant," "marked impairment," and "excessive involvement in . . . ," all requiring judgment based on experience to make a determination. Even some counseling and therapy professionals, if they have not trained in a setting where they have had the opportunity to see very sick patients, may not really have an appreciation for what constitutes "severe"— simply because they have never seen and worked with "severely" depressed or manic patients. Nonprofessionals will, of course, usually have even less experience with the range of normal and abnormal moods. Without the experience of seeing many patients with severe mental illnesses and treating them, it is impossible to accurately separate normal from abnormal mental experiences or "clinically significant" mood changes from those that are within the range of the normal. In psychiatry as perhaps in no other field, the dictum "A little learning is a dangerous thing" holds quite true!

Moreover, as we shall see in chapter 18, many *medical* conditions can mimic abnormal mood states, dozens of pharmaceuticals can cause depression or euphoric states in some persons, and drugs of abuse can cause all kinds of mood states and psychoses in almost anyone. Almost all the *DSM* diagnoses contain "exclusion criteria" for medical conditions, such as "the symptoms are not due to a general medical condition." A physician will probably notice the abnormalities in the facial appearance of a patient with Graves' disease or Cushing's syndrome as soon as the patient walks into the room; the nonphysician probably has never heard of these illnesses and doesn't know that they can cause psychiatric symptoms practically identical to those of a major depression episode. The physician knows well the typical walk of the patient with Parkinson's disease, the subtle language problems of the patient who has had a silent stroke—both neurological conditions that can cause mood symptoms. Obviously, only a clinician trained in the diagnosis and treatment of physical illness will be able to pick up these sorts of problems.

Finally, just as the range of normal experiences and behaviors is enormous, so is the range (and complexity) of abnormal mental experiences and behaviors; they cannot be contained in any one book and certainly cannot all be described in a few dozen diagnostic categories. Another great student of human behavior, the pioneering researcher on sexuality Alfred Kinsey, once said, "The world is not divided into sheep and goats . . . Nature rarely deals with discrete categories. Only the human mind invents categories and tries to force facts into separated pigeonholes."[2] To paraphrase Kinsey a bit, bipolar disorder is probably not divided simply into type I and type II, either—and patients often don't fit into *DSM* pigeonholes.

For these reasons I am not going to list here the *DSM* diagnostic criteria for the bipolar disorders. I don't want to tempt nonclinicians to engage in self-diagnosis or diagnosis of family members. The *DSM* is easily available in libraries, but it should be considered a reference book for clinicians, not a textbook of psychiatry.

A "Multiaxial" Diagnostic System

A formal *DSM* diagnosis always lists five types of diagnoses and other pieces of clinical information on patients in five separate categories, each of which is called an *axis:*

Axis I   Clinical disorders
Axis II   Personality and intelligence
Axis III   General medical conditions
Axis IV   Psychosocial and environmental problems
Axis V   Assessment of level of functioning

The reason for this complexity is, to put it plainly, that people are complex creatures, and to understand their mental life requires looking at them from several different angles.

Axis I lists the psychiatric illness or condition that is being treated or studied. This is where a mood-disorder diagnosis would go, as would diagnoses like "schizophrenia" or "panic disorder" or "alcohol abuse." This diagnosis will often include additional descriptive terms such as *chronic, acute, severe,* or *recurrent.*

Because symptoms of a mental illness might be expressed differently depending on a person's personality and intellectual ability, these two factors are also recorded in every patient, on axis II. Because these factors will affect how a person copes with a particular psychiatric illness, they are very important in developing plans for treating the disorder. This is also where a diagnosis of a *personality disorder* goes. A personality disorder is diagnosed when patients' personality—a complex mix of temperament, attitudes, and habits, their way of approaching life's problems, their attitudes toward themselves and those around them—causes problems for them in relationships and functioning. For example, persons with *antisocial personality disorder* show a chronic disregard for the rights of others that starts in childhood and continues throughout life. They manipulate and take advantage of others, break the law repeatedly, and show no remorse. This pattern of thinking, relating, and behaving seems to be something ingrained in their personality from an early age rather than the expression of an illness that is imposed upon them at some point. A diagnosis of mental retardation would also be listed on axis II.

Axis III is for any medical problem the individual may have. Examples would be high blood pressure, asthma, kidney failure, or migraine headaches. As we shall see in chapter 18, the axis III diagnosis is sometimes very important in treating a patient with a mood disorder because mood symptoms can be caused or affected by medical conditions such as stroke, Huntington's disease, and thyroid problems, to name only a few.

On axis IV are listed problems in and stresses from the patient's environment that may contribute to his or her difficulties: recent marriage or divorce, job stress or unemployment, chronic poverty, living in an unsafe neighborhood. These factors can also affect how individuals cope with illness as well as their response to treatment. Axis IV information is especially important in the mood disorders, since environmental stressors can be an important precipitating factor for an episode of illness (see chapter 20).

On axis V the clinician records an assessment of the patient's functional level. Using a 1–100 rating scale called the Global Assessment of Functioning (GAF) scale, a judgment is made as to how impaired (or unimpaired) the patient is on the basis of his or her symptoms in everyday life. On this scale, a score of 80 or above means basically normal everyday functioning; below 50 means serious impairment, such as recurrent unemployment due to psychiatric impairments; below 20 pretty much means that the person is in need of psychiatric hospitalization. This axis is perhaps more useful to researchers and statisticians than to clinicians, but it serves to round out a picture of the patient, capturing the person's strengths as opposed to his or her afflictions. For example, an individual might suffer from a severe psychiatric disorder like schizophrenia, have a low IQ, suffer from diabetes, and live at the poverty level but despite all these handicaps be a good parent who contributes to her community; an axis V rating would indicate that despite her psychiatric, intellectual, medical, and environmental problems, this person is functioning rather well. This hypothetical patient's *DSM IV* diagnoses would be as follows:

Axis I	Schizophrenia, paranoid type
Axis II	Mild mental retardation
Axis III	Diabetes
Axis IV	Poverty
Axis V	GAF = 80

Bipolar Categories in *DSM IV*

Only two subtypes of bipolar disorder have been characterized well enough, as to symptoms and course of illness, to have been assigned their own *DSM* categories: *bipolar I* and *bipolar II*. As we saw in chapter 2, in the section on bipolar spectrum disorders, there are probably other forms of the illness that will eventually be described and understood well enough to be demarcated with their own label as well, but for now a patient having another of

TABLE 3-1 Bipolar Disorders in *DSM IV*

Bipolar disorder I: Mania and depression
Bipolar disorder II: Depression and hypomania
   Severity specifiers for bipolar disorders:
      —mild, moderate, severe (with or without psychotic features)
      —in partial or full remission
   Special syndrome specifiers for bipolar disorders:
      —with catatonic, melancholic, or atypical features
      —with postpartum onset
   Longitudinal course specifiers for bipolar disorders:
      —with or without full interepisode recovery
      —with seasonal pattern
      —with rapid cycling
Bipolar disorder NOS: "Soft" bipolar and bipolar spectrum disorders
Cyclothymic disorder: Depressive symptoms and hypomanias
Substance-induced mood disorder
Mood disorder due to a general medical condition

these "soft" bipolar disorders would be diagnosed with *bipolar disorder not otherwise specified (bipolar disorder NOS)* according to *DSM. Cyclothymic disorder* is included in the *DSM IV* as an axis I diagnosis as well (see table 3-1).

For bipolar I patients, the clinician using the *DSM* is supposed to specify the type of the patient's latest episode, as in "bipolar I disorder, most recent episode manic," or "bipolar I disorder, most recent episode depressed."

The *DSM* also provides several other descriptive terms called *specifiers* that can be added to the main diagnosis to describe the current episode better. The clinician can call the episode *mild, moderate,* or *severe.* If the patient had not had any episodes in two months, the disorder is said to be *in remission* (in *full* remission if there have been no symptoms for two months, in *partial* remission if there have been only a few symptoms or if the remission has been less than two months).

The specifier *with psychotic features* can be added if the patient has hallucinations or delusional beliefs (such as those described in chapter 1) during his or her illness. The specifier *with catatonic features* is added if the patient shows symptoms of catatonia, a rare syndrome in which the patient lies (or sometimes sits or stands) motionless for long periods of time staring into space and has other bizarre physical mannerisms such as rigid posturing, grimacing, or meaninglessly repeating whatever is said to him or her. The specifier *with melancholic features* can be added when the patient's depressive episode is dominated by loss of ability to experience pleasure (anhedonia), the presence of guilty feelings, a loss of appetite, and the classic daily fluctuation of mood (early-morning awakening with the mood lifting slightly as the day progresses)—in short, the "textbook" depressive syndrome so eloquently described by William Styron in *Darkness Visible*. Another clinical syndrome, more common in depressive disorders than in bipolar disorders, has been called *atypical depression*. These patients retain reactivity in their mood (their mood brightens when good things happen); in fact, they seem to have a "hyper-reactive" mood and an especially difficult time with rejection in interpersonal relationships, even when not in an episode of depression. As noted before, this mood syndrome, called depression *with atypical features*, is not usually seen in bipolar disorder. If the mood episode occurs within four weeks of the birth of a child, it is called depression *with postpartum onset*.

There is another set of specifiers that describe the course of the illness over time, called *longitudinal course specifiers*. Bipolar disorders may be *with* or *without full interepisode recovery* depending on whether or not patients are completely free of symptoms between episodes.

In chapter 16 we shall learn about a form of bipolar disorder in which patients have repeated depressive episodes occurring regularly in winter and hypomanic or manic symptoms in the summer that has been called *seasonal affective disorder*. In *DSM IV* these patients are diagnosed with bipolar I or bipolar II, and the specifier *with seasonal pattern* is added. Finally, patients who have had at least four episodes of the disorder in twelve months have a disorder *with rapid cycling*.

When drug intoxication or medical problems mimic manic, hypomanic, or depressive episodes (see chapters 15 and 18), the *DSM* diagnoses *substance-induced mood disorder* or *mood disorder due to a general medical condition* are used. When the mood problem is due to a medical condition, the medical condition and type of mood change are specified in the diagnosis (as in, for example, "mood disorder due to hyperthyroidism, with manic features"). When the problem is due to substance abuse, the type of mood change and whether the symptoms came on during intoxication or withdrawal are specified. (Examples would be "cocaine-induced mood disorder with manic features, onset during intoxication," or "alcohol-induced mood disorder with depressive features, onset during withdrawal.")

CHAPTER 4

The Mood Disease

HAVING REVIEWED THE MANY SYMPTOMS OF BIPOLAR DISORDER AND the many forms the illness can take, I want to take a moment to review just how far we've come in our understanding of this illness—and where we've come *from*. I think that the understanding of any subject is incomplete unless you know a little about its history; and the history of the development of our current thinking about bipolar disorder is not only a fascinating story in its own right but also will provide valuable insights into how psychiatrists think about the diagnostic process and approach the treatment of disorders.

Before "Bipolar"

The ancient Greeks believed that all maladies of mind and body were caused by imbalances among four vital bodily fluids, or "humors." One of the terms we still use to describe depression, *melancholia,* is derived from the Greek word for one of these humors: black bile. According to humoral theory, depression was thought to be caused by an excess of black bile and mania by an excess of yellow bile. In a way this approach to explaining bipolar disorder was remarkably insightful. Modern scientists explaining abnormal mood states might talk of "dysregulation of neurotransmitter systems" rather than too much bile, but the idea that normal physiology is disrupted in the disease still rings true.

Although they were incorrect about the causes of the two opposite mood states of bipolar disorder, several ancient physicians had remarkable insight into the connection between them. Aretaius of Cappadocia (ca. 150) described the syndrome of depression in which patients became "peevish, dispirited, sleepless," and "complain[ed] of life and desire[d] to die." In other patients he described manic symptoms: "At the height of [their] disease [they] have impure dreams, and irresistible desire[s] . . . if roused to anger by admonition or restraint, they become wholly mad." But most remarkably, he stated that "in my opinion, melancholia is without any doubt the beginning and even part of the disorder called mania."[1] Paul of Aegina (625–90) made a similar connection between the two syndromes and based his thinking on humoral theory. Paul also assumed that melancholia was caused by too much ordinary black bile but postulated that mania was caused by an excess of "yellow bile which, by too much heat," had become burned black bile.[2]

Considerations of possible physical causes for the symptoms of bipolar disorder more or less ceased during medieval times, and the symptoms and behaviors that we now recognize as arising from psychiatric conditions were usually attributed to witchcraft or demonic possession rather than to disruptions of a person's physiology. When the Dark Ages gave way to the Renaissance and the Enlightenment, mental illness again became the purview of physicians rather than priests, and modern attempts to understand and classify diseases began. Melancholia and mania were often considered to be two separate disorders by these early physicians. However, a few insightful clinicians, such as the English physician Robert James (1705–76), connected the two syndromes:

> There is an absolute Necessity for reducing Melancholy and Madness [mania] to one Species of Disorder, and consequently considering them in one joint View . . . we find, that they both arise from the same common Cause and Origin, that is, an excessive Congestion of the Blood in the Brain . . . We find that melancholic Patients . . . easily fall into Madness, which, when removed, the Melancholy again discovers itself.[3]

Melancholia and "madness" were thought by most early physicians who wrote about mental disease to predispose to one another, but nevertheless to be entirely different conditions.

It was not until the middle of the nineteenth century that the idea that depression and mania might be expressions of a single mental illness was first proposed. It was proposed by two French *alienists* (a term—from *aliéné*, the French word for "insane"—that was used in France and in English-speaking countries at one time to denote physicians specializing in mental disorders). Jules Baillarger (1809–90) published a paper in 1854 describing an illness he called *la folie à double forme*, and two weeks later Jean-Pierre Falret (1794–1870) rushed a paper into print in the same journal in which he insisted that he had been teaching his students about *la folie circulaire* at the

Salpetrière hospital for ten years. (This was, incidentally, the same hospital where several years later the young Sigmund Freud would begin to formulate his own theories about mental phenomena.) Both men described a mental illness characterized by alternating periods of melancholia and mania that were often separated by periods of normal mood. After the appearance of their original papers, Baillarger and Falret wrote several "me first!" "no, *me* first!" letters to the *Bulletin* of the Imperial Academy of Medicine, each claiming to be the originator of this idea. Which of them deserves credit for being first to describe bipolar disorder is a matter upon which scholars still disagree.[4] But medical historians do *not* disagree about the identity of the psychiatrist who published the first comprehensive description of the mood disorders and established the basis of the classification system for mental illnesses that we still use today.

Dr. Kraepelin and "Manic-Depressive Insanity"

It was the German psychiatrist Emil Kraepelin (1856–1926) (see figure 4-1) who, in 1899, solidified the modern concept of bipolar disorder in the sixth edition of his enormously influential textbook on mental illnesses, *Psychiatrie: Ein Lehrbuch für Studirende und Ärzte*. Kraepelin had been working for several years to develop a logical and comprehensive classification system for major mental illnesses, and successive editions of his *Textbook of Psychiatry* document the development of his thinking.

In the fifth edition he divided severe forms of mental illness into two broad categories: those that had a deteriorating course of illness and those that were "periodic." These two groups are still recognizable in modern classifications of psychiatric disorders, the "deteriorating" group containing the various forms of schizophrenia and related disorders and the "periodic" group containing the mood disorders. Although he was not the first to suggest that mania and depression were both expressions of one disorder, Kraepelin was the first to articulate, clearly and convincingly, the idea that *all* disorders of mood were related to one another:

> Manic-depressive insanity . . . includes on the one hand the whole domain of so-called periodic and circular insanity, on the other hand simple mania, [and] the greater part of the morbid states termed melancholia . . . In the course of the years I have become more and more convinced that all the above-mentioned states only represent manifestations of a single morbid process.[5]

Kraepelin's "manic-depressive synthesis"[6] was a major breakthrough in the understanding and classification of major mental illnesses.

But Kraepelin was more than an academic and theoretician; he was a

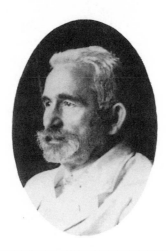

FIGURE 4-1 Emil Kraepelin
Source: Hulton Getty Images

clinician who saw enormous numbers of patients and recorded his observations of their illnesses in superb detail. As you know from reading them in
previous chapters, his descriptions of the symptoms of bipolar disorder are
vivid and insightful, and they have really never been surpassed. A former professor once told me that "anyone who thinks they've discovered something
new in psychiatry simply hasn't read the German psychiatric literature." I
think it's fair to say that anyone who thinks he or she has discovered something new about bipolar disorder—at least, about its symptoms and diagnosis—simply hasn't read Kraepelin.

Kraepelin's contributions, although tremendously significant for those
interested in the classification of mental disorders, offered little practical
benefit in his time to those afflicted with them. I would imagine that Dr.
Kraepelin's patients were more accurately informed about their illness than
most patients of that time, and had more reliable prognostic information,
but there was really nothing he could do to help them with their symptoms.
There was still no treatment for *any* psychiatric condition that offered much
hope of alleviating the symptoms or altering the course of the disease. Although the English translation of the chapter on "manic-depressive insanity" in the eighth edition of Kraepelin's textbook is over two hundred pages
long, the "Treatment" section is less than five pages long—and most of that
consists of warnings about the suicidal behaviors of depressed patients and
against discharging them too soon from hospital. In the absence of treatments for manic-depressive illness, patients spent months, even years, in
hospitals and asylums.

As the study of mental disorders entered the twentieth century, hopes for more effective treatment of psychiatric disorders rose when scientific discoveries shed some light on the causes of several mental illnesses. In 1906 the German microbiologist August Wassermann discovered a method to detect antibodies in human spinal fluid to the microorganism that causes syphilis. Syphilitic infection of the central nervous system was at the time one of the most common causes of severe psychiatric symptoms, and many patients in mental institutions suffered from "general paresis of the insane," as syphilis with psychiatric manifestations was known. With the development of the Wassermann test, it became possible to diagnose the illness with a very high degree of reliability. For the first time a cause of a form of "madness" had been discovered. That same year another German microbiologist, Paul Ehrlich, developed the first effective treatment for syphilis using arsenic compounds. Although the treatment was crude and dangerous, it was effective enough in the early stages of the disease to reduce the incidence of the illness by 50 percent in several European countries.

We hardly think of syphilis as a mental illness today, but patients with syphilitic infection of the brain can suffer hallucinations, delusions, and mood changes not very different from those seen in bipolar disorder and schizophrenia. An early-twentieth-century psychiatric text describes the mania-like excitement that was sometimes seen in persons with central nervous system syphilis: "The intensity of the excitement is extreme; there is absolute sleeplessness [and] incessant restlessness. The grandiose delusions are the controlling feature of the paretic's thought. The patient . . . comes before us tremulous with emotion, his eye bright, as the overpowering visions of wealth and grandeur float before his mind."[7] The discovery of reliable and effective diagnostic techniques for general paresis of the insane—unfortunately, arsenicals had little effect on the advanced central nervous system disease—was seen by many as an enormous advance in the understanding of psychiatric disorders. Clinicians charged with the care of psychiatric patients had great hopes that the causes of other psychiatric disorders would soon be found.

As more and more powerful microscopes were invented and special tissue stains were developed for brain tissues, various microscopic structures of the brain—the many different types of neurons and the microscopic architecture of the different parts of the brain—became visible for the first time. Anatomical and chemical abnormalities were found to characterize several other diseases with prominent mental symptoms. In 1906 the Swiss neuropathologist Alois Alzheimer, who was a student of Kraepelin, discovered abnormal microscopic plaques and tangles of cellular debris in the brains of persons who had died from the progressive brain disease that was eventually named for him. Individuals with *cretinism,* a particularly severe form of mental retardation, were found to have abnormally low levels of thyroid hormones. In 1915 *pellagra,* another mysterious disease, characterized by skin lesions and gradual mental deterioration, was discovered to be caused by a deficiency of vitamin B.

But blood tests and brain studies revealed nothing about manic-depressive illness. Try as they might, pathologists and anatomists could find nothing different or abnormal in the brain structures of individuals with bipolar disorder.

New ways of thinking seemed necessary to understand the mental illnesses for which no physical cause could be found, and shortly after the beginning of the twentieth century, new theories were advanced—by, among others, Sigmund Freud in Europe and Adolf Meyer in the United States (see figures 4-2, 4-3)—that seemed to have considerable power to explain the basis of these still mysterious illnesses. These theories, boiled down to their essence, held that mental symptoms were reactions to life events in vulnerable individuals—not disease states caused by disruptions in biological functioning. The new theories of mental illness instructed psychiatrists to use "talking cures" to treat their patients.

By carefully exploring patients' biographies in minute detail, physicians attempted to understand what conflicts and life events their patients were reacting to with symptoms of depression or mania. It was the expectation that

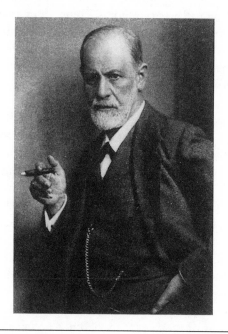

FIGURE 4-2 Sigmund Freud
Source: National Library of Medicine

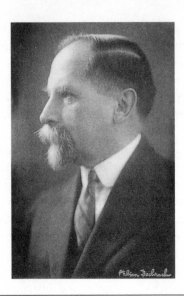

FIGURE 4-3 Adolf Meyer
Source: Alan Mason Chesney Medical Archives and Bachrach Photography

the proper combination of understanding, reinterpretation, and encouragement could alleviate patients' symptoms. Freud, more than any other early psychiatrist, developed elaborate theories about normal and abnormal childhood psychological development that he felt could explain why some people developed extreme psychological symptoms in response to difficult life situations and events while others did not. Manic-depressive illness and schizophrenia came to be called *functional illnesses* because it was believed that patients with depression or mania or symptoms of schizophrenia had *normal* brain and nervous system functioning. Although Freud and Meyer did not totally discount biological agents as having some role in the causation of these problems, they did not see their patients as suffering from *diseases*. A "functional illness" was believed to be an illness of the mind, not of the brain. These concepts dominated American psychiatry until well into the 1960s.

During these decades most psychiatrists believed that abnormal mental phenomena were caused by traumatic childhood events, poor parenting, repressed sexual feelings, and interpersonal conflicts. They lost interest in the classification and categorization of psychiatric illnesses; the very idea of trying to make a diagnosis in a psychiatric patient seemed a waste of time because the form as well as the cause of a psychiatric problem was as individual as the biography of the patient in whom it occurred. Then in 1949 an unknown Australian psychiatrist published an article in the *Medical Journal of Australia* called "Lithium Salts in the Treatment of Psychotic Excitement."

Dr. Cade and Lithium

By the 1930s and 1940s most physicians interested in the treatment of mental disorders had joined psychoanalytic institutes to learn the theory and practice of psychiatry according to the teachings of Freud and his followers. They trained and practiced mostly in the big cities, mostly treating patients with mild depression or anxiety, patients who had the time, motivation, and money to attend therapy sessions four or five days a week, to explore their past and reinterpret their present in order to become healthier, happier, and better "adjusted." The theories of Freud revolutionized the understanding of many aspects of human behavior, and they continue to form the basis for the practice of psychotherapy. But there were many patients who benefited little from these new ideas. They were the patients Dr. Kraepelin had cared for: the victims of schizophrenia and manic-depressive illness.

For these patients, housed for months or years in (mostly public) hospitals and asylums, the therapeutic armamentarium had not changed much in two hundred years: bed rest for the depressed; physical restraint for the agitated; baths, tranquilization with morphine and bromides, and the use of a number of other substances thought to have beneficial effects, among them quinine and even cod-liver oil. None of these interventions had any but the most insignificant effects on serious mental illness.

John F. J. Cade, M.D., senior medical officer in the Mental Hygiene Department of Victoria, Australia, was convinced that manic-depressive illness was a biological disorder, not a psychological one. Working in his laboratory to determine if some toxin might be present in the urine of patients with manic-depressive illness, Cade became especially interested in urea and uric acid, byproducts of protein metabolism found in urine, and was testing the toxicity of these compounds by injecting small amounts of them into guinea pigs.

One of the technical problems with this work was that uric acid is rather insoluble in water, making preparation of injectable solutions difficult at higher concentrations. Looking for a soluble urate salt to use instead of uric acid, Cade consulted prior research and discovered that uric acid was easiest to dissolve in water when it was combined with a lithium ion as lithium urate. He injected small amounts of lithium urate into the guinea pigs and noticed that uric acid seemed to be much less toxic in this form. This suggested to Cade that the lithium component of the compound might have some sort of protective effect against urate toxicity. To determine what the effect of the lithium ion might be, he injected lithium carbonate—the carbonate ion is a harmless compound found in things such as baking soda—and discovered that "after a latent period of about two hours the animals, although fully conscious, became extremely lethargic and unresponsive to stimuli for one to two hours before once again becoming normally active."[8]

Cade admits in his original paper that "it may seem a long distance from lethargy in guinea pigs to excitement in psychotics," but asylum doctors of the time were desperate for new treatment possibilities, so Cade decided to administer lithium preparations to several patients who were chronically agitated. The effect on patients with mania was dramatic:

Case I—W.B., a male aged fifty-one years, who had been in a state of chronic manic excitement for five years, restless, dirty, destructive, mischievous and interfering, had long been regarded as the most troublesome patient in the ward. His response was highly gratifying. From the start of treatment on March 29, 1948, with lithium citrate he steadily settled down and in three weeks was enjoying the unaccustomed surroundings of the convalescent ward. As he had been ill so long and confined to a "chronic ward," he found normal surroundings and liberty of movement strange at first. He remained perfectly well and left the hospital on indefinite leave with instructions to take a dose of lithium carbonate, five grains, twice a day. He was soon back working at his old job. However, he became more lackadaisical about his medicine and finally ceased taking it. His relatives reported that he had not taken any for at least six weeks prior to his readmission on January 30, 1949 and was becoming steadily more irritable and erratic. On readmission to the hospital he was at once started on lithium carbonate, ten grains three time a day, and in a fortnight had again settled down to normal. He is now (February 28, 1949) ready to return to home and work.

Case VIII—W.M., a man of fifty years, was suffering from an attack of recurrent mania, the first of which he had had at the age of twenty. The present attack had lasted two months and showed no signs of abating. He was garrulous, euphoric, restless and unkempt when he started taking lithium. Two days later he was reported to be quieter. By the ninth day he was definitely settling down and the following day commenced work in the garden. By the end of two weeks he was practically normal—quiet, tidy, rational, with insight into his previous condition. This was in marked contrast to his condition a fortnight before when he had to be locked in a single room at night . . . and was too restless to eat in the dining room owing to his unsettling effect on the other patients.[9]

Dr. Cade had treated ten manic patients with lithium, and all ten had shown the same dramatic improvement. He had also given lithium to six patients with "dementia praecox" (schizophrenia) and three patients with "chronic depressive psychoses," but with less effect. The agitated patients with schizophrenia became less agitated but had "no fundamental improvement"; the depressed patients had "no improvement."

It is often emphasized in textbooks and articles on the history of lithium treatment that Cade's discovery of lithium's efficacy in bipolar disorder was pure accident—an observation that misses an important point. Cade, like many hospital psychiatrists, but unlike perhaps many other psychiatrists of his time, was pursuing a biological intervention for what he believed was a biological disorder. His case descriptions reveal that even though he had little specific therapy to offer them, he had taken a complete history of his patients' course of illness, carefully examined them, and, following in the footsteps of Emil Kraepelin, made a *diagnosis* based on his examination and history taking. Cade's approach to these severely ill patients—his assumption that they suffered from diseases rather than from emotional reactions—provided the theoretical underpinning that made his discovery possible. A psychiatrist who believed in "reactions" and "functional illness" would have been unlikely to divide patients into the diagnostic categories of mania, schizophrenia, and depressive psychosis and report on differential efficacy of a pharmaceutical in each group (let alone have been looking for toxins in the urine of patients with mania).

One would think that the news of Cade's discovery would have spread like wildfire. It did not. In fact it was several decades before lithium was approved for the treatment of bipolar disorder by the United States Food and Drug Administration. Why this incredible delay?

Part of the reason was the state of world psychiatry following the end of World War II. German psychiatry was in ruins, literally and figuratively. The German psychiatric establishment, which had produced superb clinicians like Kraepelin and Freud and many other pioneers in the science of mental disorders, had been mesmerized by the Nazi movement. Prominent German psychiatrists had enthusiastically participated in the expulsion of Jewish colleagues from the profession and in the murder of the patients they had been charged to care for. Thousands of mentally retarded and mentally ill individuals were gassed in the years leading up to the war and during the war. When Cade wrote of his work with lithium, Germany was no longer providing leaders in psychiatric medicine; rather, German psychiatry was in dire need of rehabilitation.[10]

In the United States and England, psychoanalytic theories had replaced the traditional medical practices of evaluation, diagnosis, and treatment with the prescription of the "talking cure" for all emotional problems. Accurate psychiatric diagnosis simply didn't exist; any patient with severe symptomatology was usually called "schizophrenic" and admitted to a state psychiatric hospital for little more than custodial care. Ronald Fieve, the American psychiatrist who would champion the use of lithium in the United States in the

1970s and who was instrumental in getting American psychiatrists to prescribe it for their patients, observed that during the late 1940s and the 1950s in New York, he "rarely met with the diagnosis of manic-depression . . . It had virtually disappeared. Most cases of excitable, talkative, and elated behavior were being diagnosed as schizophrenia."[11]

But a Danish psychiatrist, Morgans Schou, realized that Cade's discovery represented a real breakthrough, noting in a 1954 paper that "it is rather astonishing that [Cade's] observation has failed to arouse greater general interest among psychiatrists."[12] Schou and his colleagues did the careful clinical trials that eventually resulted in the development of recommended dosages and preparations of lithium for the treatment of symptoms of bipolar disorder. Perhaps more than any other clinical researcher, Schou established the efficacy of lithium treatment for mania. Even more important was his discovery of lithium's ability to *prevent* the reoccurrence of symptoms in patients with bipolar disorder.

In 1957 another breakthrough occurred in the treatment of mood disorders when Roland Kuhn, a Swiss psychiatrist, discovered that a compound originally developed as an antihistamine had remarkable therapeutic effects on depressed patients. He reported his results in a Swiss medical journal in a paper reprinted the next year in English as "The Treatment of Depressive States with G 22355 (Imipramine Hydrochloride)." But Kuhn also noticed that in some patients imipramine simply replaced one mood problem with another: "In marked manic-depressive psychosis, i.e., if the depressions are easily and frequently replaced by manic-like phases or actual manic states, the reaction is less favorable . . . the tendency arises for the depression to switch over into a manic phase."[13]

In one of their first papers on the use of lithium in manic patients, Schou and his colleagues had pointed out that "the beneficial effect of lithium in cases of mania appears to offer new possibilities for a study of the *pathophysiology* of the manic-depressive psychoses."[14] The discovery of the therapeutic effects of imipramine on depressed patients and the observation that it could precipitate mania in patients with "manic-depressive psychosis" were two more clues that bipolar disorder might be more than a psychological "reaction."

The fact that a chemical (lithium) made the symptoms of mania go away indicated that mania had at least some biochemical basis. The discovery of the different effects of imipramine on depressed persons with and without a history of mania reinforced the disease model for bipolar disorder. Persons with a history of mania became manic if they took imipramine; persons who did not have a history of mania (usually) did not. Imipramine was not simply a "manio-genic" drug, a drug that produced euphoria in everyone who took it. The fact that only bipolar individuals became manic from it suggested that their illness had a different biochemical basis from depression. The distinction between *bipolar* and *unipolar* depressions became established in psychiatric diagnosis. The modern age of psychiatry had begun, as had the search for more and better pharmaceutical treatments and for the physical basis of these disorders.

PART II

TREATMENT

Several years ago I heard a classical guitarist being interviewed on the radio. He said that he was often asked by strangers, usually people who didn't know much about classical music, whether he played the *electric* or the *acoustic* guitar. "I hate that term, *acoustic guitar*. I'd rather just say I played the guitar," he said. "But after the electric guitar was invented, I suppose somebody had to come up with a term for a non-electric guitar."

There is a term for psychiatric problems that many nonpsychiatrists use that I dislike, and that's *chemical imbalance*. It's a term that we started hearing used in the 1970s to describe psychiatric problems that were not psychological reactions or "functional" problems (as I described them in chapter 4) but rather were illnesses caused by some malfunction of brain physiology. To paraphrase the guitarist, I suppose somebody had to invent a term for psychiatric illnesses as opposed to purely psychological conditions, but *chemical imbalance* implies several things about psychiatric illnesses that are very misleading.

First is the idea that all disturbances of mental life fall into two mutually exclusive categories: "chemical" and "nonchemical" (or perhaps "chemical" and "psychological" might work better). As we shall see in this next group of chapters, such a division is not possible, for the "chemical" and "psychological" aspects of mental life interact and overlap in many ways. Second, to say that a psychiatric problem like bipolar disorder is simply an "imbalance" of brain chemicals is a monumental oversimplification of what really lies at the root of these problems. The fantastically complex human brain is not simply a cantaloupe-sized organ bathed in a soup of "chemicals" that can be adjusted by the addition of medications to achieve a "balance" (as a chef adds a little more salt or another pinch of cayenne to make a favorite recipe come out right).

In the first chapter in this part of the book I'll do my best to explain what causes bipolar disorder (without using the term *chemical imbalance*) and also touch on how we think the medications used to treat the illness work. The details here are a bit complicated, but the basics are not difficult to grasp. This chapter might require a slower, more careful reading pace for those unfamiliar with terms like *neurotransmitters*, but this effort will pay off later, allowing you to understand the use of medications in bipolar disorder much better.

Then we'll start talking about treatment more specifically, beginning with a review of the pharmaceuticals used in the treatment of the disorder. We'll also cover electroconvulsive therapy—still a very valuable resource for the treatment of mood syndromes—and, last but certainly not least, the important role of counseling and psychotherapy in the treatment of the illness. We'll end with a brief overview of the treatment approaches and some principles of treatment that I think are important to remember.

The Brain: Neurons,
Neurotransmitters, and More

I'M ABOUT TO DISCUSS SOME RATHER COMPLICATED SCIENCE. NOW, IF that sentence sends shivers up your spine, you can skip this chapter. You'll still be able to understand the chapters that follow. Although no one really knows for sure exactly what causes bipolar disorder, we have some theories, based on research, that make sense. If you are interested in those theories, read on. If you're not, you can skip ahead to the medication chapters.

Some years ago, the psychiatrist and neuroscientist Nancy Andreasen wrote a book, *The Broken Brain*,[1] about the new discoveries in biological psychiatry. The title makes the point that psychiatric illnesses such as bipolar disorder and schizophrenia are caused by biological and chemical malfunctions of the brain, not by repressed memories or traumatic childhoods. Although we still don't know exactly what these malfunctions are, we are getting very close to understanding some of the biological mechanisms that might be involved. In this overview of brain functioning, I want to tell you about what scientists think might be "broken" in bipolar disorder.

Many people imagine that the human brain is a kind of wonderful computer. Although this is a vast oversimplification of the true capabilities of the brain, it's a good place to start in trying to understand how this fantastic organ of the mind works.

Like the computer that I'm using to write these words, a human brain receives input, processes the information it receives, and then delivers output. Like a computer, it stores information and often uses this stored information to help process further input. The human brain receives its input from the sense organs—the eyes, ears, taste buds, touch receptors, and so forth—and delivers output in terms of behavior.

You may know that a computer computes by means of many thousands of microscopic switches embedded in its processing chip. It is the pattern of "on" and "off" in the switches that stores information; the control of the flow of signals through these switches is the processing. The human brain contains about eleven billion nerve cells, or *neurons*—but as powerful as a computer with eleven billion switches might be, our brain is many orders of magnitude more impressive than that. This is because the neuron is not just a switch that is either "on" or "off," but rather is an impressive microprocessor in its own right. Each neuron receives input from many other neurons, processes this information, and sends output to many others. The brain, then, is not like a computer with billions of switches; it is more like a network of billions of computers, all capable of being individually programmed. Each neuron in the brain may receive input and then transmit signals to up to fifty thousand other neurons. The number of all the possible connections in the human brain is incomprehensibly large, a hyper-astronomical number on the order of the number of molecules in the universe! (Even if we could figure out how to build such a computer, there'd be no place on the planet big enough to put it.)

I'm going to jump the gun a little and tell you that there is a lot of evidence that bipolar disorder (and perhaps all mood disorders, as well as anxiety disorders) is caused by some defect in the mechanisms by which the individual neurons are programmed. Neurons have the ability to be "reprogrammed" in response to various situations (stress is one); this capability is called *neuroplasticity* (remember that the original meaning of *plastic* refers to a material that can be shaped and reshaped, like modeling clay). But before we get to that, we need to talk about neurotransmitters.

Although the human nervous system uses electrical signals to do much of its work, it uses chemical signals as well; molecules called *neurotransmitters* are the means by which nerve cells communicate with each other. Neurons send these chemical signals to each other at the *synapse*, an area where two neurons nearly touch, separated only by an ultramicroscopic space called the *synaptic cleft*. The first ("presynaptic") neuron releases packets of neurotransmitters, which flow across this narrow space to link up with targets called *receptors* on the next ("postsynaptic") neuron (figure 5-1). When enough of the receptors are occupied by neurotransmitter molecules, which fit into the receptors like keys fit into locks, the recipient nerve cell is activated and fires off its own signal. There needs to be some mechanism for this signaling system to be turned off and reset, of course. After neurotransmitter molecules link up with receptors across the synapse, they must somehow be removed in preparation for the next batch. This happens in a variety of

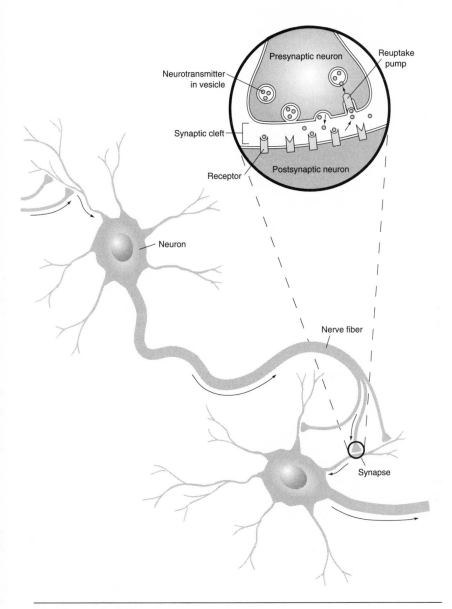

FIGURE 5-1 Synapse

ways in different cells, but one of the most important mechanisms is by re-uptake into the neuron that released them. A *reuptake pump* on this neuron removes neurotransmitter molecules from the synapse and transports them back into the interior of the cell, where they can be repackaged for rerelease.

Neurons are continually communicating with each other. Neurotransmitter molecules passing from one neuron to another across synapses maintain a steady tone of chemical signal, with the signal getting stronger, or pulsing up, at times and the neuron detecting and reacting to these pulses. Thus, as I noted earlier, neurons are not just switches that can only be set to "on" or "off" but rather are tiny information-processing units that are constantly communicating with other neurons to which they are functionally linked.

Soon after Roland Kuhn discovered that G 22355 was an effective antidepressant (see chapter 4), neuroscientists started to investigate the effect of this pharmaceutical on brain chemistry. They discovered that imipramine is a powerful inhibitor of one type of reuptake pump, blocking the reuptake of a group of neurotransmitters called *neurogenic amines* (or *neuroamines*), of which *norepinephrine* was thought to be the most important. Remember that neurons turn off their chemical signals ("turn down" is probably more accurate) by scooping up neurotransmitter molecules from the synapse and repackaging them. Just as partly closing the drain in a bathtub while the water is running will cause the tub to begin to fill, if you block the reuptake of neurotransmitter molecules into cells, the net effect will be an increase of neurotransmitters in the synapse. Neuroscientists later found that nearly all the medications that are effective antidepressants cause blockade of neurotransmitter reuptake in brain cells. This observation led to the "amine hypothesis" of the mood disorders. This theory basically stated that depression was caused by an abnormally low level of neurotransmitters and that mania was caused by too high a level. (This may be where the unfortunate term *chemical imbalance* had its origins.)

Further work soon indicated, however, that too little norepinephrine was too simplistic an explanation. As more antidepressant medications were discovered, researchers found that some very effective ones seemed to have little effect on norepinephrine. Fluoxetine (Prozac) is one of a family of pharmaceuticals that are powerful inhibitors of the reuptake of a different neurotransmitter, *serotonin;* they have very little direct effect on norepinephrine. Other antidepressants seem to affect yet other neurotransmitters.

Another argument against a simplistic theory involving too much or too little norepinephrine is an observation about the time course of the antidepressant-induced chemical changes in the brain. Antidepressant-induced changes in neurotransmitter levels at the synapse occur almost immediately after the drug is taken—in a matter of hours. But, as is well known, it takes several weeks for these agents to start alleviating the symptoms of depression. If the problem were simply too little neurotransmitter in the synapses of certain brain circuits, why would it take several weeks after the drug raised neurotransmitter levels at the synapse for the symptoms of depression to improve?

It has been suggested that the neurons respond to these higher levels of neurotransmitters by changing their receptor molecules, either making them more sensitive to the neurotransmitter or putting more of them in the synapse. The idea is that antidepressants work by triggering an "up-regulation" of receptor sensitivity in the neuron. This hypothesis continues to be popular among neuroscientists interested in the chemistry of mood disorders, but there is increasing recognition that this, too, is only part of the story.

Because of the unique therapeutic effects of lithium in bipolar disorder, there has naturally been a lot of effort to figure out where this medication is active in the brain and what its effect on brain chemistry is. In fact, investigating lithium's effect on brain chemistry is leading scientists closer to the "broken" mechanism of bipolar disorder than ever before.

Lithium doesn't seem to affect neurotransmitter levels in the synapse and doesn't interact with neurotransmitter receptors or affect the reuptake pumps. In fact, it has none of the types of direct effects on cells that the antidepressants have. Only in the last few years has the probable site of lithium action been found, and it's not at the synapse at all. Lithium (and perhaps the newer mood stabilizers as well) seems to work at a different cellular level: *inside* the neuron.

Although the precise fit between a neurotransmitter and its receptor molecule has often been compared to the precise fit of a key in a lock, it has become apparent that the receptor is much more than just a lock. Starting in the 1970s, scientists were able to elucidate the structure of cellular receptors and discover the details of these complex and elegant mechanisms. Receptors on the surface of the cell are coupled with structures called *G proteins* that extend through the cell membrane (the covering of the cell) and link up with a complex array of other proteins and enzymes in the cell that regulate various cellular functions. The G proteins act as transducers, converting data from outside the cell into functional changes inside the cell. They don't do this directly, but by a complex cascade of chemical events that probably also include turning the cell's genes on and off.

There is evidence that lithium has direct effects on G proteins, but scientists have recently started to focus on several other groups of molecules that work inside the cell as "second messengers." The neurotransmitters, the molecules that bring messages from other cells to the neuron, are considered the *first* messengers. The *second* messengers are molecules inside the cell that are activated by G proteins, travel within the neuron, and activate various cellular switches in the cell membrane and in the main control center of the neuron, the nucleus.

You can think of the G protein/second-messenger system as a communications and activity-monitoring system for the neuron, constantly assessing the level of neurotransmitter activity and, perhaps by turning genes on and off, constantly altering and adjusting the functioning of the neuron in

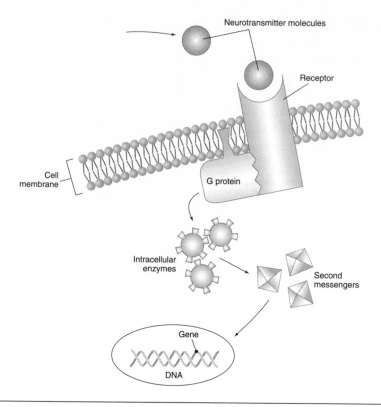

FIGURE 5-2 Receptors and G proteins

response to this activity. This is the neuroplasticity I mentioned earlier in this chapter—the ability of the neuron to react and reshape itself, perhaps "tuning" itself to certain levels of signaling. Several small molecules inside the neuron, with odd names like BDNF (for brain-derived neurotrophic factor) and CREB (for cAMP response element binding protein), are thought to be very important for this "programming and reprogramming" of neurons.

There is also increasing interest in another neurotransmitter, *glutamate*, which doesn't seem to be affected by antidepressants at all, but is affected by lamotrigine and other mood stabilizers; glutamate seems to be very important in neuroplasticity.

You can think of neuroplasticity as the neurons' responsiveness and ability to react to change and stress. It is also thought to be involved in memory and learning. If you consider the symptoms of bipolar disorder, which include thinking and concentration problems in addition to mood changes, and about how episodes of the illness can be triggered by stresses of various types, this idea that neuroplasticity is disrupted in bipolar disorder begins to make sense. Neuroplasticity may be a necessary part of maintaining mood within a normal range, somehow "tuning" the responsiveness of our mood state to experiences and environment. Perhaps bipolar disorder is the result of problems with neuroplasticity in the neurons that make up the norepinephrine and serotonin circuits that we know are important in regulating mood; perhaps in bipolar disorder, the sensitivity of these circuits is incorrectly tuned too high or too low, and abnormal changes of mood result.

Another interesting area of research in mood disorders concerns the *growth* of cells in an area of the brain called the *hippocampus*. It was thought for many decades that the brain stopped producing new neurons shortly after birth—that the adult brain was not capable of growing new nerve cells. We now know this is not the case; in fact, new cells are constantly being produced in certain areas of the brain. One of these areas is the hippocampus, a very specialized area that is involved in memory and emotion. Studies of humans with depression, using specialized imaging techniques that allow the size of brain structures to be measured in living persons, show that the hippocampus is smaller in individuals with chronic depression. Animal studies indicate that lithium, antidepressants, and electroconvulsive therapy all increase the growth of neurons in the hippocampus. There is also evidence that chronic stress interferes with this cell growth in research animals. This last finding is extremely interesting because it may explain why stress triggers mood episodes in persons with mood disorders.

Taken together, these new findings on the importance of the cell plasticity and growth may explain why medications that help with symptoms of bipolar disorder often take several weeks to do so. Antidepressants may artificially change neurotransmitter levels in the synapse, which in turn sets off a cascade of events, through the G protein/second-messenger system, to turn on genes that start making molecules like CREB and BDNF or other cell components that are needed to retune existing neurons and grow new ones. This would explain why treatments for symptoms of bipolar disorder, especially bipolar depression, take several weeks to work.[2]

It may be a while before we understand how all the molecular and cellular pieces of this complicated story fit together, but the work to unravel the basic cause (or causes) of bipolar disorder is proceeding very rapidly. And when we understand exactly what is "broken" in bipolar disorder, the job of fixing it will become much easier.

Mood-Stabilizing Medications

MOOD STABILIZERS ARE MEDICATIONS THAT HAVE BOTH ANTIMANIC and antidepressant effects. Perhaps an even more important effect of this class of medications is their ability to decrease the frequency and severity of episodes of the illness. Thus, the vast majority of patients with bipolar disorder are treated with one or another of these medications, and sometimes with several.

Lithium

We've already learned about the discovery of the therapeutic effects of lithium in bipolar disorder by John Cade in the 1940s. But lithium has an even older history as a pharmaceutical that is just as interesting as the story of Dr. Cade and his guinea pigs. In the second century A.D. the Greek physician Seranus Ephisios recommended that physicians treating patients suffering from mania should prescribe "natural waters, such as [from] alkaline springs."[1] We now know that the water from many alkaline springs is rich in lithium. Roman physicians recommended that their patients "take the waters" at various springs for a number of physical and mental ailments. Down through the centuries centers for healing grew up around natural springs all over Europe, from the little town in eastern Belgium called Spa to Bath in England, Wiesbaden in Germany, and dozens of other towns in Italy and Greece. As the science of analytic chemistry developed, curious chemists and physicians evaluated these various springs and found that the waters of many were rich in lithium.

In the middle of the nineteenth century, lithium compounds were tried as treatments for gout and kidney stones. Gout is a painful arthritic condition caused by abnormally high levels of uric acid in the body; the uric acid is deposited in the form of urate crystals in the joints and other tissues. Kidney stones are also usually made up of urate compounds. It was hoped that lithium would somehow dissolve the urate crystals in the joints of gout patients as well as urate kidney stones. (Remember that Dr. Cade picked lithium urate to work with because it is the most soluble of the urate compounds.) Unfortunately lithium did not turn out to be helpful for these problems, and the approach was abandoned. But this work led to the formulation of pharmaceutical preparations of lithium compounds and to information on the range of safe doses for lithium preparations in humans.

In the late 1940s lithium came to medical attention again when lithium chloride was introduced as a salt substitute for patients with medical problems, like heart disease and high blood pressure, that required them to be on a low-sodium diet. But when heart patients were given salt shakers full of lithium salts to sprinkle on their food, the results were catastrophic for some. Because lithium is toxic in surprisingly low concentrations, substituting lithium chloride for sodium chloride turned out to be a disaster. There were many reports of severe lithium poisoning and even several deaths among these patients. The use of lithium as a salt substitute ended. This episode had the effect of giving lithium a very bad reputation among physicians, and it was perhaps another factor that explains the delay in the acceptance of Cade's discovery of lithium's efficacy in bipolar disorder.

In the 1950s the Danish psychiatrist Morgans Schou began what was to be his life work: the development and refinement of the therapeutic use of lithium for the treatment of bipolar disorder. Schou very quickly became convinced of the effectiveness of lithium in treating acute mania, and he was one of the first clinical researchers to become convinced of another therapeutic effect of the drug: its ability to prevent further episodes of illness (lithium's preventative or *prophylactic* effect). Schou had a more difficult time convincing his colleagues around the world that lithium could prevent recurrences of bipolar disorder, and that patients should take it even after their acute symptoms had subsided. In 1967 Schou and his colleague Paul Christian Baalstrup reported on eighty-eight patients who had taken lithium for several years and who had a dramatic reduction in the frequency and duration of their mood episodes (figure 6-1 shows a sample of their results). Several patients who had been sick for several weeks out of every year experienced a complete remission of their illness that lasted for over five years; their illness had essentially stopped.[2]

As they treated more and more patients with the medication, it became so apparent to Schou and his colleagues that lithium favorably altered the

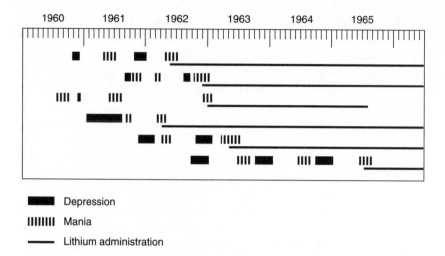

Depression

Mania

Lithium administration

FIGURE 6-1 This graph illustrates data from six patients in Baalstrup and Schou's early study on the prophylactic effects of lithium on bipolar symptoms. Each line represents the symptom course of one patient. In all these patients, when lithium was started, episodes of mania and depression stopped completely.

Source: Data from Paul Baalstrup and Morgans Schou, "Lithium as a Prophylactic Agent: Its Effect against Recurrent Depressions and Manic-Depressive Psychosis," *Archives of General Psychiatry* 16, no. 2 (1967): 162–72.

course of bipolar illness that they had ethical qualms about doing a more rigorous placebo-controlled study—one in which bipolar patients would be divided into two groups, some to receive lithium and the others a placebo. In a rather cranky 1968 article titled "Prophylactic Lithium: Another Therapeutic Myth?" several British psychiatrists scolded the Danes for reporting their results without a placebo group.[3] So Baalstrup and Schou did a lithium discontinuation study in which they took patients who had been stable on lithium for at least a year, divided them into two roughly equal groups, and in one group substituted a placebo for the lithium.

This was a *double-blind study*, the most powerful type of clinical trial possible—and now pretty much a required test for new medications. In this type of study, patients who are similar as to age, diagnosis, severity of illness, and so forth and who agree to be in the study are divided into two groups. One group gets the medication that is being tested, and the other group (the *control* group) gets a placebo (or in some studies the control group receives a standard medication for the disorder being studied). The patients do not know whether they are taking the new medication or the placebo, and neither do the clinicians who examine them for improvement; hence the term *double*-blind. It is only after the trial is over that the group membership of the patients is revealed and the results of the two groups compared. Improvement is measured objectively by using checklists of symptoms and various rating severity scales that have been verified as being reliable and valid.

The results of the Baalstrup and Schou study were dramatic: of the thirty-nine patients whose lithium was replaced with the placebo, twenty-one relapsed within five months; of the forty-five other patients, those whose lithium was not replaced, *none* had a relapse. In 1970 Baalstrup and Schou published their results in the same British journal in which their critics' paper had appeared,[4] establishing once and for all that lithium's prophylactic effect on bipolar disorder was no myth.

THERAPEUTIC PROFILE

It has now been shown in many more studies that lithium is not only effective in the treatment of acute mania and acute bipolar depression but also that it reduces the severity, duration, and frequency of manic and depressive episodes of bipolar patients.

Lithium is a naturally occurring element found in mineral springs, seawater, and certain ores. Like its close cousin sodium, it is never found in its pure form in nature but only combined with other ions as a salt of one type or another. It is mined on an industrial scale for use in the manufacture of ceramics and batteries. Therapeutic lithium preparations usually contain lithium carbonate (the carbonate ion combined with lithium; when the carbonate ion is combined with the closely related sodium, it forms sodium carbonate, which is common baking soda).

Because it is an element, lithium is not chemically transformed (metabolized) within the body, and because lithium atoms are so similar to sodium atoms, the body handles lithium in much the same way it handles sodium. Lithium is rapidly absorbed through the gastrointestinal tract, enters the bloodstream, and is eliminated from the body by being filtered out by the kidneys. (Table 6-1 summarizes the therapeutic profile.)

Descriptions of the effects of a pharmaceutical in the body always include one vital statistic: the medication's *half-life*. This is a measure of how quickly the body gets rid of a pharmaceutical. Specifically, it is the time required for half the amount of the drug to be eliminated or metabolized by the body. Put another way, it is the time it takes for the body to reduce the level of the medication by half. The half-life of lithium in adults is between fourteen and thirty hours.[5] Another useful number that can be derived from the half-life statistic for any medication is the time it takes for the level of medication to build up to a constant level in the body, or in other words the time it takes for the amount being taken in to equal the amount being eliminated: the *equilibrium point*. By a series of mathematical steps that we don't

TABLE 6-1 Therapeutic Profile of Lithium

Medication class:	Mood stabilizer
Brand names:	Eskalith, Eskalith CR, Lithobid, Lithonate, Lithotabs
Half-life:	14–30 hours
Metabolism:	None
Elimination:	Kidneys
Birth control:	Probably mandatory
Other considerations:	Blood levels extremely important

need to detail here, it can be shown that the equilibrium point is always the same for all medications: five half-lives. This means that since the half-life of lithium is roughly one day, it will take roughly five days for a patient who starts on lithium to reach a steady level of lithium in the bloodstream. It also means that if the lithium dose is changed, it will take about five days for the blood level to stabilize at the new level.

Because of the toxicity and even deaths that were reported when heart patients sprinkled it freely on their food as a salt substitute, there was a significant delay in the acceptance of lithium as a therapeutic agent. Lithium is a powerful pharmaceutical, one that must be treated with respect. It has a very low *therapeutic index,* meaning that the difference between the therapeutic dose and a toxic dose is small.[6] Fortunately, lithium can be measured in the bloodstream accurately and fairly cheaply, and the dosage adjusted according to the results.

It is important to pay attention to lithium blood levels not only to prevent toxicity but also because it has been clearly demonstrated in clinical studies that lithium needs to be present in the bloodstream at a certain level to be effective in most patients. (We speak of a "therapeutic level" in discussing the effective range of lithium in the bloodstream for treatment, not a "normal level." Lithium is a trace element in the body, normally present in undetectable concentrations. Bipolar disorder is not a lithium deficiency!) Just what that level should be has been a matter of debate, and the definition has shifted over the years. But an important study from Massachusetts General Hospital found that a level of between 0.8 and 1.0 meq/L (this stands for milliequivalent per liter and is a chemical measure of concentration) was most effective.[7] In this double-blind study, bipolar patients were divided into two groups, a "standard-dose" group, whose lithium levels were kept between 0.8 and 1.0 meq/L, and a "low-dose" group, whose levels were maintained between 0.4 and 0.6 meq/L. The researchers found that the relapse rate in the "low-dose" group was more than double that in the "standard-dose" group (see table 6-2).

TABLE 6-2 Comparison of Higher and Lower Lithium Levels in Relapse Rates of Bipolar Disorder

Treatment Group	Any Relapse	Depressed	Manic/ Mixed	Hypomanic	Withdrew from Study
Standard range (0.8–1.0 meq/L)	6 (12%)	3 (6%)	3 (6%)	0	24 (51%)
Low range (0.4–0.6 meq/L)	21 (44%)	1 (2%)	17 (36%)	3 (6%)	11 (23%)

Source: Data from Alan Gelenberg, John Kane, Martin Keller, Phillip Lavori, Jerrold Rosenbaum, Karyl Cole, and Janet Lavelle, "Comparison of Standard and Low Levels of Lithium for Maintenance Treatment of Bipolar Disorder," New England Journal of Medicine 321, no. 22 (1989): 1489–93.

There's more to these data than may initially meet the eye, however. Many more patients from the "standard-dose" group than from the "low-dose" group dropped out of the study because of side effects. The take-home message seems to be that levels closer to 1.0 meq/L are more protective—but that many people have trouble taking that high a dose because of side effects. Many psychiatrists compromise and try to maintain their patients at levels between the "standard" and the "low" range. Dr. Schou, whom many consider to be the father of lithium therapy, has recommended levels of 0.5 to 0.8 meq/L.[8] However, it's very clear that some people have good control of their symptoms on even lower levels—elderly patients, for example. Lithium levels thus need to be individualized to the patient, and Dr. Schou also points out that "changes in lithium levels as small as 0.1 to 0.2 [meq/L], upward or downward, may substantially improve patients' quality of life during maintenance treatment."[9]

The lithium level in the bloodstream rises after every dose, peaks in about two hours, then begins to fall again. If a patient takes his or her lithium two or three times a day, there will be several peaks and valleys. Because the level is rising and falling throughout the day, it is important that the blood be drawn at a time when it can be correctly interpreted. The convention that has been adopted is to use a twelve-hour level, making it convenient to draw blood in the mornings. For most patients this means getting to the lab twelve hours after their bedtime dose—for example, at 11 A.M. if the bedtime dose was taken at 11 P.M. the night before—with their usual morning dose in their pocket or purse.

Individuals vary widely in their sensitivity to the side effects of lithium (and to all medications, for that matter). Some patients will have none, others will have several. Fortunately, almost all the side effects of lithium can be eliminated or managed (see table 6-3).

Many of lithium's side effects are *dose-related,* meaning that the higher the dose, the more severe side effect. One side-effect management strategy, then, is simply to lower the lithium dose. The advantages of higher levels are clear, as noted above, but most physicians will try to maintain patients at the lowest possible dose that controls their symptoms.

Because of its similarity to sodium, lithium has some of the same effects that an increased sodium (salt) intake would have: increased thirst, increased urination, and water retention. These side effects are often temporary and subside as the body adjusts to the medication. Many patients notice this slight and temporary increase in urination and thirst when they start taking lithium. For some patients, however, it's after taking lithium for many years that they notice they need to urinate much more often and are frequently thirsty. This occurs because lithium can affect the functioning of the kidneys over time. Remember that the kidneys' job is to remove waste products from the bloodstream; they filter nearly twenty gallons of blood every hour to do this, and they recycle nearly all of this fluid back into the bloodstream. When taken for many years, lithium can impair this recycling function, resulting in the production of large amounts of urine. The term for this problem is *diabetes insipidus* (which has nothing to do, incidentally, with diabetes mellitus, the common "sugar diabetes"). This problem develops very slowly and is easy to diagnose with a few laboratory tests. When caught early it is usually com-

TABLE 6-3 Treatable Side Effects of Lithium

Side Effect	Remedy
Nausea, diarrhea	Take immediately after meals
	Switch preparations
Weight gain	Diet and exercise
Thirst, frequent urination	Diuretics may help, but must be prescribed by an M.D. (see text)
Tremor	Beta-blocker medications
Flareup of preexisting dermatologic conditions	Dermatologic preparations
Hypothyroidism	Thyroid medications

pletely reversible, so it's very important that patients taking lithium let their doctor know if they find themselves awaking more often to urinate during the night.

When lithium was first being prescribed, some concern arose, based on a few case reports, that lithium disrupted the kidneys' filtering system, causing the kind of damage that can result in the need for dialysis. This has now been shown to be extremely rare, probably occurring in persons who are at risk for kidney damage from other causes. Fortunately this problem is also very slow to develop.[10]

Because of these potential problems, blood tests that measure kidney functioning are routinely ordered for patients taking lithium, in addition to blood tests to monitor their lithium blood levels.

Lithium is irritating to the gastrointestinal tract and can cause nausea or diarrhea. Taking it on a full stomach can ease these problems considerably. A fine shaking in the hands (tremor) can occur at higher levels. Medications used to treat tremors, called *beta blockers,* are frequently prescribed and can be very helpful. Weight gain can be a very annoying side effect and unfortunately has an equally annoying remedy: diet and exercise.

Between 5 and 35 percent of patients treated with lithium develop depression of thyroid gland functioning (hypothyroidism).[11] When hypothyroidism develops, it seems to be able to cause an increase in mood cycling in addition to the symptoms of too little thyroid hormone (low energy, dry skin, sensitivity to heat, and puffiness around the eyes are some of the early signs). If a person's lithium seems to "stop working"—that is, if the person suddenly seems to have an acceleration in his or her illness—the development of hypothyroidism should be suspected. When it does occur, hypothyroidism can be treated by thyroid replacement medications. A test of thyroid functioning is the third in the battery of blood tests routinely ordered for lithium patients.

Lithium can cause flareups of preexisting skin conditions but only rarely causes the onset of new dermatological problems. Patients with psoriasis, acne, and other dermatological problems may need closer follow-up from their dermatologist.

Lithium has been associated with birth defects. Remember that by the time a woman misses her period after conceiving, development of many of the embryo's major organs is already well on its way. Stopping a medication after a woman *knows* she is pregnant may well be too late to prevent a birth defect. Women of childbearing age should practice birth control while taking lithium if there is any chance of becoming pregnant. Lithium is secreted in breast milk, and patients taking lithium should not breast-feed. (See chapter 14 for a more complete discussion of medications and pregnancy.)

Another side effect that troubles a significant number of patients taking lithium is a noticeable dulling of mental functioning and coordination. Patients complain that their ability to memorize and learn is affected, and that they have a difficult-to-explain sense of mental sluggishness. For years these complaints were downplayed by clinicians, many of whom tossed them off as coming from patients who simply weren't used to feeling "normal," who missed the mental alacrity of hypomania. This view seemed to be supported by research using psychological tests on bipolar patients taking lithium, research that has been basically inconclusive. But when nonpatient volunteers were administered lithium and similarly tested, there was a small but definite drop-off in their performance, proving that lithium-induced mental sluggishness is a very real problem for some patients.[12] This is a dose-related side effect and is another reason to strive for the lowest possible maintenance dose of lithium that still controls mood symptoms adequately. Fortunately these problems also often get better with time.

Valproate (Depakote, Depakene, Epival)

The development of valproate (brand names include Depakote and Depakene) for the treatment of bipolar disorder is another convoluted study in serendipity. Valproic acid is a carbon compound similar to a number of others that are found in animal fats and vegetable oils: a fatty acid. It was first synthesized in 1882 and was used for many years as an organic solvent for a variety of purposes. (Remember that a solvent is a liquid that other substances easily dissolve into.) Many decades ago pharmacists used it as a solvent for bismuth salts, which were used to treat stomach and skin disorders.

In the early 1960s scientists looking for treatments for epilepsy were working with a group of new pharmaceutical compounds that appeared promising but were difficult to dissolve. (Is this beginning to sound familiar?) They discovered that valproic acid was an effective solvent for the compounds they were testing, and they started using it to dissolve their test drugs for animal experimentation. As they tested their various new pharmaceuticals, the results they obtained seemed to be confusing—until someone realized that it didn't matter *which* of the new pharmaceuticals was used. As long as *any* of them was dissolved in valproic acid, the drug was found to be effective in stopping epileptic seizure activity. It soon became obvious that it was the valproic acid that was stopping the seizures, not what was dissolved in it. By 1978 valproate had been approved by the Food and Drug Administration for use in treating epilepsy.[13]

In the 1960s there were some reports that valproate might be helpful in treating mood disorders, and throughout the late 1960s and early 1970s a French psychiatrist named Lambert published a series of papers about using it to treat bipolar disorders. After the discovery that another antiepilepsy medication, carbamazepine, was effective in treating mania (we'll cover this story in the next section of this chapter), interest in the possibilities of valproate as a mood stabilizer grew. In the mid-1980s several studies by American psychiatrists of the use of valproate in treating bipolar disorder appeared, and ten years later valproate had become firmly established as an effective antimanic medication and a mood stabilizer.

Valproate's therapeutic action in bipolar disorder—or in epilepsy, for that matter—is still completely unknown. It is known to improve neuronal transmission in the brain that is mediated by the neurotransmitter gamma amino butyric acid (GABA). GABA seems to have an inhibitory or modulating effect on many brain circuits, and valproate's effect may be to enhance this modulator in some way.

THERAPEUTIC PROFILE

Valproate has been established to be effective in the treatment of acute mania. It also appears to be effective in preventing the recurrence of, and to reduce the severity of, episodes of bipolar disorder. Its effectiveness in the treatment of acute depressive episodes of bipolar disorder has been less impressive.

In reading about this medication, you may become confused by the many names it goes by: valproate, valproic acid, divalproex sodium, not to mention the brand names Depakote and Depakene. Many chemicals, many medications included, consist of two parts called ions, one of which is positively charged and the other negatively charged. When the two parts exist together as a *compound,* the charges cancel each other out and the system is stable. Valproate is actually the name of the ion. When it is associated with a hydrogen atom, the result is valproic acid. In combination with a sodium ion, it becomes sodium valproate. Depakote is a preparation manufactured by Abbott Laboratories consisting of a stable combination of sodium valproate and valproic acid that is called divalproex sodium. Depakene is Abbott's brand name for its valproic acid preparation.

The half-life of valproate is between six and sixteen hours in adults (see table 6-4).[14] Thus, it reaches equilibrium in the body more quickly than lithium, in two to three days. Valproate seems to have a number of advantages over lithium in the treatment of acute manic episodes. First, it appears to work more quickly. Whereas lithium may take up to three weeks to have its full effect, valproate has been shown to start working within five days, especially if a "loading-dose" strategy is used.[15] This strategy consists of calculating a valproate dose (based on a patient's weight) that should cause the patient to reach a therapeutic blood level and then starting at that dose immediately; this differs from the usual practice of beginning with a lower "starting dose" that is gradually raised. This method of treating acute mania

TABLE 6-4 Therapeutic Profile of Valproate

Medication class:	Mood stabilizer (anticonvulsant)
Brand names:	Depakene, Depakote, Epival
Half-life:	6–16 hours
Metabolism:	Affected by other antiepilepsy drugs
Elimination:	Liver
Birth control:	Probably mandatory
Other considerations:	Blood levels helpful; blood tests for liver inflammation are needed

has been reported to be highly effective, well tolerated in many patients, and very fast acting.[16] Valproate also seems to be more effective than lithium for certain subgroups of manic patients: patients with rapid cycling (four or more mood episodes per year) and patients with mixed mania (a mixture of manic hyperactivity and pressured thinking with depressed or unpleasant mood).[17] Valproate is much less toxic than lithium.

One big disadvantage of valproate is that it does not seem to be as helpful in acute depression as lithium is. Neither is it very effective in preventing recurrences of depression.[18] This suggests that valproate may be a better choice for patients with rapid cycling or with mixed mania, but that patients with classic euphoric mania and major depressions may have better control of their symptoms with lithium.[19]

Like lithium, valproate can be measured in the bloodstream; unfortunately, it is more difficult to measure, and the test is therefore more expensive to perform. Blood levels above 45 mcg/ml (micrograms per milliliter) have been shown to be necessary for the therapeutic effect to occur, and side effects become more problematic at levels greater than 125 mcg/ml.[20] Several studies show that valproate is helpful in cyclothymia, bipolar II, and "soft" bipolar disorders, and that lower doses and lower blood levels are required than in the treatment of bipolar I with valproate.[21] As with lithium, blood for valproate levels should be drawn twelve hours after the last dose of medication.

SIDE EFFECTS

Valproate has a milder side-effect profile than lithium and is not nearly as toxic in overdose. Side effects that are common as a patient starts taking the medication include stomach upset and some sleepiness. These problems usually go away quickly. Increased appetite and weight gain have been reported, though in my own experience this is an uncommon problem. Mild tremor occurs as well and can be treated with beta-blocker medication. A few patients report hair loss, usually temporary, which resolves even more quickly with vitamin preparations containing the minerals zinc and selenium.[22]

Several cases of severe liver problems have been reported in patients taking valproate, but these have occurred almost exclusively in children taking the drug for control of epilepsy, most of whom had other medical problems and were taking several different medications. A 1989 review article states that no fatalities from liver problems caused by valproate had ever been reported in patients over the age of ten who were taking only valproate. Just to be on the safe side, however, a blood test that can detect liver inflammation is done on patients taking valproate for the first time and is repeated at appropriate intervals while they are taking it. Since valproate can also in rare cases cause a drop in blood counts, a complete blood count is usually done as well. These are very rare problems, and even when they do occur, they develop slowly and usually during the first six months of therapy. Thus, they can be picked up with routine blood tests. Nevertheless, patients on valproate should be on the lookout for signs of liver or blood count problems, which include unusual bleeding and bruising, jaundice (yellowing of the eyes and skin), fever, and water retention.

Valproate has been associated with birth defects, and as with lithium, women in childbearing years should practice birth control while taking valproate if there is any possibility of becoming pregnant.

Carbamazepine (Tegretol, Equetro, Epitol)

After the introduction of carbamazepine for the control of epilepsy in the 1960s, several reports appeared indicating that epilepsy patients taking carbamazepine who also had mood problems not only had good control of their seizures but had improvement in their psychiatric symptoms as well. It was a small step to test carbamazepine in patients with mood problems who did not have epilepsy. Much of the earlier work on the use of carbamazepine in bipolar disorder was done by Japanese clinicians looking for an alternative to lithium, which was not approved for use in Japan until years after it was available in the United States. In 1980 a study appeared in the *American Journal of Psychiatry* titled "Carbamazepine in Manic-Depressive Illness: A New Treatment,"[23] and the race was on to refine the use of this medication in bipolar disorder and to define the group or groups of patients whom it helped the most.

THERAPEUTIC PROFILE

Although carbamazepine has been used to treat bipolar disorder for several decades, much less research has been done on its efficacy in this illness than for other medications such as lithium and valproate. This gap is slowly being filled, however, and newer studies have appeared, prompted by the development of a sustained-release preparation of carbamazepine.

Every once in a while a patient of mine requests that I prescribe the "best" mood stabilizer or antidepressant medication there is. I usually respond by saying that if there were a "best" medication in a particular class of medications, it would be the only pharmaceutical manufactured and prescribed. What would be the point of using anything else? The reason there are so many drugs of a particular type is that some work better or have fewer side effects in particular patients. Many newer medications don't seem to be more effective than available ones when studied in large groups of patients, but they are clearly better for certain patients who can't take or don't respond to an older agent.

Carbamazepine is one such medication: it doesn't seem to have any big advantage in most studies of groups of patients but works *very* well—in fact, works when other medications do not—for some patients. In one well-designed double-blind study, manic patients who took carbamazepine actually seemed to do worse than patients taking lithium.[24] But most psychiatrists have had a patient like "Ms. B.," whose case history was reported in a paper from the National Institute of Mental Health (NIMH) in 1983:

> Ms. B., a 53-year-old woman, had a history of treatment resistant, rapid cycling manic-depressive illness that required continuous state hospitalization from 1956 to her admission to NIMH in 1978. She had been non-responsive to [antipsychotic medications, tricyclic antidepressants] and lithium . . . After institution of carbamazepine, both mood phases improved dramatically and she was able to be discharged . . . During a subsequent hospitalization her severe mania again did not respond to [antipsychotic medications] and she was not able to leave the hospital until she was treated with carbamazepine.[25]

In this study the authors noted that "additional improvement appeared to occur when [antipsychotic medications] were used in conjunction with carbamazepine or when lithium and carbamazepine were used in combination." This had become carbamazepine's niche: a second-line mood-stabilizing agent used for patients who did not respond to other agents, and often used in combination with other agents. This may be changing, however, and new research, such as a placebo-controlled study using carbamazepine alone to treat patients hospitalized with mania,[26] is supporting the idea that this medication may be underused and can be helpful for many patients.

Like the other mood-stabilizing medications, carbamazepine can be measured in the bloodstream, and blood levels can be used to adjust the dose. Unfortunately not much work has been done on carbamazepine blood lev-

TABLE 6-5 Therapeutic Profile of Carbamazepine

Medication class:	Mood stabilizer (anticonvulsant)
Brand names:	Tegretol, Equetro, Epitol
Half-life:	18–55 hours (shortens after time)
Metabolism:	Complex; affects and is affected by other drugs
Elimination:	Liver
Birth control:	Probably mandatory
Other considerations:	Blood levels helpful; blood tests for liver inflammation and blood abnormalities needed

els in bipolar patients, so the therapeutic range used for the treatment of epilepsy is usually the target that psychiatrists aim for in their patients.

Carbamazepine is metabolized in the liver (see table 6-5), and like some other drugs it causes the liver to increase the level of the enzymes that metabolize it. This means that the longer a person takes carbamazepine, the better the liver becomes at getting rid of it. So after a few weeks the blood levels may go down and the dose may need to be increased. This increase in liver enzymes can also affect other medications that the patient might be taking, including certain tranquilizers, certain antidepressants, other epilepsy medications, and some hormones. The change in hormonal levels is very important for women using birth control, since some oral contraceptives that use very low hormone levels lose their effectiveness if taken with carbamazepine. It is very important that all physicians involved in a person's care know when he or she has started taking carbamazepine so that dosage adjustments for other medications can be made.

SIDE EFFECTS

Carbamazepine can cause the sort of general side effects that many medications affecting the brain can cause: sleepiness, lightheadedness, and some initial nausea. These problems tend to be short-lived and dose-related.

As with valproate, there have been rare cases of liver problems associated with carbamazepine, so blood tests for liver inflammation are routinely done. There have been even rarer reports of dangerous changes in blood counts, so blood cell counts are also done, especially in the first several weeks of therapy. Some cases of a rare but dangerous skin reaction called Stevens-Johnson syndrome have occurred. Although all these problems are very, very rare, patients should be on the watch for the development of a rash, jaundice, water retention, bleeding or bruising, or signs of infection.

Oxcarbazepine (Trileptal)

As its name suggests, oxcarbazepine (brand name Trileptal) is very similar to carbamazepine. It is another medication used to treat epilepsy, and it seems to work similarly to, but has several advantages over, carbamazepine. Oxcarbazepine is not associated with the blood-count problems that can be caused by carbamazepine or with the changes in liver enzymes that affect the metabolism of other drugs. This makes it significantly easier to take, with less need for monitoring blood tests and changes in dosage. Much of the earlier work on oxcarbazepine in bipolar disorder was done in Europe, and studies by German investigators in the mid-1980s suggested it was as beneficial as carbamazepine in treating mania. More recently American clinicians have also published favorable reports on its safety and efficacy.[27]

Many clinicians have been reluctant to prescribe oxcarbazepine's parent compound, carbamazepine, because of the possibility of severe adverse reactions. Given the much less significant problems associated with oxcarbazepine, we will probably see it prescribed more often and studied more closely.

Lamotrigine (Lamictal)

Lamotrigine (brand name Lamictal) is something of a child prodigy among medications used to treat bipolar disorder. Unlike other medications, which became common treatments for bipolar disorder only after many years on the market, lamotrigine proved its usefulness very quickly. As a result it went from an uncommonly used drug prescribed mostly at research medical centers to a mainstay of the treatment of bipolar disorder in only a few years. Like several other medications already discussed, lamotrigine is also an antiseizure medication. The first studies on lamotrigine began to appear in the 1980s, describing it as a useful "add-on" therapy for epilepsy patients who were already taking other antiseizure medications. During the early investigations of this use, researchers noted that patients who took lamotrigine for seizure control reported an improvement in their mood and sense of well-being—even if it hadn't helped much with their seizures. These observations led to clinical trials in patients with mood disorders, which quickly revealed that lamotrigine is an effective medication for many such patients.

Lamotrigine has several effects on the brain that might explain its efficacy in bipolar disorder. It seems to inhibit release of the neurotransmitter glutamate, an amino acid that causes stimulation of various neural circuits. Lamotrigine is also thought to affect at least one of the same second-messenger systems that lithium affects, the inositol triphosphate system.[28]

The most exciting aspect of lamotrigine's profile is its apparent effectiveness in bipolar depression. One of the first reports on its use in the treatment of bipolar disorder described a patient who had suffered from rapid-cycling bipolar I disorder since he was fourteen years old.[29] In the year before starting lamotrigine, he had been either depressed or manic continuously with no period of normal mood. When he was first seen by the research team, he had been severely depressed and had not responded to lithium or carbamazepine or an antidepressant. After beginning to take lamotrigine, his depressive symptoms gradually improved, and as of eleven months later he'd had no recurrence of either depressive or manic symptoms. Case reports and studies of lamotrigine as a medication added to other agents started to accumulate and continued to look promising.

In 2003 two large studies were published that compared the efficacy of lamotrigine with lithium (and also with placebo) in keeping patients with bipolar disorder from having another mood episode over a period of eighteen months. In one study patients were recovering from a manic or mixed episode as they entered the study;[30] in the other, patients were recovering from a depression.[31] In my discussion of early research in the section on lithium, I mentioned that the best way to tell whether a medication is truly effective is to do a double-blind, placebo-controlled study. Both these studies comparing lamotrigine with lithium and placebo were carried out in just this way; they also were large studies that included hundreds of patients, and they lasted for a year and a half—much longer than most medication trials. So when both studies reported that lamotrigine was just as effective as lithium in keeping patients well, this new medication suddenly came into the spotlight and quickly became one of the foundations of the treatment of bipolar disorder.

The exciting finding from these studies is that lamotrigine is especially effective against depression in bipolar disorder, which is extremely good news.[32] This is such an important finding because, as you will see later, the depression of bipolar disorder is much more difficult to treat than manic or mixed states (see "Treating Bipolar Depression" in chapter 7). You may remember that individuals with bipolar II disorder have more problems with depression than with mania and that these depressions can be especially long, debilitating, and difficult to treat. Some experts are suggesting that lamotrigine may fill an important, as yet unmet therapeutic need for these patients.[33]

Lamotrigine has a half-life of about twenty-four hours, and its metabolism is affected by taking carbamazepine and valproate (see table 6-6). Blood levels are not routinely ordered for lamotrigine because of its low toxicity and

TABLE 6-6 Therapeutic Profile of Lamotrigine

Medication class:	Mood stabilizer (anticonvulsant)
Brand names:	Lamictal
Half-life:	15–24 hours
Metabolism:	Affected by carbamazepine, valproate
Elimination:	Liver
Birth control:	Recommended
Other considerations:	Rarely causes severe skin rashes, but has good side-effect profile

because therapeutic effects have not been correlated with a particular blood level range.

SIDE EFFECTS

In contrast to the other mood stabilizers, lamotrigine has a very low side-effect burden. It can cause some initial nausea or gastrointestinal upset and the sort of side effects that many medications affecting the brain can cause: sleepiness, light headedness or dizziness, and headache. At higher doses, some patients complain of concentration problems similar to those often reported by patients taking lithium. In my experience, lowering the dose usually takes care of this problem.

The most serious problems that have been associated with lamotrigine are very dangerous types of allergic skin rashes called Stevens-Johnson syndrome and toxic epidermal necrosis (TED). These problems were reported early on, when the drug was given to patients with epilepsy. When research was done to see which patients were at highest risk for these serious reactions, it was discovered that children, and patients who started the drug at high doses, were more likely than others to develop a serious rash. Subsequently, the drug's manufacturer recommended against prescribing lamotrigine to children except under special circumstances and also changed the dosing recommendations for starting the drug in adults. Now patients start lamotrigine at a very low dose and gradually increase it over a period of weeks. This means that it may take five weeks or more to get to the usual therapeutic dose of 200 to 400 mg/day (even longer if the patient is already taking a drug, such as valproate, that raises lamotrigine levels in the body; in these cases the dose must be increased even more slowly). Since these recommendations were put into effect, the number of patients developing serious rashes has dropped dramatically. In clinical trials in which lamotrigine was prescribed to several thousand patients for the treatment of bipolar disorder, none of the patients developed a serious rash.[34]

TABLE 6-7 The Stanford Protocol for Patients Starting Lamotrigine

Do not start lamotrigine within 2 weeks of any rash, viral infection, vaccination
During first 3 months of treatment, avoid new
  Medicines, foods
  Soaps, cosmetics, conditioners, deodorants
  Detergents, fabric softeners
During first 3 months of treatment, avoid
  Poison ivy/oak, sunburn

Many individuals develop skin reactions to medications (and lots of other things as well), so it's important when starting on lamotrigine to take precautions against developing a rash from another source. This would make it impossible to know for sure that the rash was *not* caused by lamotrigine; the patient might need to stop the drug unnecessarily, perhaps missing out on a medication that might be very effective. For this reason, patients starting on lamotrigine should consider the protocol developed at Stanford University to prevent skin rashes (see table 6-7).

Other Mood Stabilizers

Several other agents show promise for the treatment of bipolar disorder. For the most part the promise of these medications is based on a few case reports of a therapeutic effect, or in some cases they are medications in the same class as other pharmaceuticals already shown to be helpful.

Gabapentin (Neurontin) is another antiseizure medication that may be a mood stabilizer in some patients. As with the other antiseizure medications, reports of beneficial effects on mood-disorder symptoms in patients who were taking it to treat epilepsy were the first indications that gabapentin might be a useful agent. Then several reports of its use in bipolar disorder appeared. One of these concerned a man with bipolar disorder who had refused to take lithium and who had liver disease and low blood counts caused by alcoholism.[35] Since he wouldn't take lithium and his medical problems made the use of valproate or carbamazepine risky, gabapentin was tried. The patient had a "dramatic" decrease in manic symptoms, his sleep pattern returned to normal, and best of all he reported no side effects. When more scientifically rigorous studies were done, however, enthusiasm for gabapentin waned dramatically. In two placebo-controlled studies, it was no more effective than placebo in treating symptoms of bipolar disorder. In one of these studies, gabapentin was the only medication the subjects were taking;[36] in the other, gabapentin was added to lithium, valproate, or both.[37]

Because of these and other conflicting data, it's impossible to say exactly how gabapentin should fit into the treatment of bipolar disorder. Some points in its favor are that it is not metabolized in the liver and so does not affect the blood levels of other medications; it doesn't need blood-level monitoring; and it has a very good side-effect profile.

Case reports and small studies suggest that *topiramate* (Topamax), another antiepilepsy medication, may be effective in bipolar disorder. As is usually the case with new medications, topiramate has so far been used mostly to treat patients with difficult-to-control symptoms who have not benefited from other available drugs. In many of these reports, patients were taking several other medications at the same time they started on topiramate. A good example of this kind of study is one in which fifty-eight patients were prescribed topiramate in addition to their other medications for various symptoms of bipolar I and bipolar II.[38] Researchers thought that almost two-thirds of these individuals had at least moderate improvement. But since so many different factors are involved—different diagnoses, different combinations of medications—it is very difficult to make a confident assessment of the results. There have been reports of topiramate helping with both the depressed and the manic phases of bipolar disorder, but there have also been reports of the medication making depression worse and triggering mania and mixed states.[39]

The side-effect profile of topiramate is favorable; the most serious problems are attention and concentration problems that become troublesome at higher doses. Topiramate has one common side effect that, for once, is usually considered an advantage: weight loss. Patients vary in this response, but most lose several pounds and some a significant amount of weight. If topiramate turns out to be a useful medication in bipolar disorder, it will be a welcome addition to our list, but the final word on efficacy and safety is not yet in.[40]

Tiagabine (Gabitril) and *zonisamide* (Zonegran) are other antiepilepsy drugs that have attracted the interest of clinical researchers on bipolar disorder. Ongoing work may result in these drugs also being introduced as mood-stabilizing medications.

Another promising agent is *riluzole* (Rilutek), a medication approved for the treatment of amyotrophic lateral sclerosis (ALS, sometimes known as Lou Gehrig's disease, after the famous baseball player of the 1930s who suffered from it). Riluzole has a protective effect on neurons, explaining why it helps slow the progression of ALS, a disease characterized by progressive deterioration of the nerve cells that control muscles. (Lithium has long been known to have a similar protective effect.) Riluzole works through the same chemical pathways that lamotrigine does. Not surprisingly, some of the most promising studies on the use of riluzole in bipolar disorder have been those showing that it is helpful in bipolar depression.[41]

Antidepressant Medications

ANTIDEPRESSANT MEDICATIONS ARE HIGHLY EFFECTIVE IN TREATING the depression of bipolar disorder. They must be used carefully and judiciously, however, because these medications can push a bipolar patient from depression into a manic state and cause other problems as well. In fact, the observation of manic symptoms in patients being treated for tuberculosis with a medication called iproniazid led to the development of the class of antidepressants called monoamine oxidase inhibitors (MAOIs). Despite these findings and the risks associated with antidepressants for persons with bipolar illness, antidepressant medications have become very important in the treatment of patients with bipolar disorder.

Tricyclic Antidepressants

Although tricyclics are now less frequently used as antidepressants, our discussion starts with this group because these were the first antidepressant medications developed and because they still provide the standard by which all promising new pharmaceuticals for the treatment of depression are judged.

These drugs are called tricyclics because of the three rings in their chemical structure (see figure 7-1). Although some tricyclics have an effect on serotonin systems in the brain, their primary effect in the brain seems to be an inhibition of reuptake of the neurotransmitter *norepinephrine* by neurons. Remember that reuptake of neurotransmitters into the neuron after they

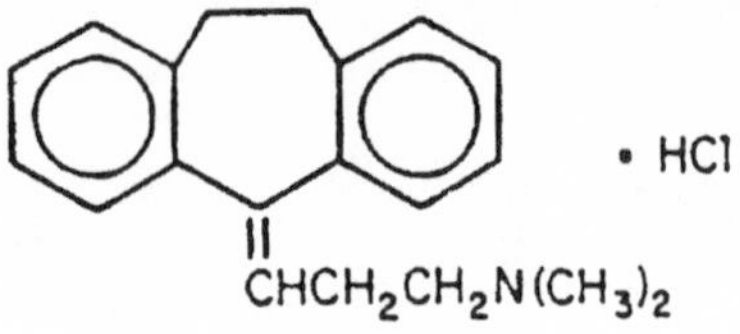

FIGURE 7-1 Chemical structure of two tricyclic antidepressants, showing their characteristic three-ringed structure

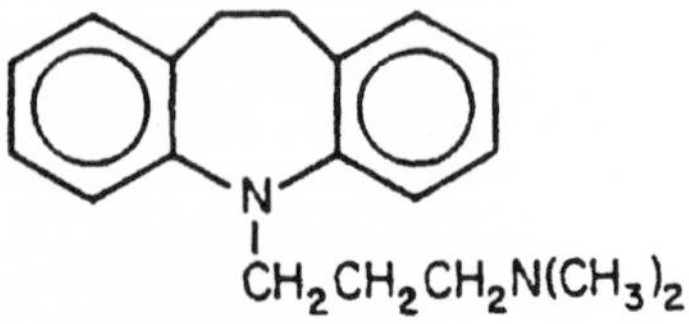

have been released into the synaptic cleft, and have done their work signaling the next cell, is the means by which the synapse is "reset." Norepinephrine is usually quickly removed from the synapse and pumped back into the cell that released it in order to turn off and reset the system. By blocking the removal of norepinephrine, tricyclics seem to prolong or intensify norepinephrine's message to the next cell in some way.

This effect of tricyclics on norepinephrine in neurons was one of the first chemical effects of a medication active in the brain to be measured in the laboratory. The observation that tricyclics *increased* the amount of norepinephrine in the synapse, along with the discovery that certain other medications used to treat high blood pressure *reduced* norepinephrine—and were observed to cause depression in some patients—led to the early amine hypothesis of the mood disorders: the theory that depression was caused by too little norepinephrine, and mania, presumably, by too much. However, further research indicated that tricyclics increased amines in the synapse within *hours* of taking them but took *weeks* to begin to help with depressive symptoms, and this led to a search for an alternative explanation. That search is still going on. The fundamental biochemical effect of antidepressants that is responsible for alleviating the symptoms of depression remains a mystery. It is thought that the change in signaling at the synapse that antidepressants cause may set off a cascade of events, probably involving a second-messenger system, that eventually results in an improvement of the symptoms of de-

TABLE 7-1 Tricyclic Antidepressants

Pharmaceutical Name	Brand Name
Amitriptyline	Elavil
Amoxapine	Ascendin
Clomipramine	Anafranil
Desipramine	Norpramin
Doxepin	Sinequan
Imipramine	Tofranil
Maprotiline	Ludiomil
Nortriptyline	Pamelor
Protriptyline	Vivactil

pression. Unfortunately, the question of how these medications work remains largely unanswered. (Table 7-1 lists the common tricyclics.)

The principal reason that tricyclic antidepressants are now less frequently prescribed is their many side effects. As with all medications, some patients can take tricyclics easily and without unpleasant side effects, but many patients have to put up with a few days or even weeks of troublesome side effects in order to get the benefits. Fortunately all the side effects are dose-related, and most are temporary.

You may remember that Roland Kuhn found imipramine, the first tricyclic, among a group of compounds that had some antihistamine effects. It's not surprising, then, that these medications affect some people the way antihistamines do, causing mild sleepiness and sometimes what some of my patients have called a "weird" or "spacey" feeling for the first day or two of starting them. Tricyclics block another neurotransmitter called *acetylcholine*, which is used in the part of the nervous system that regulates many "automatic" functions of the body such as digestion. These *anticholinergic* side effects include a slowing down of the gastrointestinal tract, causing constipation and dry mouth. The focusing of the lens of the eye and emptying of the urinary bladder are also controlled by this system, and tricyclics can cause blurry vision and urination difficulties also, although usually only at high doses. Patients with a history of glaucoma or urinary tract problems should be monitored closely by their physician while taking these medications. Tricyclics also cause weight gain in many patients.

Tricyclic overdoses are very dangerous and are responsible for many of the completed suicides by overdose in people with mood disorders. Although the lethal overdose is up to twenty times the normal dose for an adult, children are more sensitive to the toxic effects of these medications, and just a handful of tablets can be fatal in a small child. For this reason, these medications must be scrupulously safeguarded in households with children.

Selective Serotonin Reuptake Inhibitors (SSRIs)

It will come as no surprise that a new pharmaceutical that had none of the tricyclic side effects listed above and was not toxic in overdose caused something of a sensation when it was introduced in 1988. That pharmaceutical was fluoxetine (Prozac), and for a time it seemed that everyone you talked to was either taking Prozac or reading about it: in *Listening to Prozac* or *Talking Back to Prozac* or *Prozac Nation*. A Prozac capsule showed up on the covers of *Newsweek* and *New York* magazines, and the drug was featured in innumerable other magazine and newspaper articles.

Unlike the tricyclics, this class of antidepressants has little direct effect on norepinephrine in the brain but instead blocks the reuptake of another neurotransmitter, *serotonin,* into neurons. The very potent and specific serotonin-reuptake blocking effects of these agents give this class its name: *selective serotonin reuptake inhibitors,* or *SSRIs* (see table 7-2).

The main side effect of these medications is gastrointestinal discomfort. Many patients experience nausea for the first couple of days after starting one of the SSRIs, and a few have diarrhea or vomiting. Fortunately these side effects tend to pass quickly. These medications (especially fluoxetine) are also somewhat stimulating in some people, and while this is just what is needed by some depressed patients, others feel unpleasantly nervous or "wired" when taking these medications. The converse can also be seen, and sleepiness can sometimes be a side effect. Many patients report that SSRIs seem to curb

TABLE 7-2 Selective Serotonin Reuptake Inhibitors

Pharmaceutical Name	Brand Name(s)
Citalopram	Celexa (Cipramil)
Escitalopram	Lexapro (Cipralex)
Fluoxetine	Prozac, Sarafem (Erocap, Fluohexal, Lovan, Zactin, and others)
Fluvoxamine	Luvox
Paroxetine	Paxil, Paxil CR* (Aropax, Seroxat, and others)
Sertraline	Zoloft (Altruline, Aremis, Gladem, Besitran, Lustral, Sealdin, and others)

Note: Names in parentheses are brands marketed outside the United States.
*Slow-release preparation.

their appetite a bit and notice some weight loss, especially early on in taking an SSRI. Weight gain can also be a problem, however. All of these side effects are usually noticed by patients pretty much immediately, if they are going to occur, and none of them sneaks up after a person has been on an SSRI for weeks or months.

One problem that might not be noticeable to patients until they've been taking an SSRI for weeks or months is a change in sexual functioning, specifically a noticeable decrease in sexual interest (loss of libido) or a difficulty in reaching or inability to reach orgasm. The frequency of these problems is difficult to gauge, because these sorts of side effects were often not asked about during clinical trials with these medications. But as more patients have been treated with SSRIs during the last decade, it has become apparent that this is a significant problem affecting about one-third of patients. A variety of strategies are available for dealing with these problems when they occur, so they should be reported to the physician. Weekend "vacations" from the medication have been reported to be helpful, as well as the addition of other medications that seem to block these effects, but sometimes a switch to an antidepressant in another class is the only solution.

When I asked one of my male patients whether he was having any sexual dysfunction from his new antidepressant he replied that he thought fluoxetine had *improved* his sex life: increasing his sexual stamina and causing him to have more intense orgasms—a reminder that a list of potential medication side effects should never be a reason not to try a particular medication. Pleasant surprises sometimes do occur. Also, a medication effect that causes problems for some patients can actually be helpful for others; for example, SSRIs have been reported to be helpful in treating premature ejaculation.[1]

Other New Antidepressants

Since the early 1990s many other new antidepressants have come onto the market that aren't tricyclics and aren't SSRIs. Since most of these pharmaceuticals don't really share many common features, there isn't a very good class name for them, although you'll sometimes see many of these new agents listed as "atypical" or "second-generation" antidepressants (see table 7-3). They have a variety of effects on norepinephrine, serotonin, and other neurotransmitters. Some have more than one effect on these systems, and so they are thought to provide different ways of manipulating the chemical systems in the brain that are concerned with mood. Venlafaxine and duloxetine, for example, inhibit the reuptake of both norepinephrine and serotonin and are referred to as "dual reuptake inhibitors" or "SNRIs," for *serotonin and norepinephrine reuptake inhibitors.* Bupropion is most active on a different neuro-

TABLE 7-3 More Antidepressants

Pharmaceutical Name	Brand Name(s)
Bupropion	Wellbutrin, Wellbutrin XL,* Wellbutrin SR*
Duloxetine	Cymbalta (Davedax, Xeristar, Yentreve, and others)
Mirtazapine	Remeron (Remergil, Zispin, and others)
Nefazodone	Serzone† (Dutonin)†
Trazodone	Desyrel (Azona, Molipaxin, Sideril, Thombran, and others)
Venlafaxine	Effexor, Effexor XR* (Efexor, Efexor XR,* and others)

Note: Names in parentheses are brands marketed outside the United States.
*Slow-release preparation.
†Brands withdrawn by manufacturer because of reports of liver failure.

transmitter altogether, one called *dopamine.* The side-effect profiles of these medications vary widely. Some have a profile more like tricyclics, others more like SSRIs.

Monoamine Oxidase Inhibitors (MAOIs)

In the early 1950s a new drug that had been developed for the treatment of tuberculosis was observed to cause mood elevation in some patients who took it for their lung disease. After several more years of investigations, mostly in England, several papers appeared that confirmed the therapeutic effects of iproniazid in patients suffering from depression. Shortly afterward it was discovered that iproniazid causes inactivation of an enzyme in the body that metabolizes amine compounds in the nervous system. This enzyme, called *monoamine oxidase,* is responsible for gobbling up molecules of norepinephrine, serotonin, and several other neurotransmitters. Inactivating monoamine oxidase has the effect of increasing the amounts of these compounds in the nervous system, and this effect—in some as yet poorly understood way—may be the mechanism by which these medications alleviate the symptoms of depression. This effect on the enzyme gives this class of pharmaceuticals their name: *monoamine oxidase inhibitors,* or *MAOIs* (see table 7-4).

There are two forms of monoamine oxidase in the body, MAO-A and MAO-B. Until recently, all of the pharmaceuticals used to treat depression were active in blocking MAO-A. In addition to its activity in the nervous system, MAO-A is also present in the lining of the intestine. Some naturally occurring substances in foods are close enough chemically to norepinephrine to need deactivation before they are absorbed into the bloodstream, and in-

TABLE 7-4 Monoamine Oxidase Inhibitors (MAOIs)

Pharmaceutical Name	Brand Name(s)
Phenelzine	Nardil
Tranylcypromine	Parnate
Selegiline	Eldepryl, Emsam transdermal system*

*The selegiline patch.

testinal MAO-A serves this purpose. The importance of this becomes clear when I tell you that another name for norepinephrine is *adrenaline*—a name you probably find more familiar. Tyramine, an amino acid that has adrenaline-like effects on blood pressure and heart rate, is present in high enough concentrations in some foods to cause dangerous cardiovascular problems in individuals taking MAOIs. A number of pharmaceuticals, including the ingredients of many over-the-counter remedies, also have adrenaline-like effects. People taking MAOIs therefore need to observe certain dietary restrictions and, even more importantly, must *scrupulously* read the labels of any over-the-counter medication they are considering—or better yet, consult their pharmacist before taking any pharmaceutical they buy over the counter.

MAOIs also interact with other medications that are prescribed or commonly used in emergency rooms for various problems. People taking MAOIs must be sure to inform all their treating physicians that they are on this medication. And they should consider wearing an alerting bracelet so that, should they be brought into an emergency room unconscious or otherwise unable to communicate, the bracelet can communicate to ER personnel that they are taking an MAOI.

Recently a pharmaceutical has been developed that blocks primarily MAO-B, the other form of MAO in the body. MAO-B is present almost entirely in the brain and is not involved in blocking tyramine absorption in the intestine. The big advantage of an MAO-B inhibitor over an MAO-A inhibitor, then, is that persons taking it wouldn't have to be on a special diet. This drug, called *selegiline*, has been used for the treatment of Parkinson's disease for several years. There were early attempts to use it as an antidepressant, but it was discovered that the required doses were so high when taken in pill form that selegiline affected *both* forms of MAO (A and B)—that is, the specificity for MOA-B is lost. This meant that patients taking it would still need to watch their diet for sources of tyramine—no advantage there! Then someone came up with the idea of making a selegiline *patch*, whereby the drug is absorbed through the skin rather than taken orally. The patch turns out to have two important advantages. First, because the selegiline is more directly absorbed into the bloodstream, it can be given at a lower dose and maintain its specificity for MAO-B. Second, since it doesn't travel though the intestine, it doesn't affect the MAO-A located there nearly as much as the older MAOIs. Thus, the selegiline patch is an easier way of taking an MAOI, with fewer side effects and less worry about tyramine-rich foods.

MAOIs can have other side effects, too. They can be stimulating and cause insomnia. For this reason, taking the oral preparations at bedtime should be avoided. Dizzy spells, especially when suddenly getting up from lying down, can occur. MAOIs block a blood-pressure reflex that usually maintains blood pressure when we stand up, and the sudden drop in blood pressure on standing (called *orthostatic hypotension*) causes lightheadedness. Weight gain and sexual dysfunction are other side effects.

Because of these issues, MAOIs are most often prescribed to patients who have failed to benefit from other antidepressants. This said, they are sometimes uniquely effective, indeed are "miracle drugs," for some patients who have been helped by no other antidepressants. I think every psychiatrist I've ever spoken with has had the experience of effectively treating a particular patient with an MAOI after no other antidepressant had helped.

Treating Bipolar Depression

The observation that antidepressants can cause manic symptoms in persons with bipolar disorder has been confirmed again and again. Perhaps more worrisome is the observation that antidepressants may cause an acceleration of the illness in some patients. Some persons with bipolar disorder experience increased cycling of their mood episodes and can even switch to a period of rapid cycling. Yet, antidepressants can be safely taken for symptoms of bipolar depression by many patients. When a bipolar patient gets depressed, how does the psychiatrist decide whether or not to prescribe an antidepressant?

Studies on the issue of precipitation of mania and rapid cycling indicate that some patients are at more risk than others for a worsening of their situation with antidepressant treatment. Unfortunately it is not possible to say with certainty who is and who is not at risk. Bipolar I patients seem to be at greater risk than bipolar II patients; women are at greater risk than men; and patients who already have a history of more rapid cycling—either more full-blown episodes or a tendency toward cyclothymia (continuous low-amplitude cycling) between full-blown episodes—are at greater risk. Moreover, some antidepressant medications seem to be riskier than others. A few studies indicate that bupropion, paroxetine, and MAOIs may be safer than other antidepressants—that is, less likely to precipitate mania (and, by implication, perhaps less likely to increase cycling).

In later chapters in this part of the book I discuss two treatments for depression that do not have these risks. These are electroconvulsive therapy (ECT) and psychotherapy. These treatments are often avoided or overlooked in the treatment of bipolar depression: ECT often thought of as "too drastic," and psychotherapy dismissed because "talking can't help." As I hope to convince you, neither of these attitudes is justified by the research.

Perhaps more than any other treatment issues, the questions surrounding the use of antidepressants in bipolar disorder emphasize the need for individualization of treatment for every patient. There are no hard-and-fast rules for when, why, or how to use antidepressant medications for bipolar patients. Patient and physician need to communicate clearly and honestly about every aspect of symptoms and treatment in order to achieve the best treatment outcome.

CHAPTER 8

Antipsychotic Medications

A DIFFICULTY THAT IMMEDIATELY ARISES IN DISCUSSING THE ANTI-psychotic medications is their unfortunate name. *Psychotic* is an imprecise term at best, and these medications have many more uses than simply treating psychotic symptoms.

When I was training at Johns Hopkins, all the residents knew better than to describe a patient as "psychotic" within earshot of Hopkins' chairman of psychiatry, Paul McHugh. "What does *that* word mean? You might as well call the patient 'crazy!'" I can hear him say. "What are you trying to say: Is the patient delusional? Hallucinated? Disoriented? Does he have a disorder of thinking? *What?*" Dr. McHugh's point was that we have very good words to describe the various symptoms of major mental illnesses and that describing a person as suffering from "psychosis" simply doesn't say very much. Nevertheless, *psychosis* is such a frequently used word in works on psychiatric disorders that we need to agree on some sort of definition in order to understand what is usually meant by it.

A psychosis can be thought of as a mental state or disorder in which the affected person's ability to comprehend his or her environment and react to it appropriately is severely impaired. The layman's definition of *psychotic* might be "out of touch with reality." The person who is hearing voices (having hallucinations) or who has bizarre idiosyncratic beliefs (delusions) is psychotic. The word also connotes a severe disorganization of thinking and behavior, usually with restlessness and agitation. The manic syndrome is a good example of a state of psychosis, and we have already talked about "psychotic features" in depression.

In the 1930s a group of pharmaceutical compounds called *phenothiazines* were synthesized in Europe and were found to have antihistamine and sedative properties. One in particular, chlorpromazine, was found to be very useful in surgical anesthesia because it deepened anesthetic sedation more safely than other available agents. In the early 1950s two French psychiatrists carried out several clinical trials using chlorpromazine to treat highly agitated patients suffering from schizophrenia and mania. They had hoped the drug would provide sedation for these very sick patients, which it did—but these astute clinicians noticed that this medication did much more.

In addition to its quieting and sleep-promoting effects, chlorpromazine made the hallucinations and bizarre delusional beliefs of many patients with schizophrenia practically disappear. It also decreased the severity of the disorganization of thinking and agitated behavior seen in patients with acute mania. Chlorpromazine, in other words, had a *specific* effect on the cluster of symptoms usually referred to as "psychotic" symptoms, and thus the name for this group came about: *antipsychotic medications.* Occasionally they are still referred to as *neuroleptic medications* (or *neuroleptics*), from *neuroleptique,* the French word (coined from Greek roots) that roughly means "affecting the nervous system." The term *major tranquilizers* was frequently used for these medications at one time (with the term *minor tranquilizers* used for sleep and anxiety medications), but these agents are much more than just "tranquilizers," and this term has, fortunately, fallen out of favor.

In the 1980s a new antipsychotic medication was developed that had much more effect on the neurotransmitter serotonin than the other antipsychotics did. In the years since, many more of these drugs have been developed. This group of medications has been a very important development in psychiatry, for reasons I'll discuss below. Now antipsychotic medications are usually divided into two groups, the original group of medications being called the *typical antipsychotics* and the newer group the *atypical antipsychotics,* which have more effect on the serotonin system than their predecessors. In this chapter we'll take a look at each group in turn.

The Typical Antipsychotic Medications

As we saw in part I of this book, episodes of bipolar disorder—both depression and mania—can sometimes include extremely frightening mental symptoms and dangerously disturbed behaviors. And, as we saw in chapters 6 and 7, mood stabilizers and antidepressants sometimes take weeks to begin working. What can be done to slow down the racing thoughts, the pressured, bursting overactivity of the manic patient, before lithium starts working? What can be done to help the psychotically depressed patient tormented by hallucinations, before the antidepressant starts working? This is where the

Table 8-1 Typical Antipsychotic Medications

Pharmaceutical Name	Brand Name
Chlorpromazine	Thorazine
Fluphenazine	Prolixen
Haloperidol	Haldol
Loxapine	Loxitane
Molindone	Moban
Perphenazine	Trilafon
Thioridazine	Mellaril
Thiothixene	Navane
Trifluoperazine	Stelazine

Note: Side effects include sedation, anticholinergic effects, and extrapyramidal effects (see text).

typical antipsychotic medications have been useful (see table 8-1). Because their calming effects begin almost immediately, these medications are especially useful in acute mania and are frequently part of the treatment for the severely ill manic patient. In cases of depression where the patient is highly restless and agitated, they can have similar beneficial effects.

The main chemical effect of all antipsychotics is a blockade of *dopamine* receptors in the brain. Neural circuits that use dopamine as their neurotransmitter may be dysfunctional in some way in people with schizophrenia, causing the bizarre hallucinations and disorders of thinking typical of that illness, and antipsychotic medications may work by affecting these systems in some as yet unknown way. Whether or not these medications alleviate in a similar fashion the psychotic symptoms that sometimes complicate bipolar disorder is as yet unknown.

SIDE EFFECTS

The typical antipsychotic medications were once called "major tranquilizers" because they are, well, tranquilizers—in a major way. Some are more sedating than others, but all can be pretty powerful sedatives, especially in higher doses. They can cause some of the same anticholinergic side effects as tricyclic antidepressants: dry mouth, constipation, blurred vision. People seem to accommodate to these side effects after a period that ranges from days to weeks.

The main problem with most of these medications is their effect on muscle tone and movement, side effects that are caused by the dopamine blockade that these agents cause. In textbook discussions of these medications you will see these problems referred to as *extrapyramidal symptoms,* or simply *EPS.* Dopamine is the main neurotransmitter used in a complex circuit of brain areas called the *extrapyramidal system,* which coordinates movement. (The term *extrapyramidal* contrasts this system with another system, called the *pyramidal system* because its main fibers are carried in triangular-shaped bundles into the spinal cord [the "spinal pyramids" or "pyramidal tract"].) The pyramidal system controls the quick, accurate execution of fine muscle movement, and the extrapyramidal system makes sure that the rest of the body moves as needed for the smooth and graceful execution of these movements. Antipsychotic medications, by blocking the dopamine receptors in these centers, cause several movement problems. One is *pseudo-parkinsonism.* In Parkinson's disease there is a degeneration of part of the extrapyramidal system: the death of dopamine neurons in one of its crucial components (a brain area called the *substantia nigra*). You may know that persons suffering from Parkinson's disease have a slowed and shuffling walk, seem to lose facial expression because of stiffness of their face muscles, and also have trembling of their hands. Pseudo-parkinsonism consists of these same symptoms. The neurons don't die as they do in Parkinson's disease, but their chemical messenger, dopamine, is blocked from doing its work by a pharmaceutical agent.

Another set of extrapyramidal side effects is the *acute dystonic reactions.* These are muscular spasms that usually involve the tongue and facial and neck muscles, and they are more common in young males than in other patients. People taking antipsychotic medications can also develop a very uncomfortable restlessness called *akathesia.* This is felt mostly in the legs, and the individual feels the need to walk or pace.

Fortunately, all these side effects are treatable, either by lowering the dose of medication or by adding one of several medications that are also used to treat Parkinson's disease. Although uncomfortable, these side effects are not dangerous and usually respond quickly to treatment once they are encountered and identified.

Most of these medications can, over years, cause a side effect called *tardive dyskinesia,* or *TD* for short. This consists of repetitive involuntary movements, usually of the facial muscles—usually chewing, blinking, or lip-pursing movements. There is no good treatment for TD other than discontinuing the medication. We used to worry a lot about TD because some patients who developed it seemed to continue to have these movements even after the medication was stopped. But two factors are calming these worries: the discovery that most TD symptoms *do* eventually go away with time and, more importantly, the development of the atypical antipsychotic medications, which do not seem to cause TD. We'll talk about these medications in the next section of this chapter.

I want to emphasize that extrapyramidal symptoms are usually easily treated, and are not dangerous. On the other hand, the symptoms of bipolar disorder that the antipsychotic medications are usually used to treat *are* extremely dangerous. These medications are powerful agents, and they need to be used carefully and for the shortest period of time possible, but for the present, at least, they are nearly irreplaceable in treating the most dangerous and most terrible symptoms of severe mania and psychotic depression.

Atypical Antipsychotic Medications

As is probably apparent after reading the foregoing paragraphs, there is room for improvement in the antipsychotic medications. Not only are the extrapyramidal symptoms uncomfortable until treated, but it is usually necessary to add another medication to control them—and the more different medications a person takes, the more likely he or she is to have problems with side effects and drug interactions. So it created quite a stir when a new group of antipsychotic medications was introduced, antipsychotics that don't seem to cause EPS. Even more good news: these medications seem to work better than their predecessors. One article in the *American Journal of Psychiatry* called the first of these new agents "arguably the most significant development in antipsychotic drug therapy since the advent of chlorpromazine."[1]

These agents are called *atypical antipsychotic medications* (see table 8-2), designated *atypical* because, although they block dopamine receptors just as their predecessors do (though not as potently), they differ from the typical antipsychotics in that they are also active at serotonin receptors. This double action seems to have two effects: extrapyramidal symptoms do not appear nearly as often, and these medications seem to have significant mood-stabilizing effects.

The first atypical antipsychotic, *clozapine,* was synthesized in the laboratory in the 1960s but was not marketed in the United States until 1990. One

TABLE 8-2 Atypical Antipsychotic Medications

Pharmaceutical Name	Brand Name(s)
Aripiprazole	Abilify
Clozapine	Clozaril
Olanzapine	Zyprexa, Zyprexa Zydis
Quetiapine	Seroquel
Risperidone	Risperdal
Ziprasidone	Geodon

of the reasons it took so long for clozapine to get onto the market is that, in about 1 percent of patients who take it, it causes a very dangerous drop in the number of white blood cells (called *agranulocytosis*).[2] This problem might have meant the end for clozapine as a new medication were it not for the fact that it was found to be highly effective in treating patients with schizophrenia who had derived little benefit from traditional antipsychotic medications. Dramatic case studies of patients with chronic treatment-resistant schizophrenia who basically "awakened" from years of unrelenting psychotic symptoms after they started clozapine sustained the interest of clinicians and pharmaceutical researchers. When it was discovered that the risk of agranulocytosis could be substantially reduced if the patient had his or her white blood cell count monitored weekly, clozapine treatment became more available to larger groups of patients, and before long, treatment-resistant mood-disorder patients were treated with it as well.

There are now many studies of the use of clozapine for people with treatment-resistant bipolar and schizoaffective disorder. A year after clozapine came onto the market, a letter to the editor of the *Journal of Clinical Psychopharmacology* reported that clozapine had been effective in treating two rapid-cycling bipolar patients "who were resistant to all conventional treatment."[3] One patient was a forty-eight-year-old woman who had been very ill for more than thirty years, had started rapid cycling about five years previously, and had been almost constantly cycling between delusional depressions and dysphoric mania for a whole year before starting on clozapine. The authors stated that after the woman had been taking clozapine alone for three months, "her mood swings completely stopped." The case report indicates that there were episodes of breakthrough manic and depressive symptoms, but the patient had done remarkably better on clozapine. (This case illustrates why, for some patients at least, weekly blood tests are a price they are willing to pay.)

Another study looked at the use of clozapine in twenty-five acutely manic patients "for whom lithium, anticonvulsants and [traditional] neuroleptics had been ineffective, had produced intolerable side effects, or both."[4] Almost three-quarters of the patients had "marked improvement" in their manic symptoms. The answer to the question posed in a 1995 article title, "Is Clozapine a Mood Stabilizer?"[5] seems to be an emphatic yes.

In the years since the introduction of clozapine, several other atypical antipsychotic medications that do *not* cause blood count problems have come along, and their introduction has substantially expanded the number of treatment options for bipolar disorder. More and more evidence is emerging that the atypical antipsychotic medications are helpful in all phases of bipolar disorder—mania *and* depression—as well as for ongoing treatment to prevent relapse (sometimes known as maintenance treatment). This

TABLE 8-3 Weight Gain Risks of Atypical Antipsychotics

Higher risk	Clozapine
↑	Olanzapine
	Quetiapine
	Risperidone
	Ziprasidone*
Lower risk	Aripiprazole*

Source: T. Baptista, N. M. Kin, S. Beaulieu, and E. A. de Baptista, "Obesity and Related Metabolic Abnormalities during Drug Administration: Mechanisms, Management, and Research Perspectives," *Pharmacopsychiatry* 35, no. 6 (2002): 205–19.
*Negligible effect on weight.

means that some patients will take atypical antipsychotic medications over the long term.

SIDE EFFECTS

Of the atypical antipsychotics, only clozapine causes the blood-count problem that requires frequent blood counts. None of the atypical antipsychotics cause EPS except at high doses. High doses can also trigger the other side effects that the traditional antipsychotic medications cause: anticholinergic side effects and sedation.

The most significant side-effect problem with the atypical antipsychotic medications has been their tendency to make some individuals gain weight and develop such obesity-related problems as high cholesterol and even diabetes. Not all individuals develop these problems, but attention to diet and weight issues is very important for persons taking these medications, especially for patients who take them over the longer term. The primary mechanism for the weight gain associated with the atypical antipsychotics seems to be stimulation of the appetite center of the brain, although it has also been suggested that these medications affect several hormones that control how the body handles calories and stores fat.[6] Some of the atypical antipsychotics are more likely to cause weight gain than others; in fact, several seem relatively weight neutral—that is, they seem to have little or no effect on weight (see table 8-3). These weight-neutral agents would seem to be preferable for already obese patients and for patients with diabetes or a family history of diabetes. Blood tests for diabetes and high cholesterol should be done at the beginning of treatment and regularly thereafter in patients taking antipsychotics for maintenance treatment. All patients taking atypical antipsychotics should take steps to control possible weight gain by paying attention to their diet and getting regular exercise.

CHAPTER 9

More Medications, Hormones, and Dietary Supplements

A NUMBER OF OTHER PHARMACEUTICAL AGENTS HAVE ATTRACTED AT-
tention because they have been proven helpful in the treatment of bipolar
symptoms. Others seem to show promise—or have promised more than
they have delivered—and warrant a discussion as well.

Benzodiazepine Medications

The benzodiazepine medications represented a major advance in the
treatment of psychiatric symptoms when they were first developed, and they
continue to be widely prescribed (see table 9-1). They often have a place in
the treatment of bipolar disorder because they are highly effective for the
treatment of anxiety and insomnia and, in higher doses, are safe and effective sedatives. If this sounds too good to be true and you're wondering if
there's a hidden drawback, there is. These medications can be abused, and it's
possible to become psychologically dependent on and even physically addicted to them. (Withdrawal symptoms in persons taking high doses of these
medications can include very serious problems like seizures.) Moreover, their
sedating effects decrease over time, and after several weeks of use their effectiveness as tranquilizers decreases. For these reasons benzodiazepines are
best thought of as temporary measures.

Benzodiazepines really have two main uses in treating bipolar disorder:
in treating patients who are very sick and in treating patients who are doing
very well. This seems to be a contradiction, doesn't it? The explanation is in

TABLE 9-1 Benzodiazepine Medications

Pharmaceutical Name	Brand Name
Alprazolam	Xanax
Chlordiazepoxide	Librium
Clonazepam	Klonapin
Clorazepate	Tranxene
Diazepam	Valium
Lorazepam	Ativan

Note: These medications are best thought of as temporary agents and are frequently prescribed for occasional "as-needed" use.

the doses used and how these medications are combined with other medications. In acutely manic patients, the short-acting benzodiazepine lorazepam (Ativan) can be an effective short-term tranquilizer, especially in combination with a typical antipsychotic medication like haloperidol (Haldol). This combination is very familiar to psychiatrists working in emergency settings because it works quickly and effectively in calming even the most agitated patients. A very ill manic patient, perhaps delusional and agitated, who hasn't slept for days can be asleep less than an hour after receiving this combination, especially in injectable form. The longer-acting benzodiazepine clonazepam (Klonapin) has also been used and extensively studied in the treatment of acute manic symptoms and appears also to be an effective adjunct medication.

These medications are not mood stabilizers and are not effective in treating hallucinations or delusions, but as sedatives they are unsurpassed. Remember that before effective psychiatric medications became available, patients with severe mania died of the physical stress of the manic state. By simply slowing manic patients down for a few hours or days until antipsychotic medications and mood-stabilizing medications start working, benzodiazepines can be literally lifesaving.

At the other end of the spectrum of illness severity, patients who are not having severe mood symptoms can safely take these medications for anxiety symptoms and insomnia. As we shall see in part IV of this book, anxiety and psychological stress can make bipolar patients more susceptible to an episode of their mood disorder (as can sleep deprivation). During periods of unavoidable psychological stress, such as after the death of a loved one, benzodiazepine medications can help with the insomnia and lessen the psychological tension that can bring on mood symptoms in bipolar patients. It's important to emphasize here that these medications should not be used as substitutes for making changes to chronically stressful situations. A person who finds that he or she needs a sedative to deal with usual everyday situations is well on his or her way to psychological dependence on tranquilizers, medication abuse, and addiction. We'll discuss this in more depth in chapter 15.

There's another way these medications are used, and that is in treating patients who have anxiety disorders. Anxiety disorders (such as recurrent panic attacks) are effectively treated with benzodiazepines. The connections between the mood disorders and anxiety disorders are poorly understood, but there are certainly some people who need treatment for both. The treatment of panic disorder and other severe anxiety disorders sometimes involves taking benzodiazepine medications on a more long-term basis, but prolonged use of benzodiazepines is the exception rather than the rule in treating bipolar disorders, and any use requires close monitoring.

Calcium-Channel-Blocking Agents

Since the 1970s, scientists researching bipolar disorder have been interested in a group of medications called calcium channel blockers. The flow of calcium ions is instrumental in the electrical activity of cells, and these medications modulate this flow by blockading the channels through which the calcium ions move into the cell. These medications are widely used in the treatment of heart problems. Like nerve cells, muscle cells are active electrically, and calcium channel blockers have powerful effects on the tiny muscle cells that open and close blood vessels. Blocking the calcium channels of these cells has the effect of relaxing them, allowing the arteries to open more and blood flow through them to increase. This is a very useful effect in treating coronary artery disease and angina—chest pains caused by too little flow through the coronary arteries, the arteries that supply the heart—as well as in treating high blood pressure, heart failure, and abnormal heart rhythms. The most widely prescribed calcium-channel-blocking agents are verapamil (Calan, Isoptin, and Verelan), nimodipine (Nimotop), nifedipine (Adalac and Procardia), diltiazem (Cardizem), and amlodipine (Norvasc).

These agents can be thought of as having a calming effect on electrical cells, analogous in some ways to the effect of anticonvulsants. So it didn't take long for clinical researchers to look into the effects of calcium-blocking agents on mania. A case report appeared in 1982 describing a therapeutic effect of verapamil in treating a manic patient.[1] Since then, several more reports and series of controlled trials in several hundreds of patients have appeared.[2] These reports suggest that some of the calcium channel blockers may be effective antimanic agents for some patients, but the superiority of these agents over lithium remains unproven. Many of the studies were of only several weeks' duration, so the mood-stabilizing effects of these agents over time remain largely unknown as well. There is practically no research on the antidepressant effects of these medications.

Psychiatrists have not rushed to use calcium channel blockers on bipolar patients, possibly because there is so much more research on lithium and other agents. Since calcium channel blockers don't appear to offer any special advantages over the medications we are more familiar with and that have a longer track record, there has been little impetus to do more research on them.

Might calcium channel blockers have a place in the treatment of patients who have bipolar disorder and who also have heart or blood-pressure problems? Will one agent effectively treat both conditions in some people? The problem here is that psychiatrists aren't usually very experienced in managing heart disease, and cardiologists aren't very experienced in managing bipolar disorder, so if we attempt to manage both problems with one medication, the treatment of one or the other will suffer. Moreover, both bipolar disorder and most heart and blood-pressure disorders are long-term conditions that often require a shift in treatment approaches over time, and this can cause any number of problems. For example, if a hypertensive bipolar patient's verapamil needs to be switched to another type of blood-pressure medication because it isn't working anymore, the last thing he or she needs is to risk a manic episode by going off the mood-stabilizing medication. Should the patient be put on a new antihypertensive and a new mood stabilizer simultaneously? If side effects appear, which medication is to blame?

I include this section on the calcium-channel-blocking agents simply because most books and papers on the treatment of bipolar disorders mention them and cite a report or two on their use in some unusual group of patients.[3] But at this point, routine use of these agents is not usually recommended.[4]

Stimulant Medications

For many years the treatment of depression often included the use of powerful medications known as psychostimulants (see table 9-2). Amphetamine, the prototype compound, is perhaps the best known of this group. These medications boost energy levels, concentration, and mood, and a number of years ago they were frequently prescribed for patients with depression. As psychiatrists became more sophisticated in using antidepressants, and as more antidepressants became available in the 1970s—and perhaps more significantly, when the many problems with amphetamine-like drugs became more apparent—their use in the treatment of mood disorders fell out of favor.

The problems with these medications are their tendency to raise blood pressure and their abuse potential. Because they increase wakefulness and improve concentration and physical endurance, they were widely abused by long-distance drivers, athletes, college students cramming for exams, and other persons trying to improve their performance at any cost. Amphetamines tend to lose their stimulating effects with prolonged use, can cause symptoms of paranoia indistinguishable from paranoid schizophrenia, and when stopped after prolonged use or use of high doses frequently cause the abuser to crash into a severe, even suicidal depression.

As with a number of powerful and highly effective treatments for psychiatric symptoms, enthusiastic overuse led to abuse and discredit for these medications, which in turn led to underutilization of an effective treatment and even denial of it to patients who could benefit from it; physicians were reluctant to prescribe what had come to be seen as a "bad" pharmaceutical. But as usually happens with enough time and enough good research, the pendulum has swung back toward the center, and the legitimate and safe uses of psychostimulants have become established. (A similar chain of events unfolded for electroconvulsive therapy, as we'll see in the next chapter.)

The use of psychostimulants as adjuncts to other treatments has become established in the approach to treatment-resistant depression, depression in the elderly, and also depression associated with medical illnesses such as cancer and AIDS.[5] Their use in bipolar depression is not as well defined, but cautious use in bipolar patients with treatment-resistant depression has been recommended.[6] There have been reports of mania induced by stimulants, warranting special caution in patients with frequent or severe manic episodes.[7] Psychostimulants are safe when used as prescribed, although side effects can include headache, flushing, loss of appetite, and insomnia. The severe problems noted in the preceding paragraphs are usually associated with prolonged use of high doses.

Another interesting use of psychostimulants has recently been reported: as treatment for the sexual dysfunction caused by SSRI antidepressant medications.[8] One small study found dextroamphetamine or methylphenidate to be 80 percent effective in reversing the sexual dysfunction caused by a serotonin reuptake inhibitor in twenty-four patients. (It should be mentioned here that psychostimulants are not the only remedy for sexual dysfunction symptoms caused by SSRIs; see chapter 7.)

TABLE 9-2 Psychostimulant Medications

Pharmaceutical Name	Brand Name
Amphetamine	Adderall, Dexedrine
Methylphenidate	Concerta, Metadate, Ritalin
Pemoline	Cylert

Note: Side effects include headache, flushing, loss of appetite, and insomnia.

Thyroid Hormones

In several sections of this book we're going to talk about the interrelationships of mood and hormones. The pulsing daily rhythms of melatonin from the pineal gland that may be involved with the seasonal mood changes of seasonal affective disorder (SAD), the mood fluctuations that can follow changing levels of female reproductive hormones (important in understanding postpartum mood symptoms and premenstrual syndromes), the stress hormones secreted by the adrenal gland—all these hormonal changes seem to be important in the regulation of mood. But perhaps the most important hormones in this respect are the thyroid hormones.

The thyroid gland plays a major role in the body's energy regulation. Too little thyroid gland activity leads to sluggishness and weight gain, and too much leads to metabolic overdrive—rapid pulse, nervous energy, and anxiety. While the precise role of thyroid hormones in the regulation of mood remains unclear, it's very clear that normal thyroid functioning is essential for effective treatment of mood disorders. Put another way, if a patient's mood symptoms don't respond to the usual treatments, or if a treatment that has been effective seems to lose its effectiveness, a thyroid problem, especially abnormally low thyroid functioning (hypothyroidism), should be suspected.

Several studies have shown that hypothyroidism is surprisingly common in patients with rapid-cycling bipolar disorder.[9] One group of scientists tested for thyroid abnormalities in stored blood samples from almost four thousand patients who had been hospitalized for psychiatric problems over a period of four years. They found a high association between thyroid abnormalities and a diagnosis of rapid-cycling bipolar disorder.[10]

But it is also clear that some patients with bipolar disorder whose thyroid hormone levels prove to be in the "normal range" when blood tests are done can nevertheless benefit from treatment with thyroid medications. Studies have demonstrated that many patients with bipolar depression symptoms that are not responding to treatment have thyroid function that is "normal" by the usual criteria, but blood tests show them to be in what might be called the "low normal" or even "barely normal" range.[11] It may be that depressed individuals need a higher level of thyroid hormones than individuals who are not depressed. Perhaps thyroid medication somehow makes these patients more responsive to other treatments. Patients who have a partial response to lithium or other mood stabilizers may have better control of their mood symptoms when thyroid medication is added, even if their thyroid hormone levels are normal. As a paper on treating rapid-cycling bipolar disorder put it, "Normal thyroid [blood test results] should not discourage the clinician from pursuing thyroid supplementation" in bipolar patients.[12]

At one time very high doses of thyroid medication—enough to make the patient slightly hyperthyroid—were considered necessary to obtain this effect, but this approach seems unnecessarily risky. Patients seem to benefit just as much from usual doses. For more on thyroid hormones and mood disorders, see "Mood Disorders Due to Hormonal Problems" in chapter 18.

St. John's Wort

Hypericum perforatum, commonly know as St. John's wort, is one of about three hundred species of shrubby perennial plants (of genus *Hypericum*) with bright yellow flowers that grow in most temperate regions of the world. Teas and other extracts of St. John's wort have been recommended by herbalists for centuries to treat everything from insomnia to the painful viral skin infection called shingles. In the late 1980s hypericum (*H. perforatum*) was investigated as a possible treatment for HIV infection when it was found to have activity against retroviruses, activity that unfortunately did not translate into clinical usefulness against HIV infection.

Most of the early scientific work on hypericum was done in Germany, where there is intense interest in herbal medicine, herbal preparations are more widely available, and, perhaps, herbal preparations are more seriously regarded as valid treatment options for serious illnesses. Several studies were done comparing hypericum extracts with placebo and with a standard antidepressant. The results of these earlier studies were generally quite encouraging and indicated that hypericum extracts had an antidepressant effect that is clinically significant in some people. A 1996 article in the *British Medical Journal* that systematically reviewed twenty-three different studies involving a total of 1,757 patients concluded that "extracts of hypericum are more effective than placebo for the treatment of mild to moderately severe depressive disorders."[13] This paper indicated that patients taking hypericum preparations generally reported fewer and less severe side effects than those taking standard antidepressants.

More recent studies have been less encouraging. When St. John's wort was compared with placebo in two hundred patients who had been rigorously evaluated and diagnosed with major depression, the herbal preparation was no better than the placebo in treating depression. This study concluded that "the results do not support significant antidepressant or anti-anxiety effects for St. John's wort when compared to placebo in a clinical sample of depressed patients" and that "persons with major depression should not be treated with St. John's wort, given the morbidity and mortality risks of untreated or ineffectively treated major depression."[14] In a follow-up study, the same researchers reported that when the individuals who had not responded to St. John's wort were given standard antidepressants, most of them improved, suggesting that the herbal preparation had failed not because these were "treatment-resistant" patients but simply because St. John's wort wasn't effective against their depression.[15]

It is difficult, then, to recommend hypericum preparations for persons with bipolar disorder. There are simply not enough rigorously controlled studies of its therapeutic effects in persons with major mood disorders—and, as we have seen, antidepressants are not without risk in bipolar disorder. People who suffer from mild unipolar depression symptoms might prudently attempt treatment of their symptoms with hypericum preparations under the supervision of a physician; people with bipolar disorder, however, are well advised to hold off using hypericum until more information about its use in bipolar disorder becomes available.

Nevertheless, the fact that St. John's wort is helpful for at least some patients, perhaps patients with uncomplicated depression (and, by definition, this does not include patients with bipolar disorder), is encouraging. The discovery of a pharmacologically active plant compound has often formed the basis for development of a much larger number of useful new drugs and led to other exciting discoveries. The chemical isolation of opium from the poppy plant, for example, led to the development of dozens of safer and more potent pain medications, and also to the discovery of similar compounds in the brain (called endorphins), which have become the basis for practically an entire new branch of neurochemistry. As we learn more about hypericum, it may turn out that a safer and more effective medication will derive from the active compounds found in St. John's wort.

Omega-3 Fatty Acids and Fish Oil

There are some nutrients that we must include in our diet in order to remain healthy. These are compounds that our body cannot manufacture but are nevertheless necessary for normal cellular functioning. The most familiar of these are, of course, the *vitamins*, compounds manufactured by some plants and animals but not by humans. Their name, from the Latin word *vita* meaning "life," indicates just how important to health they are. Unless we eat foods that contain the vitamins we need, serious illness results. Scurvy, beriberi, and pellagra are three—now, thankfully, unfamiliar—illnesses that result from deficiencies of, respectively, vitamin C, vitamin B_1, and niacin. All these illnesses have significant central nervous system symptoms, especially B_1 deficiency, which causes severe central nervous system degeneration.

Another group of essential nutrients is the *essential fatty acids*, a collection of complex fat molecules that are found in some vegetables and other plant sources (such as flaxseed) and in large amounts in some fish (see table 9-3). Nutritionists have long touted the health benefits of diets rich in

TABLE 9-3 Omega-3 Fatty Acids in Fish

	Omega-3 Fatty Acid Content (per serving)	
High (>100 mg)	*Moderate (500–900 mg)*	*Low (<500 mg)*
Anchovies	Halibut	Catfish
Herring	Rockfish	Cod
Mackerel	Sea bass	Flounder
Salmon	Smelt	Mahi mahi
Sardines	Swordfish	Perch
Trout	Whitefish	Sea trout
Tuna	Yellowfin tuna	Shellfish, shrimp, crab, lobster

seafood, and the lower incidence of breast cancer and heart disease in the Japanese population has been attributed to a diet rich in seafood.

Some evidence suggests that essential fatty acids, especially a subgroup called *omega-3 fatty acids*, may be useful in the treatment of mood disorders, especially bipolar disorder. The particular compounds thought to have the most health benefits have tongue-twisting names typical of complex organic compounds: eicosapentaenoic acid (EPA) and docosahexaenoic acid (DHA).

Some preliminary studies indicated that omega-3 fatty acids, taken as fish-oil capsules, are beneficial for individuals with mood disorders. A 1999 study showed that some patients who took fish-oil capsules in addition to their usual treatments for bipolar disorder had less relapses of mood symptoms over a period of four months than a group of patients who took placebo capsules containing olive oil.[16] Both groups of patients were on a number of other medications during the study, and there were other problems with the design of the study,[17] but despite these limitations, the results point to a new approach to the treatment of mood disorders with a new set of compounds. Other than very mild gastrointestinal discomfort and a fishy taste, there were no significant side effects.

Studies show that omega-3 fatty acids are incorporated into cell membranes in association with molecules that are known to be involved in cell signaling. They seem to be active at some of the same points in cellular signaling mechanisms where lithium and valproate are thought to work. Since valproate is, after all, a *synthetic* fatty acid, the idea that natural fatty acids might have benefits in mood disorders shouldn't seem strange at all. Other circumstantial evidence has been cited to support the importance of omega-3 fatty acids for good mental health. Archeological and epidemiological studies suggest that modern humans consume much less food that is rich in fatty acids than ancient peoples did and that we may be deficient in these important compounds compared with our ancestors. This fact, combined with the evidence that the prevalence of depression is increasing and the age of onset of mood disorders is decreasing, has been cited as further evidence of a link between these important compounds and mental health. Omega-3 fatty acid therapy is at this point an unproven treatment for mood disorders, so it should *not* be substituted for proven treatments. However, given the apparent low risk of these compounds, supplementation of standard treatments for mood disorders with fish-oil capsules, under the supervision of one's physician, may be an option some patients will want to explore.

CHAPTER 10

Electroconvulsive Therapy and Related Treatments

Electroconvulsive therapy (ECT) is a highly effective treatment for both phases of bipolar disorder, often providing dramatic and rapid relief of symptoms even when other treatments have failed. Unfortunately ECT is also often thought of as a "last resort" by physicians, and patients and their families resist its use because of myths and misconceptions about it.

Too often the popular media refer to ECT as "shock treatments," with all the unpleasant connotations of that term: *shock* defined as an unpleasant jolt or blow, or reminding you of the painful spark of static electricity that comes from touching a doorknob after crossing a carpeted room on a dry winter day. Calling ECT "shock treatments" is a bit like referring to modern surgery as "knife treatments"—accurate in a crude sort of way, but doing injustice to what is now a safe and effective treatment that can be literally lifesaving. That's not to gloss over the fact that ECT was crude and unpleasant in its early days—though not nearly as unpleasant as surgery was in *its* early days—but modern anaesthetic techniques have changed all that.

Although the effectiveness of ECT in mood disorders was not a completely accidental discovery, its original theoretical basis has been shown to have no validity, so the development of modern ECT was a kind of happy accident. In the early 1930s the Hungarian physician Joseph Ladislas von Meduna proposed that there was a mutual antagonism between epilepsy and schizophrenia: patients who suffered from epilepsy did not suffer from schizophrenia and vice versa. Modern research has shown that this is not the case, but von Meduna—convinced of the truth of this idea on the basis of his examination of the microscopic appearance of the brains of persons with the two conditions—conducted animal experiments attempting to find a way to produce seizure activity artificially. In 1935 he published a paper reporting a dramatic improvement in symptoms after artificially inducing seizures in several patients with schizophrenia. Von Meduna had used injections to produce seizures, but several years later two Italian psychiatrists reported that seizures could be produced by briefly passing a low-voltage electrical current through the skull by means of electrodes applied to the scalp. Ugo Cerletti and Lucio Bini had developed their technique in animals and then tried it with several patients with schizophrenia, and they also reported remarkable success.

Although patients with some forms of schizophrenia did indeed often show improvement in some of their symptoms after these treatments, it quickly became apparent that severely depressed patients showed improvement that was little short of miraculous. Decades previously Emil Kraepelin had described patients in a catatonic state from depression: "The patients lie in bed taking no interest in anything. They betray no pronounced emotion; they are mute, inaccessible; they pass their [bowel movements] under them; they stare straight in front of them with [a] vacant expression of countenance like a mask and with wide open eyes."[1] With "electroshock" treatments, such patients had complete recovery from their symptoms within a matter of days. The last major breakthrough in the treatment of psychiatric problems—the discovery of the Wassermann test for syphilis more than thirty years earlier—now seemed almost insignificant compared with this astonishing new therapeutic technique. Naturally, interest in ECT spread quickly around the globe.

But ECT's success was also its near downfall. Like many seemingly miraculous treatments, it was overprescribed at first and probably administered to many hundreds of persons it had little chance of helping. It's important to remember, however, that these were desperate times in psychiatry. With the discovery of antipsychotic medications nearly a decade off and the discovery of antidepressants nearly two, "little chance" of helping was better than no chance at all. Since, as we shall see, ECT is a highly effective treatment for mania, some institutions were inclined to use it for any and all highly agitated patients, and sometimes on merely uncooperative ones (a misuse that was dramatized—with a few inaccuracies unfortunately thrown in—in the film One Flew over the Cuckoo's Nest). Another negative factor was that in the first decade or so after its development, ECT had very serious complications. An epileptic seizure is a violent event: all the muscles of the body contract simultaneously for a few moments, sometimes with such force that broken bones result. Breathing stops as well, and heart rhythm irregularities occur which can be fatal.

The nearly indiscriminate overprescription of a therapy that had serious potential side effects led to a backlash against ECT. By the late 1960s and 1970s, although modern anaesthetic techniques were making ECT safer, and more careful research was being done to determine which psychiatric disorders the treatment helped with and which it did not, the damage to ECT's reputation had already been done. (*Cuckoo's Nest,* awarded the Oscar for best movie in 1975, depicted ECT as it would have been administered circa 1945, and certainly didn't help.) State hospitals drew up regulations sharply curtailing its use, and legislation was in effect briefly in California banning the procedure completely.

Fortunately the pendulum has swung back to center. ECT is now safer than most surgical procedures, side effects are minimal, and indications for its use have been clarified. A 1980 survey of 166 ECT patients reported that about half of them thought a trip to the dentist was more unpleasant than an electroconvulsive treatment.[2]

Modern ECT

The major improvements in ECT have been due to developments in anaesthetic techniques. ECT is usually done in the recovery room of the surgical suite of a hospital, the area where patients waking up from surgery are taken for observation. This makes sense when you realize that the actual ECT treatment is over in about sixty seconds, and that most of the "treatment" time is actually the ten minutes or so it takes for the patient to awaken from general anaesthesia. Some large psychiatric hospitals have their own treatment suites that are similarly equipped.

ECT is now done under general anaesthesia just as surgery is. The crucial anaesthetic advance for ECT was the introduction in the 1950s of agents called *muscle relaxants,* or more properly *neuromuscular blocking agents.* These medications, also given intravenously, temporarily paralyze the patient by blocking nervous center transmission to the muscles. This prevents the violent muscle contractions during seizures that characterized early ECT.

Immediately before the treatment, patients sometimes receive an injection of a medication that prevents abnormal heart rhythms (atropine or glycopyrrolate). Then an IV is started, and the patient is given the anaesthetic and the muscle relaxant. The patient is asleep and completely relaxed in less than five minutes. Electrode disks similar to those used to take cardiograms are applied to the scalp. Modern ECT equipment designed for the purpose delivers a precisely timed and measured electrical stimulus, usually of a half-second to several seconds' duration. In *bilateral* treatments, an electrode is applied over each temple. In *unilateral* treatments, wherein the object is to stimulate only half the brain, one electrode is placed in the middle of the forehead and the other at the temple. (Unilateral treatment causes less post-ECT confusion and memory problems and is now used almost exclusively. In some rare cases it doesn't work as well, and those patients must therefore receive bilateral treatments.)

The "seizure" in modern ECT is pretty much an electrical event only, with little or none of the jerking movements that usually characterize seizures. Most ECT machines used today also record an electroencephalogram (a measurement of the electrical activity of the brain), so that the physician can see how long the induced "seizure" lasts—usually twenty-five to forty-five seconds. There might be a few brief muscle contractions observed during this time, but the muscle relaxant keeps the patient nearly motionless. There is usually a brief quickening of the heart rate and an increase of blood pressure that also signal that the "seizure" has occurred. The anaesthetist uses a face-mask breathing device to deliver oxygen until the patient wakes up five or ten minutes later and the treatment is over.

About the only patients who absolutely can't receive ECT are those very few individuals with medical conditions so severe that even ten to fifteen minutes of general anaesthesia is too dangerous—people with really severe cardiac or lung diseases, for example. ECT is safe in the elderly and even during pregnancy.

Patients awakening from anaesthesia are a bit groggy, of course, and many are also slightly fuzzy-headed and feel "spacey" for another hour or so. This effect is probably related to the treatments themselves, not just the anaesthesia, and it resembles the mild postseizure confusion that patients with true epilepsy sometimes experience. Occasionally a more severe period of confusion called *delirium* is seen, especially after bilateral treatments and especially toward the end of a course of treatments. Sedatives can treat this problem quickly, but when it occurs, consideration should be given to stopping the treatments or giving them less often.

The most troublesome possible side effects of ECT relate to its effect on memory: about two-thirds of patients report that ECT affects their memory in some way. The most common memory loss seen with ECT is for events occurring during the several weeks when the patient was actually receiving ECT. Since treatments are typically given three times a week and a patient typically needs six to twelve treatments for complete recovery, a course of ECT will last two to four weeks. Patients not infrequently lose memory for some events that occurred during those weeks. Patients sometimes also suffer *retrograde amnesia* as well: memory loss for a period of time before they actually started ECT. This is thought to occur because ECT somehow disrupts the process by which shorter-term memories become incorporated into longer-term memory. (If you've ever lost an hour's worth of computer work because you didn't save your work before something untoward "froze" your computer, you get the idea of what retrograde amnesia is. The short-term memories that are still in the brain's memory "buffer" are lost because of the ECT.) Patients who have successfully completed a course of ECT may report not remembering checking in to the hospital, or they might not recollect a home visit or a trip they took with their family during the treatments. This problem seems to be worst just after a patient receives ECT. In a study of forty-three patients interviewed about their memory a few weeks after completing ECT, some reported difficulty remembering events for a period up to two years before their ECT. But when these patients were tested again seven *months* after their treatment, these more distant memories had been almost completely recovered.[3]

In addition to these sorts of memory problems, patients report a loss of isolated memories that occurs in an almost random fashion. It's as if some snippet of memory were edited out by the ECT. One of my patients went into her kitchen soon after ECT to bake her husband's favorite dessert, a pastry that she had made for years without a recipe, only to discover that she didn't have the recipe in her head anymore. As you might suspect, these kinds of memory problems are almost impossible to pick up on tests, and so despite many years of memory research on ECT patients it has been difficult to quantify very precisely the effect of ECT on these long-term memories. Another factor that confuses the issue is the effect that severe depression has on memory. Several studies indicate that complaints of memory problems after ECT correlate better with the severity of the patient's depression than with how they do on memory tests.[4] Unilateral ECT appears to reduce sharply the number of memory complaints.[5]

Although many patients report no memory problems whatsoever after ECT, and most who do report problems say that their memory problems are temporary and minor, there are a very few who report that their memory has never been quite the same. My impression is that memory problems are not significant difficulties for my patients, the vast majority of whom are grateful that such an effective treatment as ECT is available to them.

The mechanism by which ECT works continues to be profoundly mysterious. During seizure activity, the neurons of the brain fire simultaneously and rhythmically, and there is a massive discharge of many neurotransmitters. We used to compare ECT to cardiac defibrillation: just as applying a current to the heart muscle "resets" abnormal rhythms in cardiac muscle, perhaps ECT "resets" rhythmic discharges in the brain in some way. But newer work seems to indicate that, as with other treatments for bipolar disorder, the effect occurs at the level of the individual neurons. Animal experimentation indicates that ECT, like lithium, affects G proteins within the neurons. It may be that ECT, like lithium, works on the neuronal "tuning" mechanisms, the G protein/second-messenger system discussed in chapter 5.

ECT for Bipolar Disorder

ECT can be thought of as a symptomatic treatment for both phases of bipolar disorder: although it can quickly interrupt an episode of depression or mania, it does not have a long-term effect as a mood stabilizer (a *symptomatic* treatment treats *symptoms* but not the underlying disease process). Medication treatment will still be necessary to sustain the benefit of ECT and to keep the patient's mood state stable after the treatments are finished.

Typically, when the decision is made to give a course of ECT, all medications are stopped. (Sedative medications often shorten and otherwise interfere with the ECT "seizure," and so do the anticonvulsant mood stabilizers—they are anticonvulsants, after all! Lithium, meanwhile, seems to make patients more prone to episodes of confusion after their treatments.)

ECT is generally considered to be the most effective antidepressant treatment available. Naturally, it should be a treatment consideration whenever a bipolar patient continues to be severely depressed despite antidepressant medication treatment. It is also *rapidly* effective. Often, patients are dramatically improved after just three or four treatments—that is, after five to seven days. Severely suicidal patients or those who have stopped eating and drinking and are in danger of malnutrition and dehydration—any patients for whom profound depression has become an imminently life-threatening illness—are candidates for ECT. Pregnancy is also considered to be an indication for use of ECT to treat bipolar depression because of the risk most mood-stabilizing medications pose to the fetus.[6] Because depression can be highly resistant to antidepressant medications and also very dangerous in the elderly, ECT is frequently recommended as a first-line treatment for severe depression for older people as well. Depressed bipolar patients who receive ECT can become slightly hypomanic. When this occurs, obviously it's time to stop the treatments. Unlike the antidepressants, however, ECT does not seem to increase the cycling of the illness.[7]

ECT is also a highly effective treatment for mania. A 1994 review in the *American Journal of Psychiatry* of fifty years' experience of the use of ECT for treating mania found that it provided complete symptom remission or marked improvement in 80 percent of the manic patients studied. Many of the patients in these studies had failed to respond to many other available treatments—making this success rate all the more impressive.[8] ECT seems to work more quickly in mania than in depression. One study found that patients recovered after an average of six treatments, about half the usual requirement for the treatment of depression.[9] Severely manic patients whose highly agitated state becomes physically dangerous are obvious candidates for ECT, as are pregnant manic patients.

ECT is a valuable therapeutic tool for any bipolar patient who is very sick and seems to be getting sicker despite aggressive treatment with medication. It is also helpful for that small group of bipolar patients whom I call "brittle." These are patients, often with a rapid-cycling illness, who are poorly responsive to mood stabilizers and prone to adverse effects of other medications as well. They seem to start having manic symptoms if they so much as hold a Prozac capsule in their hand, but they crash into severe depression only days after getting a bit of relief from agitated mania with huge doses of antipsychotic medications; medications seem to do them more harm than good. Patients who have been either manic or severely depressed for months often have a dramatic response to ECT after everything else has failed, and once ECT has treated their acute symptoms, they can go on to have sustained periods of normal mood on medication.

ECT is perhaps the most effective treatment there is for severe depression and severe mania, and it often works more quickly than medications.[10] If you're beginning to wonder why ECT isn't used more often in bipolar disorder, you're in very good company. It is certainly much more complicated to go through general anaesthesia two or three times a week for two to four weeks than it is to take medication, but ECT may well still be underutilized, especially for patients sick enough to need hospitalization. We also know that bipolar depression can be less responsive to medication treatment, and there is the risk of antidepressants accelerating the cycling of bipolar illness. These facts make the use of ECT for severe bipolar depression even more compelling.

Transcranial Magnetic Stimulation

Transcranial magnetic stimulation (TMS) is a new experimental therapeutic technique similar to ECT that appears to be effective in treating mood disorders. TMS is currently a research technique only, but preliminary results with it are very encouraging. The great advantage of TMS over ECT is that TMS is much simpler to administer: no seizure activity is induced by the treatment, and therefore no anaesthesia is necessary.

This novel technique takes advantage of a principle of electromagnetism called *induction* to deliver an electrical stimulus to the brain without applying electrical energy to the scalp (as in ECT). During TMS treatments, a magnetic coil is held against the scalp (see figure 10-1), and the magnetic field that develops in the coil causes electrical current to flow through nearby neurons within the skull. No electricity passes through the skull, as in ECT; rather, the magnetic field "induces" a tiny electrical current in the underlying brain tissue. Since the electrical current that is generated in the brain tissue by TMS is so small, a seizure does not occur; thus, no anaesthesia is necessary. Pulses of magnetic energy are delivered over a period of about twenty minutes while

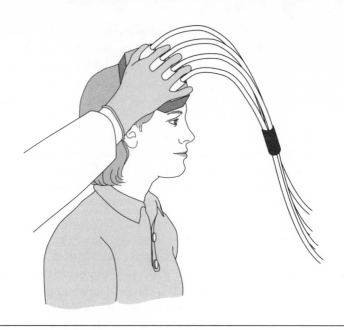

FIGURE 10-1 Transcranial magnetic stimulation

the patient simply sits in a chair, awake and alert throughout the whole procedure. Other than some soreness from muscle stimulation, there appear to be no side effects of any kind.[11]

TMS has been used for a number of years to do brain mapping. The mapping of motor areas of the brain involves stimulating an area and then measuring electrical activity in the muscles controlled by that area. Stimulating a sensory area of the brain can cause a person to feel tingling in the part of the body that sends sensory nerves to that area. Sophisticated TMS techniques are also being used to study language functions and the organization of complex movements as well.

It is possible to give a placebo TMS treatment, making it easier to do valid research on the efficacy of TMS in depression. (A true placebo-controlled study of ECT would mean giving two groups of patients anaesthesia but giving the electrical stimulus only to patients in one of the groups. Risking anaesthesia to receive a fake ECT treatment is something few people would volunteer for, and ethically it is a rather dubious idea.) When the TMS coil is applied to the scalp at a slightly different angle from that normally used to give treatments, it does not cause electrical current to flow through the brain tissue and thus will not have the usual TMS effect. However, because stimulation of the muscles still occurs, the slight muscle soreness associated with the treatment occurs as well, and research subjects will have no way of knowing whether they are getting a sham treatment or the real thing. This makes the all-important double-blind placebo-controlled studies fairly easy to do.

As we shall see in chapter 18, various studies indicate that the left prefrontal lobes of the brain are less active than normal in depression. This finding has led researchers to try TMS treatments on depressed patients by stimulating the left prefrontal lobes. Early results have been very promising. One of the first studies on TMS in the treatment of depression appeared in the *American Journal of Psychiatry* in 1997.[12] In this study from the National Institutes of Mental Health, twelve patients received twenty two-second TMS stimulations over a period of twenty minutes every weekday for two weeks. Either before or after the two weeks of therapy, the patients were given two weeks of "sham" treatments (the placebo), during which the TMS coil was held at an angle that would not cause brain tissue stimulation. The patients were tested for depressive symptoms by trained investigators using a standardized questionnaire. Neither the patients nor the investigators giving the mood questionnaire knew whether the patients were receiving real or sham TMS (making the study *double* blind). There was a statistically significant mood improvement in these patients after the real TMS treatments, but not after the sham treatments. Several patients continued TMS after the completion of the study and experienced even further clinical improvement in their depressive symptoms. In several studies, depressed patients with drug-resistant depression showed improvement after TMS.[13]

TMS is in its infancy. The strength of the magnetic stimulation that is most beneficial, the exact placement of the coil, the number of treatments, and the duration of therapy are all under investigation at various centers around the world. Will TMS, like ECT, be effective in bipolar depression as well as in unipolar depression? How about in mania? These and many other questions remain to be answered.

Perhaps the biggest unanswered question is, How does TMS work? It has always been thought that the seizure is the necessary therapeutic factor in ECT. Does TMS work in a different way? Or is TMS some kind of "gentler" ECT that works by a similar mechanism but without causing a seizure? (If the TMS coil is made to generate a strong enough magnetic field, a seizure can indeed be triggered with this technique, perhaps suggesting the latter explanation.)

It is clear, however, that TMS is a very promising development in the treatment of mood disorders and may open up a whole new array of treatment options.

Vagal Nerve Stimulation

Vagal nerve stimulation (VNS) is another new approach for treating depression that has now been approved by the FDA.

The vagal nerve (or *vagus*) is a long nerve that emerges from the base of the brain, travels down the neck and into the chest and abdomen, and regulates some vital bodily functions such as digestion and heart rate. Its connections in the brain occur through important centers thought to be involved with emotional regulation and specifically with mood regulation. VNS is done by means of a pacemaker-like device that must be surgically implanted; it then constantly delivers tiny electrical signals that stimulate the vagus nerve.

Animal studies done as early as the 1930s demonstrated that electrical stimulation of the vagal nerve produced changes in the electrical activity of the brain, and studies in the 1980s demonstrated that VNS could control epileptic seizures in dogs.

In the 1990s VNS became available for the treatment of intractable epilepsy in humans, first in Europe and then in the United States. By the end of 2000, about six thousand patients worldwide had received VNS, almost all of them for the treatment of epilepsy. As with antiepileptic medications that later turned out to be effective mood stabilizers, VNS was noted to have beneficial effects on mood in several patients who had received it to treat their seizures. Some had substantial antidepressant effects from VNS even though the treatment didn't improve their seizure control.

In one of the first studies of the VNS treatment of depression, thirty adults received VNS for severe treatment-resistant depression; nine of the patients had a diagnosis of bipolar I or bipolar II disorder. Some of these patients had taken dozens of different medications and undergone ECT, with little benefit. About half of the patients benefited from VNS.[14] In a follow-up study, most of the patients who had shown a response were continuing to do well, and several were found to have experienced continued improvement when they were evaluated after one year of VNS treatment.[15]

CHAPTER 11

Counseling and Psychotherapy

ALTHOUGH MEDICAL TREATMENTS SUCH AS PHARMACEUTICALS ARE the foundation of the treatment of bipolar disorder, counseling and psychotherapy are important, perhaps indispensable additional therapeutic interventions for this illness. Some people still picture psychotherapy as something that happens in a richly paneled, dimly lit office where a bearded psychiatrist sits taking notes in a high-backed leather chair behind a patient lying on a couch who is trying to remember what he or she dreamed about last night. Or perhaps they think of talk-radio therapists, dispensing sound-bite-sized advice to the lovelorn and lonely between car commercials on the AM dial. Well, all this is psychotherapy of a sort, though it's not usually the sort of therapy that does people with bipolar disorder much good.

But many types of counseling and therapy *are* enormously helpful in bipolar disorder. If you've read this book to this point, you've already had several hours of therapy of a kind. You've allowed an objective but sympathetic individual with knowledge and experience about mental illness and psychological processes (that's me) to present facts about bipolar disorder to increase your understanding of the illness. This understanding has, I hope, helped you make sense of your thoughts and feelings about this problem as it affects you, and helped prepare you to make decisions based on knowledge rather than on emotions such as fear of or anger about the illness. This is, in large measure, what therapy is all about: not interpreting dreams, not simply doling out advice, and certainly not supplying all the answers, but providing good information, objective feedback, and solid encouragement in a supportive, confidential setting.

Brain and Mind

In chapter 2 I described how manic-depressive illness came to be called a "functional" psychiatric illness in the early twentieth century. After the discovery of the biological causes of mental illnesses like general paresis (central nervous system syphilis) and cretinism (mental retardation due to thyroid deficiency), psychiatric illnesses came to be divided into two categories: *organic* and *functional.* Organic psychiatric illnesses were "real" illnesses, caused by germs or abnormal hormone levels or something else that could be seen under a microscope or measured in a blood test. In functional illnesses, on the other hand, it was assumed that there wasn't anything wrong with brain functioning in a physical sense. Patients with manic-depressive illness or schizophrenia were having some kind of abnormal reaction to life events.

The question then became, Why do some people have these very abnormal reactions while others do not? It was at this point that the attempt to understand and treat these illnesses turned away from medicine and toward psychology. Sigmund Freud spent his lifetime treating and trying to understand patients who were unhappy in their relationships, disappointed in themselves for the choices they had made, perhaps confused and anxious about decisions they were facing. Freud and his followers developed a large and sophisticated system for understanding human behavior based on understanding childhood development. They developed treatments that basically consisted of helping patients understand themselves better, let go of grudges, resentments, and fears rooted in their past, and learn better, more mature coping mechanisms. This approach has come to be called *dynamic* psychology or psychiatry and is based on the belief that mental life is best understood as a dynamic interplay between emotions and intellect, present circumstances and unconscious memories of past experiences, and many other psychological factors.

Although this approach was extremely successful in helping people with a wide variety of problems and symptoms, practitioners of dynamic psychotherapy soon discovered that it didn't make much of an impact on the symptoms of illnesses like schizophrenia or bipolar disorder. These patients were thought by most traditional psychotherapists to be too disturbed or too immature or their families too dysfunctional for them to benefit from therapy. Then a revolution occurred: lithium, chlorpromazine, and other effective medications for "functional" illnesses came along. In the 1970s, persons with bipolar disorder and schizophrenia left the many therapists who had been blaming them and their families for their illnesses and made tracks for a new kind of doctor: the biological psychiatrist, the pharmacotherapist, someone who would treat them like real people dealing with a "real" illness. For a time there was a kind of schism in American psychiatry between those who believed that dynamic psychology best explained mental illnesses and those who believed that biology was the key that would unlock the mysteries of psychiatric disorders.

When I was interviewing for psychiatric training programs in the mid-1970s, this biological psychiatry/dynamic psychiatry split was at its most pronounced. Many university medical center departments of psychiatry proudly identified themselves to me as either "biological" or "psychodynamic" in their approach. Usually each camp denigrated the other: psychodynamic psychiatry was "touchy-feely" soft science based more on nineteenth-century literary theory than on medicine; biological psychiatrists were "pill-pushers" who didn't even talk to their patients and had no appreciation for the human experience. But a few departments of psychiatry—Johns Hopkins' was one— were teaching their residents that mental experiences were neither a series of chemical reactions nor simply a collection of dynamically interrelated thoughts and feelings, but both. We learned at Hopkins that people with bipolar disorder are still people, still subject to disappointments and loss, to relationship problems and blows to their self-esteem. To regard their moods as just the expression of so many chemicals to be fine-tuned with more chemicals was to do them a great disservice. (Maybe that's how I came to dislike that phrase "chemical imbalance.") Fortunately this schism has now healed for the most part, and even the most ardent biological psychiatrists understand that psychodynamic understanding of the patient is *always* important. There are also many kinds of psychological therapies now, and most do not involve the psychoanalytic couch.

Although there is certainly a place for dynamic psychotherapy in modern psychiatry—*including* traditional Freudian psychoanalysis and the psychoanalytic couch—the variety of available psychological treatments has broadened tremendously in the past twenty-five years or so. Sophisticated techniques have been developed that work for particular kinds of problems. Some involve individual sessions with a therapist, others a group setting. Some are focused on a particular problem, such as marital or family difficulties, others on a particular symptom, such as depression or panic attacks. Some are designed to last only a few sessions; others are more open-ended. Some are not "therapy" in the traditional sense at all: support groups, made up of individuals who offer guidance and support to each other, don't even include a "therapist." Moreover, a lot of research has been done on which psychological treatments work best for which problems. The prescription of a particular kind of counseling or therapy for a particular kind of problem is often backed up by as much research as is the prescription of a particular medication.

What Can Therapy Do?

No one today would even think to recommend counseling or therapy as the only treatment for bipolar disorder; to do so would constitute malpractice. But because we have highly effective medications for this illness, some doctors, and perhaps many more patients, want to turn away from counseling and therapy altogether and approach the illness as a purely "chemical" problem that has a purely "chemical" solution. This is a mistake, for several reasons.

First of all, the diagnosis of bipolar disorder is almost always a traumatic event, not only for patients but for their family members as well. In addition to the emotional turmoil that is the symptom of the illness itself, there is an emotional reeling that results from coming face to face with fears about how this diagnosis will affect one's life. Vaguely familiar terms like *manic-depression* and all too familiar terms like *mental illness* conjure up all sorts of confused and confusing ideas and feelings. "Why has this happened to me?" (or perhaps "This *can't* be happening to me!") and "My life will never be the same" and "Whose fault is this?" are only some of the thoughts and questions that start spinning through the minds of people affected by this diagnosis. Remember that I described therapy as "providing good information, objective feedback, and solid encouragement in a supportive, confidential setting." It becomes obvious, doesn't it, that this kind of psychological treatment is going to be necessary and very helpful. Some research suggests that the first year after a diagnosis of bipolar disorder is a crucial time for persons with the disorder, and that the education, support, and encouragement that psychotherapy provides are very important in making treatment successful in the long term.[1]

Another traumatic event that persons with bipolar disorder face all too frequently is relapse. The management of bipolar disorder is still far from perfect, and despite everyone's best efforts, relapse can and does occur. Many patients feel that they're "back to square one"; they blame themselves or their medication or their doctor; they become angry, disappointed, discouraged, and confused about what to do next. Again, counseling helps the person put things back into perspective, get over the setback, and move on. I shall discuss individual therapy in more detail later in this chapter.

Group Psychotherapy

Psychotherapy can be very effective in a group setting. In group therapy a therapist meets with a group of patients rather than with only one individual. The worry I often hear expressed by patients for whom group therapy is recommended is that they don't want to "sit around listening to other people's problems" week after week. But no group therapist worth his or her salt is going to let the group deteriorate into a "pity party"; instead, he or she will guide the group members onto the track of learning from, and helping solve, one another's problems—not just ventilating about them. And an excellent way to become a better problem solver is to see how other people are managing, or failing, to solve their own problems.

In traditional group psychotherapy, groups are usually made up of persons with a variety of problems. In the treatment of bipolar disorder, however, *homogeneous* groups (groups composed exclusively of persons with bipolar disorder) have been studied more and have been shown to be effective. Several studies show that bipolar-disorder patients in group therapy have fewer relapses and improved productivity at work or school.[2] The research suggests that the shared aspect of the problems seems to be very important to the therapeutic experience. Persons with bipolar disorder who are in groups with other bipolar-disorder patients report that the practical advice they receive about living with the disorder is very helpful. Their understanding of the disorder, of how it affects their relationships and self-attitudes, is enhanced, and the guidance they receive from group members is perceived as very valuable.[3] This aspect of group therapy—sharing and learning from one another—is the basis of another type of "therapy," one that doesn't require a therapist: peer support groups. We shall discuss this helping format in chapter 20.

Individual Therapy for Depression

As we saw in several earlier chapters, available pharmaceutical treatments for the depressed phase of bipolar disorder are less than perfect by a long shot. The mood stabilizers are often not very good antidepressants, and antidepressant medications carry the risk of precipitating mania or accelerating the frequency of cycles. But psychotherapy has a proven track record in helping with depression and, as far as we can tell, has no risk of precipitating mania or of accelerating the course of bipolar disorder.

"Now wait a minute," I can hear you say, "I've been reading through this entire book that the moods of bipolar disorder are caused by abnormal brain chemistry, and now you want me to believe that psychotherapy can treat the depressive phase of bipolar disorder?" Well, perhaps "psychotherapy can treat the depressive phase of bipolar disorder" overstates the case a bit, but there is some research showing—by implication, at least—that it may be very helpful.

In the 1960s Dr. Aaron Beck and his colleagues developed a theory of and psychotherapeutic treatment for depression called *cognitive therapy*.[4] This type of psychotherapy has been researched more thoroughly than most others and has a proven track record in helping with symptoms of depression; in some studies—though not in others—it has been found to work as well as, even better than, antidepressant medication for some patients.[5]

The theory of cognitive therapy maintains that people who are chronically or frequently depressed have developed a somewhat distorted view of themselves and of the world and have adopted certain patterns of thinking and reacting that perpetuate their problems. This emphasis on thinking, or *cognition,* lends the theory and the therapy its name. As we saw in chapter 1, depressed persons tend (1) to think negatively about themselves, (2) to interpret their experiences in a negative way, and (3) to have a pessimistic view of the future. Cognitive theory calls this the "cognitive triad."[6] The theory further proposes that all this negative thinking causes a person to develop a repertoire of mental habits called "schemas"[7] or "negative automatic thoughts" that spring into action and reinforce the negative thinking.

John is a thirty-two-year-old computer specialist whose idea for a new project has just been turned down by his company. He comes to his therapy session and brings along a lengthy handwritten critique of the project that the senior vice-president of his division left behind after coming by John's cubicle to tell him that the project had been turned down.

"You see, I should have known better than to take on that big a project. The senior vice-president, no less, comes by with the bad news. 'Better luck next time,' she said. Now I'm never going to move up in this company."

"Why do you say that?" I asked.

"If someone that high up thinks I'm incompetent, I'm done for. That's the last time I bother trying something I'm not cut out for."

"Did she say she thought you were incompetent?"

"Well, no, of course not."

"I see. This vice-president doesn't tell people what she thinks."

"Oh, no, that's not true at all. She's got a reputation for coming right out with her opinions about things."

"But she treats you differently from everyone else?"

John began to get a little annoyed. "Well, I wouldn't think so, but how should I know? I'd never talked with her before."

"What do you make of that?" I asked. "The fact that she came in person to give you the news about your proposal?"

"Well, I did think it was unusual."

"Could it mean she was impressed with some aspects of your proposal and wanted to meet you?"

"Well, I suppose that's possible."

I continued reinterpreting John's negative assumptions: "And how about the handwritten critique?"

"It was really negative," John went on glumly. "She went through every point and shot them down one by one."

"When had you sent the proposal to Ms. Kaiser? How long did she have to look at it?"

"Oh, I didn't send it to Kaiser; she's over the whole division. I had sent it to Bob Rodney, my team leader. I guess he sent it up to her, but I don't know how long she spent with it."

"Well, she must have spent several hours with it if she gave you back such a carefully organized critique. Don't you think?"

"Yeah, I guess she wouldn't have taken all that time and trouble if she had thought it was worthless."

"And your team leader must have thought it had some potential if he sent the proposal to *his* boss. Have you asked him for some feedback?"

"No, I assumed he'd be down on me for it, too."

"But do you see how your negative assumption stopped you from checking in with your team leader and prevented you from getting what could have been positive feedback and encouragement from him?"

"I see what you mean. If I hadn't jumped to conclusions, I might have gotten some positive strokes."

John is down on his talents and assumes everybody else is, too. In situations that can be interpreted many different ways, both positive and negative, he tends to go for the negative rather than seek alternative positive explanations. This in turn sometimes causes him to do things that reinforce his negative thinking, and the vicious cycle repeats itself. This might seem to be a trivial example, but it's not difficult to come up with a number of negative schemas that people with bipolar disorder are prone to:

Negative: "I got manic even though I was taking my lithium. It doesn't matter what I do. What's the use?"
Realistic: "Relapses occur even with medication. It might have been much worse and lasted much longer if I hadn't been on medication. Perhaps this new medication will be more effective for me."

Negative: "Everyone will be avoiding me when I go back to work. No one wants to work with a mentally ill person."
Realistic: "Some people might avoid me at work, perhaps many at first. But

when they see that I'm the same old me, they'll come around. And those who don't are people I don't want as friends anyway."

Cognitive-therapy techniques more specifically focused on bipolar disorder are being developed. Part of the treatment deals with the negative automatic thoughts that interfere with treatment with medication. For example, if a person with bipolar disorder is troubled by the negative automatic thought "Taking mood-stabilizing medication is a sign of personal weakness" every time he or she takes a dose of lithium, he or she might be more likely to skip doses or stop taking the medication altogether. Cognitive therapy works on the psychological barriers to proper treatment by replacing automatic negative thoughts with realistic ones.[8]

Cognitive therapy has been proven to be effective in the treatment of depression. Clearly it cannot replace medication treatment for bipolar disorder, but perhaps more than any other form of psychotherapy, it holds great promise for bipolar patients.

New Psychotherapies for Bipolar Disorder

For many years psychiatrists and the therapists who work with them in treating patients with bipolar disorder have had a sort of intuition that there are fewer relapses among patients who understand their illness and their treatment better, who work on learning to cope better with the stresses and difficulties that everybody faces, and whose family members are also informed and supportive. Psychiatrists have also observed that life stresses, difficult relationships at home, and even disruptions of sleep cycles seem to bring on symptoms and to impact the course of the illness. Often, though, they find it hard to persuade patients—and sometimes hard to persuade themselves, perhaps—that a course of traditional psychotherapy is what's needed.

Psychiatrists have done their best to spend time with patients and their families answering their questions about bipolar disorder and its treatments; trying to persuade patients with marital problems to get marital therapy and patients with job problems to get career counseling; and encouraging them to learn about stress management, watch their sleep habits, and steer clear of conflict and difficult situations whenever possible. But a lot of these interventions are time-consuming or expensive (or both), they are difficult to put into practice ("Steer clear of conflict? How do I do *that*, Doc?"), and until recently we have had only the impression that these are important interventions, with little hard data to back up our recommendations.

But now several research teams are developing treatment models of psychological therapy for bipolar patients that draw on these sorts of impressions. These models take into account the available research about the particular kinds of stresses that cause symptoms in bipolar patients, and they incorporate the experiences of clinicians who have treated many, many bipolar patients. These treatments emphasize things like patient and family education about the illness, stress management and conflict resolution, and close attention to the strains in family and marital relationships often caused by this illness in even the healthiest family units. These teams are testing their ideas with well-designed clinical research studies, and the results of these studies have been very encouraging. One or another or a combination of these therapies may well become standard recommendations for patients with bipolar disorder in the future.

These treatments differ from standard psychotherapy in several ways. Traditional psychotherapy is often unfocused and "exploratory"; the patient and the therapist work on the issues the patient identifies ("I want to learn to make better choices in my relationships"), and treatment is open-ended: the patient is in therapy as long as he or she finds it beneficial and has an issue to work on. These new treatments, however, are very focused. The focus varies slightly in the two current models: one focuses on family education and communication and the other on lifestyle regularization and stress management. In both kinds of treatment the therapist often acts more like a teacher or coach than a counselor, and the goals are to develop concrete solutions to real problems and to learn about and master new problem-solving techniques. Since the patient often doesn't bring "issues" to the therapy, there is a specified time course to the treatment; the main work of the treatment is "finished" within a certain time period, although there is a "maintenance" phase that can be indefinite.

Behavioral family management for bipolar disorder (BFM-BP) emphasizes the patient's family unit. It is a model that to some extent has grown out of research showing that patients with schizophrenia had more illness relapses if there were conflicts and stresses at home and within the family. This therapy works hard at family support. Educating the patient and his or her family members about the symptoms of bipolar disorder and its treatments is a priority, emphasizing that bipolar disorder is indeed an illness and that symptoms are not under voluntary control. Family sessions are held to identify difficulties and conflicts within the family unit—whether caused by the illness or by other, perhaps preexisting factors or situations. Conflict resolution and problem-solving techniques are presented and practiced, and healthy communication skills are developed through role playing and rehearsals.

Interpersonal and social rhythm therapy (IP/SRT) puts more emphasis on patients as individuals and on their "social rhythm." Based on the observation that sleep deprivation and other disruptions of body rhythms can bring on symptoms, this treatment emphasizes stability and stress management. It involves having patients track their mood states on a daily basis and also their daily routine with a sort of checklist of activities called the *social rhythm metric.*

In their sessions the patient and the therapist review these diaries and also the patient's "interpersonal inventory" (a list of the persons in the patient's social network) with an eye toward identifying conflicts and stresses in relationships. The therapist and the patient work on identifying emotional or physical stresses and factors in the environment that upset daily rhythms and emotional stability. The goal is to "find a healthy balance between daily rhythm stability, social activity, social stimulation and mood states."[9] Although it's still too soon to know the impact of IP/SRT on the course of bipolar disorder over time, early results of the research indicate that IP/SRT patients made more healthy lifestyle changes and showed greater stability in daily routines and rhythms than a control group of patients did.[10]

The research on BFM-BP and IP/SRT is still going on, and definitive results are a few years off. But for the first time research on the psychotherapeutic treatment of bipolar disorder is becoming just as scientific as research on the medication treatment of the disorder. It's only a matter of time before these results and further refinements of these therapies point the way to even better and more specific psychotherapy and counseling techniques for bipolar disorder.

"Traditional" Individual Psychotherapy

I hope I haven't given you the impression that traditional psychotherapy isn't useful for patients with bipolar disorder. Quite the contrary. Kay Jamison has written:

> At this point in my existence, I cannot imagine leading a normal life without both taking lithium and having had the benefits of psychotherapy. Lithium prevents my seductive but disastrous highs, diminishes my depressions . . . and makes psychotherapy possible. But, ineffably, psychotherapy *heals.* It makes some sense of the confusion, reins in the terrifying thoughts and feelings, returns some control and hope and possibility of learning from it all.[11]

So far in this chapter we've talked about "situational" supportive counseling focused around episodes of illness, either the first or a relapse, with the goal of helping patients deal with the acute stresses of diagnosis, hospitalization, reintegration back into their job, or other specific issues related to an episode of illness. We've discussed the cognitive therapy of depression, a course of treatment that might be recommended for chronic or smoldering depressive symptoms that medication alone doesn't seem to quite take care of. In the last section we discussed some new therapies that aim to teach patients and their families how to smooth out the bumpy spots in their relationships, improve communication and conflict resolution skills, and regularize their social rhythms. These treatments are perhaps more preventive than the others and might be thought of as providing psychological immunization against future problems as well as ways of dealing with present ones.

What, then, of traditional psychotherapy? By *traditional psychotherapy* I mean individual meetings with a therapist, usually over an extended period of time (months or years), in which the person in treatment discusses his or her past and present experiences and feelings with the goal of self-understanding, self-acceptance, and personal growth. (*Dynamic* or *insight-oriented psychotherapy* is the same thing.) Disappointments and accomplishments, affections and enmities, fears, inspirations, passions, and worries—all are, as psychotherapists are fond of saying, "grist for the mill" of therapy. Patient and therapist will, of course, talk about symptoms like sadness and anxiety too, but traditional therapy sees symptoms as indicators of underlying conflicts rather than as the focus of treatment in and of themselves. Traditional psychotherapy emphasizes exploration of the *meaning* of symptoms, the development of self-awareness and maturity.

So when would we recommend traditional psychotherapy to a person with bipolar disorder? For what types of problems would it be helpful? Basically, for the same types of problems that people without bipolar disorder go to therapists for: dealing with psychological traumas and setbacks—past and present—that cause understandable feelings of sadness, anger, or anxiety, or thought patterns, self-attitudes, and interpersonal styles that disrupt a person's ability to be happy in relationships, effective at work, carefree in play, and confident about making decisions about the future. Sounds like a tall order, doesn't it? Well, of course it is. That is why psychotherapists often study and train in their profession for almost as many years as physicians train in theirs. That is why people are sometimes in therapy for months, even for years, at a time. That is why psychotherapy is such an intense, powerful experience and the therapeutic relationship between patient and therapist a unique one.

Bipolar patients will often have had more than their share of setbacks and psychological traumas—both past and present. Because it is a genetic illness, persons with bipolar disorder often have had difficult, even traumatic childhoods. Perhaps a parent was afflicted with the illness, perhaps he or she could not or would not receive proper treatment, and the child may have suffered disruptions to family life, periods of poverty or homelessness, perhaps even physical or emotional abuse. Psychotherapy can be enormously beneficial in helping people face and work through their difficult pasts, let go of the anger, resentment, and fear that often comes out of these experiences, and move on with their lives.

The fact that a person has bipolar disorder can make ordinary life decisions seem complex and important life decisions seem overwhelming. There is no better way of dealing with these sorts of anxieties and apprehensions than traditional psychotherapy. I remember a young woman who came to see me for a routine medication-monitoring appointment when I was working in the very busy medication clinic of a community mental-health center, a clinical setting in which patients were scheduled every twenty minutes. "I've been dating a man for several months now, and I think he might ask me to marry him," she told me. She looked worried. "I haven't told him about my illness. I don't know what to tell him. How do you think I should handle this?" I stared at her helplessly for a moment and panicked just a little when I heard the nurse slipping the chart of the next patient into the bin outside the interviewing-room door. I hope I didn't sound as rushed as I felt when I tried to convince her that the situation raised an enormous number of complex issues. How, when, where, why, and with whom she discussed her diagnosis was going to need much more than one—or a dozen—twenty-minute appointments with me to get into, let alone resolve.

I doubt very much that this was the first time this young woman had been confused about what to tell someone about her diagnosis. Perhaps she had muddled through other situations at work, at church, or in her neighborhood, maybe saying nothing about her diagnosis because of feelings of shame, or maybe blurting out too much about herself and then feeling vulnerable and exposed. Perhaps being diagnosed with bipolar disorder reactivated feelings she had struggled with in childhood or adolescence about being teased for being too fat or too skinny—or perhaps, more likely in a bipolar patient, too "hyper" or "weird." I was sure that since we had discussed the fact that bipolar disorder is a genetic illness, a possible marriage proposal raised questions in her mind about having children who might be affected by the disorder. How had the diagnosis affected her identity as a potential parent, as a woman? Or perhaps none of these issues needed to be explored but instead other, completely different ones. Well, all these things are what good old-fashioned once-a-week "How do you feel about that?" psychotherapy is all about.

Psychotherapy in Bipolar Disorder: Is It Really Necessary?

All the psychiatrists I know talk about how much time they spend trying to persuade their bipolar patients to supplement their medication treatment with some form of therapy. I think there is a vast variety of reasons why persons with bipolar disorder are reluctant to do so. Some patients have made uneasy peace with taking medication for a psychiatric illness (or, as they might put it to themselves, only a "chemical imbalance"), but they see going to psychotherapy as confirmation of the "mental" aspect of their "mental illness." But if you think about it, the treatment of even the most "medical" of medical illnesses—heart disease, say, or a ruptured lumbar disk—usually requires nonmedical interventions, and sometimes these turn out to be just as important as the pharmaceutical or even surgical interventions prescribed by the doctor. The patient with diabetes would hardly regard staying on a healthy diet and watching his or her weight as unnecessary adjuncts to the management of the illness with insulin injections. The recovering coronary-bypass surgery patient wouldn't think to ignore the physician's recommendation for a cardiac-hardening exercise program. Would anyone have an operation for lumbar disk problems and skip the physical therapy sessions afterward? I don't think so.

We know that chronic psychological stresses make a whole variety of physical illnesses more difficult to treat: asthma, high blood pressure, irritable bowel syndrome. Psychological stresses will make mood-disorder symptoms more difficult to control as well.

The research results on the psychotherapeutic treatments of bipolar disorder aren't all in, so we can't yet specify particular therapies for a particular duration of time for particular mood syndromes. But the available research and many years of clinical experience indicate that psychotherapy and counseling have been enormously helpful to countless patients with bipolar disorder. If a particular type of therapy or counseling is available, is affordable, and has been recommended by the physician or treatment team, persons with bipolar disorder owe it to themselves to take advantage of the unique healing powers of these marvelous therapeutic techniques.

The Psychiatrist-Psychotherapist: An Extinct Species?

You have probably noticed that throughout this chapter I usually refer to the psychiatrist and the psychotherapist as two different individuals. Unfortunately this has become the rule rather than the exception in American psychiatry for most patients. It would, of course, be preferable for all sorts of reasons for the person prescribing medication and the person doing psychotherapy to be one and the same individual. But for a variety of complicated reasons, most people with bipolar disorder will see a psychiatrist for medication management and a nonphysician therapist—often a social worker or psychologist—for therapy. Some of the reasons for this are the changes in medication management of bipolar disorder that have come about with the development of new medications; there are now so many different pharmaceuticals used in psychiatry that staying skilled in their use has become more and more time-consuming. Perhaps even more significantly, as more and more effective medications become available for more psychiatric problems, more and more patients want (and need) to see a psychiatrist for their treatment. There simply aren't enough psychiatrists to do medication management and therapy too, especially in busy clinics. Since medical school and psychiatric training take longer and cost more than the training required to become a psychotherapist, psychiatrists are usually more expensive than other professionals. When the administrator of a busy clinic or HMO is looking to staff the organization's mental-health program, "split" treatment—psychiatric treatment split between a psychiatrist for medication management and a nonphysician therapist for psychotherapy or counseling—means more cost-effective treatment for patients.

The superior cost-effectiveness of "split" treatment allows so many more patients to receive psychiatric treatment so much more cheaply that it's difficult to envision a return to the days when psychiatrists did therapy and prescribed medications, too. Fortunately there are excellent training programs for clinical social workers, psychologists, and counseling professionals that are producing superb psychotherapists. And as we have seen in this chapter, psychotherapy is becoming more specialized, too. It has become nearly impossible to be an expert therapist and at the same time an expert psychopharmacologist. For all of these reasons, the medication management and the therapy of the person with bipolar disorder will usually be handled by two professionals rather than one.

CHAPTER 12

Treatment Approaches in Bipolar Disorder

THE BASIC CAUSE OF BIPOLAR DISORDER REMAINS UNKNOWN. TREAT-
ment approaches have been stumbled upon more or less by accident—as
with the discovery of the therapeutic effects of lithium—and although they
have been refined by decades of experience, they are still largely what physicians call *empirical*. This means that the treatment is based on experience—
on therapeutic results rather than on a true understanding of the mechanism
of the disease or symptom in question.[1]

Therapeutic Results as a Guide to Treatment

Although we have a tremendous amount of experience in the use of
pharmaceuticals to treat bipolar disorder and have data on their effectiveness
in large groups of patients, the treatment of individual patients with bipolar
disorder is often guided by treatment results rather than by the kinds of hard
data physicians use to treat other illnesses. What do I mean by this? Let me
explain by referring to a very different kind of illness, pneumonia.

A young man is rushed to an emergency room with a high fever, a pain
in his chest, difficulty breathing, and a congested cough. The doctor orders
a chest x-ray. A specimen of the young man's sputum is rushed off to the laboratory, and a tiny droplet is spread on a microscope slide, immersed in a
special dye called a Gram stain, and examined under the microscope. More
tiny droplets of sputum are spread over the surface of several flat dishes (Petri
dishes) containing mixtures of proteins and other nutrients that various bac-

teria are known to grow on. On one of the dishes are a number of little pa-per disks that have been soaked in different antibiotics.

The lab results start coming in. The young man's chest x-ray shows that one of the lobes of his right lung is filled with fluid. The Gram stain reveals that his phlegm is loaded with bacteria aligned in pairs and linked into short chains: the pneumococcus. The diagnosis is clear: pneumococcal pneumo-nia. The doctor starts the young man on penicillin, an antibiotic known to be effective against most strains of pneumococcus, and within eight hours his fever is dropping. The dose of penicillin and the length of time the young man will need to take it have been determined by years of experience, calcu-lated to the milligram and to the hour.

In a day or so the lab reports that the Petri dish containing the pneu-mococcus' favorite food is full of colonies of bacteria that other, more so-phisticated techniques now definitely confirm as pneumococcus. The best news of all is that in the dish containing the little disks of antibiotics, there is a wide halo around the penicillin disk: the penicillin is effectively inhibit-ing the growth of the strain of bacteria causing this particular case of pneu-monia. This means that the young man does not have a pneumonia caused by a penicillin-resistant bug, and his speedy recovery is assured.

The doctor treating this young man had quite a bit of hard data on which to base his or her treatment decisions. The x-ray indicated that this was prob-ably a typical bacterial lobar pneumonia rather than viral pneumonia, tuber-culosis, or any of a number of other conditions with similar symptoms but different pictures on x-ray. Also—and very important for prognostic pur-poses—the x-ray indicated that only one lobe was involved. With the results of the Gram stain, the likely identity of the bacterial culprit was determined within minutes, allowing the quick choice of a drug known to be effective most of the time against this type of germ. The identity of the bacterial culprit was solidly confirmed several days later when it grew in the culture dish and could be further tested. Most important, the lab results showed which drug would work against the germ causing the problem in this particular patient.

On the other hand, when a patient with manic symptoms comes into the ER, there are no tests to order—just the eyes and ears and experience of the psychiatrist. Fortunately, or perhaps unfortunately, full-blown mania is of-ten an unmistakable diagnosis, and effective antimanic drugs are readily available. But what of the person who comes to the office and says, "I'm de-pressed," or complains of "mood swings." There are many more diagnostic possibilities. We know that antidepressant medications can sometimes make a patient with bipolar symptoms worse. How is a physician to know whether or not a person who comes in with symptoms of depression will turn out to have a bipolar illness? There are hints, of course, such as family history, but wouldn't it be fantastic if we could order a test for bipolar disorder before considering an antidepressant for a person who is having symptoms of depression? But we can't. And how about the treatment once the acute symptoms have been controlled? Emil Kraepelin described some patients who had a remission of their bipolar symptoms that lasted for decades (apparently quite rarely, but he observed them nevertheless). Do we prescribe a mood stabilizer for a patient who might not get sick again for ten or even twenty years? Wouldn't it be great if we could stop the medication after a period of time and have the patient come in every couple of months for some kind of scan that could pick up changes in brain chemistry before symptoms became apparent? That way the patient would take medication only as it became necessary. Sometimes patients respond to one mood stabilizer but not another, or to a combination of two mood stabilizers but to neither one when used alone. How to choose? Wouldn't it be fantastic if we could take a blood sample and look for some kind of chemical reaction around little paper disks soaked with lithium or Prozac in a Petri dish to help us choose effective medications for a particular patient?

Unfortunately at the present moment we don't have any blood tests, scans, or other laboratory tests to make the treatment approach to bipolar disorder as informed and logical as the approach can be in some other illnesses. Therefore the approach to the treatment of bipolar illness can be discussed only in general terms. Patients are started on the medications that have been proven effective in many patients with similar symptoms, and if their symptoms are not effectively treated, other medications are tried.

So the bad news is that we can't test for bipolar disorder or pick from among similar agents knowing beforehand which one of them will work best. There is unfortunately a lot of "trial and error" and "wait and see" when it comes to prescribing medications for a specific patient. This can be tremendously frustrating for all involved—for the patient, of course, and for family members, and, yes, for the physician, too.

But the good news is that more and better medications are becoming available all the time. Twenty years ago there was only one mood-stabilizing medication, lithium. Ten years ago there were three. Now we have at least five and several more on the way. There are easily twice as many antidepressants on the market as there were only fifteen years ago. The newer antipsychotic medications have fewer side effects, and some seem to have mood-stabilizing properties that the older agents lacked.

Despite what you might see in the movies, electroconvulsive therapy is one of the safest medical procedures available—and probably underutilized in bipolar disorder. Transcranial magnetic stimulation may come to replace ECT if it delivers what it seems to be promising.

Don't forget counseling and psychotherapy. Research has proven how very important this unique treatment is in controlling the symptoms of mood disorders. More effective therapy programs for bipolar disorder are being refined by researchers with studies as rigorous as those used to evaluate any pharmaceutical.

And I haven't even talked about light therapy and sleep manipulation yet (that's coming in chapter 16). Researchers have discovered that exposure to bright light and changes in sleep patterns can help regulate mood and perhaps help medications work better and faster.

A Few Principles of Treatment

Every once in a while one of the medical journals publishes a "treatment algorithm" for bipolar disorder. An algorithm is a step-by-step procedure for solving a specified problem with mathematical precision. A treatment algorithm for acute mania might look something like this:

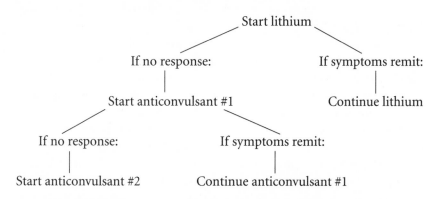

Start lithium

If no response: If symptoms remit:

Start anticonvulsant #1   Continue lithium

If no response: If symptoms remit:

Start anticonvulsant #2   Continue anticonvulsant #1

Well, you get the idea. I don't pay much attention to treatment algorithms anymore. They don't usually tell me anything new about medications, and their "if this happens, then do that" approach never captures the myriad manifestations of the disorder, the inevitable twists and turns of the world of real treatment and real patients, not to mention the specific situations and needs of the individual. That said, there are several principles of treatment that do serve patients (and their physicians) well. You'll notice, however, that these principles don't include many specifics about medications.

With so many powerful and effective medications available in psychiatry now, it's sometimes easy to become impatient when symptoms don't subside as quickly as one would wish. But in the treatment of mood disorders, a crucial principle to remember is to *take the long view.*

I saw Craig about two weeks after he had been discharged from a hospital in another city. He had been on a business trip and started to have fairly severe manic symptoms: insomnia, racing thoughts, angry irritability. He had been having good control of his symptoms on a mood stabilizer, but a series of high-stress job interviews in several different cities, jet lag, worry, and poor sleep had activated his illness, and he soon found himself hospitalized in a city several hundred miles from home.

He pulled a fistful of medication bottles out of his pocket and put them on the desk in my office. "I brought all these new medicines, but I have to admit, I've only been taking the lithium."

I picked up the bottles one by one: lithium, valproate, an antipsychotic, an anti-anxiety agent, and a sleeping pill.

"How long were you in the hospital?" I asked.

"Eight days."

"And you were discharged on *all* this?"

"That's right. I can't believe I really need all this. I was so drugged when my wife came to pick me up, I couldn't work for another week and a half. I think this is the first day I've felt safe to drive."

Craig's illness had always been very responsive to medications; it was hard for me to believe that all these medications had really been necessary. How had this happened?

When I asked Craig about his treatment in the hospital, a sadly familiar story emerged: a new medication had been added to the mix almost every other day while he was in the hospital. He was started on the antipsychotic medication as soon as he was admitted. Well, that wasn't unreasonable; I might have recommended that myself—for a while, at least. But when he didn't sleep well the next night, a sleeping pill was added. A few days later, when he mentioned that he had been worried about his finances lately, an anti-anxiety medication was added. After a week he told his doctor he was feeling less hyper but still not back to his usual self—so the valproate was added to the lithium. By the time he left the hospital, he wasn't complaining of mood problems anymore because he was too sedated to know *what* kind of mood he was in.

"Craig, you know I want you to call the clinic before you make any changes in your medication on your own," I said with a smile. "But I have to admit, in the end you did exactly what I would have recommended that you do. You certainly don't need all this."

Craig smiled back. "Well, great minds think alike—don't we?"

The medications we use to treat mood disorders usually take at least two weeks to have their full effect. When treating an episode of bipolar disorder, it usually doesn't make sense to change medications quickly. Even hospitalized patients are rarely well served by adding too many medications too quickly. And in patients having more minor mood symptoms, the four-week rule is a good one. I usually tell patients to try a medication for at least a month before they decide how it is working for them. (Intolerable side effects would, of course, cancel this advice—but even side effects usually get better with time, and sticking it out for at least a few days is often all that is needed.)

When a diagnosis of bipolar II or cyclothymic disorder is being considered, the time line should stretch out even more. The mood changes in these variations of bipolar disorder can sometimes be much more subtle than those of bipolar I. It may take three to six months of taking a mood stabilizer for its beneficial effects on a subtly unstable mood to become apparent.

In Craig's case it was the doctor who forgot to take the long view, but I think it's probably even easier for patients or their family members to fall into the trap of expecting results too quickly.

"Cindy's still having mood swings, Doctor," Jim said as he sat down beside his wife in the office. "The Depakote isn't working. Is there something else we can try?"

Jim and Cindy were a couple in their thirties. They had two small children, and Cindy usually cared for her attorney sister's little boy during the day as well as caring for her own.

Cindy was tense and quiet as her husband continued. "She's been on this medication for two weeks now, and things are no different. She started arguing with me about the television being too loud the other night, and when I tried to reason with her, she picked up the remote control and threw it at me. This has got to stop."

"What do you think, Cindy?" I asked. "Do you think the medication has helped any?"

"Well, I'm not sure, but I think maybe it has."

"Well, I'm sure it hasn't," said Jim. "The night before the remote incident she—"

"Jim," I said, "it's much too early to be sure about anything yet. Cindy's only been taking the Depakote for two weeks, and we've only been able to check the blood level once." I turned to Cindy. "What have you noticed that makes you think the Depakote might be helping?"

"Well, Jim was out of town for a few days last week, and so was my sister. I had the three kids twenty-four hours a day the whole time again. You know how keyed up I got the last time that happened."

In fact it had been a similar situation that had brought Cindy into treatment in the first place. About three weeks before our first meeting, Cindy had been with the three boys, six, five, and three years old, because of coinciding business trips taken by Jim and her sister. She had needed to call Jim and get him to fly back home because she was becoming more and more irritable with the children, snapping at them, slamming doors, starting to feel out of control.

The next week she had come to see me, and as we talked about her past history, it emerged that she had experienced episodes of depression after both her children were born, that she had had these "hyper" episodes about once a year since college, and that her mother had suffered from "mood swings" and alcoholism. A diagnosis of bipolar II or perhaps a "soft" bipolar disorder seemed likely, and we decided on a trial of a mood stabilizer.

"The kids just didn't get to me this time," Cindy continued. "First I thought they were being on their best behavior because of what had happened that last time, and maybe they were for an hour or so. But by evening I realized that they were really about as active as they usually are, and that there was something different about *me*. I wasn't as, you know, sensitive. Several times now I've noticed that I can handle things better."

"Not the other night," Jim chimed in. "I'm not noticing much difference."

"Well, maybe Jim's right," Cindy went on. "Maybe you could give me something for the times when I'm feeling really stressed? Some Valium or Xanax? I never used . . . I don't know what to call them— nerve pills? And I'm sure I wouldn't need them often."

"I don't think we should add more medication until we're sure you're getting the maximum benefit from the one you're on. And from what you're telling me, I think that's beginning to happen," I said. "The fact that you've never felt the need for tranquilizers before makes me think that the bipolar disorder explains all your symptoms and needs to be the focus of our attention. It's absolutely too early to expect the Depakote to have had its full effect. Also, your blood test indicates that we can safely raise the dose. Let's talk about this a bit more."

Cindy and Jim are very anxious for Cindy's symptoms to stop. Who can blame them? But to give up on a mood stabilizer after two weeks because it hasn't completely controlled every symptom is foolish. It's unlikely that another would work any faster—and it might not even work as well, in which case Cindy would be right back to square one after another couple of weeks.

Cindy's situation also serves to illustrate another principle of treatment:

remember the diagnosis. If the three most important words in the real estate business are *location, location,* and *location,* then the three most important words in medicine are *diagnosis, diagnosis,* and *diagnosis.* Because we have so many effective medications, it can be tempting to consider prescribing one even though there isn't really a justification for it based on diagnosis. In psychiatry especially there was a tendency at one time to see medications as *symptomatic treatments.* This means picking a medication and making the decision to use it based on identification of *symptoms,* not underlying *diagnoses.* Cindy wants to try another medication for "stress"—that is, for feeling tense and irritable. But the symptoms of our working diagnosis, bipolar disorder, include periods of tension and irritability. If Cindy's poor stress tolerance is a symptom of her mood disorder, and she takes an anti-anxiety medication to cover it up rather than getting more intensive treatment of the mood disorder, she'll end up taking a medication she doesn't really need for a symptom that isn't going to get much better because the underlying problem, bipolar disorder, isn't being properly treated. Insomnia is a similar symptom, very commonly a symptom of the mood disorder but all too commonly treated with sleeping medications as if it were an isolated symptom.

Every once in a while I see a patient with bipolar disorder who has read a magazine article about attention deficit–hyperactivity disorder and requests medication for ADHD. Some of the symptoms of ADHD—like impulsivity, impatience, fast, disorganized thinking, and poor concentration—are, of course, also seen in bipolar patients. These are distressing symptoms that deserve attention, but they deserve the right kind of attention. If they are an expression of the mood changes of bipolar disorder, then medication for ADHD won't help. (In fact the medications used to treat ADHD, stimulants and antidepressants, can make things worse.)

Making a diagnosis is the process of identifying the one disease that can explain all the patient's symptoms. This is a variation of the scientific principle called Occam's razor. Named after William of Occam (or Ockham), the medieval theologian-philosopher who developed it, this principle states that the simplest explanation for a phenomenon is always preferable to a more complex one and is most likely to be correct. Obviously a patient may have two different disorders that require two different treatment approaches. But if all the patient's symptoms can be understood as expressions of *one* disorder, treating that one will likely alleviate all the symptoms.

I see this problem of multiple diagnoses and symptomatic treatments even more commonly in depressed patients. In depression, anxiety and insomnia can be thorny and uncomfortable expressions of the mood disorder—and physical symptoms can be as well, especially in the elderly. I have seen elderly patients taking antidepressant medications (often at an inadequate dose) who are also taking sleeping pills, tranquilizers, anti-inflammatory and pain medications for arthritis, stool softeners and laxatives for constipation, and sometimes some vitamins and tonics thrown in for good measure (perhaps because of complaints of "low energy"). All these problems are symptoms of depression, but sometimes it's hard to see the forest for the trees. Before you know it, the patient is taking a dozen or so different medications for all the different symptoms of depression, and the disease that underlies them all, a mood disorder, has been missed. It is an amazing experience to see all these symptoms that have not been helped by perhaps a dozen medications disappear after a week of ECT in an elderly patient.

This leads me to another principle: *ECT should not be a treatment of last resort for bipolar disorder.* ECT should be considered whenever symptoms are very severe, or when they are severe enough to interfere with work and family life and have gone on for an extended period of time. Some geriatric psychiatrists are recommending ECT as the *first-line treatment* for serious mood-disorder symptoms in the elderly. If the patient is having symptoms day after day, has been on medical leave from work for weeks, and is still not getting relief from his or her medication, it's time to seriously consider ECT. When symptoms are disabling, ECT should probably be considered after the failure of the first medication, not after the failure of the second or third or fourth.

Finally, I can't stress enough that *every bipolar patient needs psychotherapy* at one point or another. Several weeks or months of counseling is absolutely essential after the diagnosis and initiation of treatment for bipolar disorder. Just as a person with diabetes needs to follow dietary recommendations to get the best control of his or her glucose levels, and a hip-fracture patient needs physical therapy for optimal functioning, persons with bipolar disorder need psychotherapy at times to have the best possible control of their mood symptoms.

PART III

VARIATIONS, CAUSES, AND CONNECTIONS

In this group of chapters we'll explore several variations on the theme of bipolar disorder. We'll look first at how the course and symptoms of the illness can differ in children and adolescents and then consider the differences in symptoms between men and women (with special attention to premenstrual mood symptoms, the challenge of postpartum mood disorders, and the dilemmas faced by women with the illness during the childbearing years).

In chapter 15 we'll look at the complicated relationships between bipolar disorder and substance abuse. Individuals with bipolar disorder seem to be especially vulnerable to substance-abuse disorders, so much so that it's reasonable to think of chemical dependency as a complication of the illness. The symptoms of substance abuse and bipolar disorder can become so intertwined that it is impossible to figure out which is which. In this chapter we'll look for a way out of this confusion and discuss the treatment approaches that work for individuals who have bipolar disorder complicated by chemical dependency. It's extremely important to deal with this problem head on, because research shows that alcoholism and drug abuse are often *fatal* complications of this illness.

In chapter 16 we'll learn about treating mood disorders with light, and about the intricate relationships between mood and the body's biological clock. We ignore what this clock tells us at our peril, because our sleep-wake cycle may help regulate our mood state. This is one aspect of mood regulation that we are beginning to understand in greater and greater detail. Persons with mood disorder owe it to themselves to learn as much as they can about these new findings.

In the last several chapters in this part of the book, we'll go from one extreme to the other as far as causes and connections are concerned, looking first at some very concrete scientific issues and then at some very abstract, almost philosophical ones. In chapter 17 we'll explore an area of intense interest to bipolar patients and their family members: the genetics of bipolar disorder. Chapter 18 looks at more bipolar biology: how mood disorders can be caused by medical illnesses, some of the ways we are actually picturing bipolar disorder in the functioning brain, and, finally, the possible connections between bipolar disorder and viruses.

Then, after we've finished talking about DNA molecules and chromosomes and brain chemicals, we'll leave the laboratory and go into the artist's studio, to examine some of the intriguing connections between this terrible illness and artistic genius and creativity.

Bipolar Disorder in Children and Adolescents

FOR MANY YEARS BIPOLAR DISORDER WAS THOUGHT TO BE EXTREMELY rare in young people, even though research data on adults indicated that the first appearance of the symptoms of bipolar disorder usually occurs before the age of twenty. (Emil Kraepelin found that the highest number of "first attacks" of manic-depressive illness occurred between the ages of fifteen and twenty.) Perhaps because of a reluctance to diagnose children with an illness known to be a lifelong problem and to prescribe children the powerful medications used to treat its symptoms, bipolar disorder in young children received little attention from researchers until quite recently. This means that the treatment of children and adolescents with bipolar symptoms has consisted mostly of improvised variations on adult treatments. More research has shown, however, that bipolar disorder in children and adolescents may not be the same as bipolar disorder in adults. Therefore, different treatment approaches may be necessary in younger patients.

Although research on bipolar disorder is beginning to show that it is probably not as rare in children as was once thought, the kind of large sampling study it would take to determine the prevalence of bipolar disorder in children hasn't yet been undertaken. But the studies that are available indicate that very young children can have bipolar symptoms. In one study that looked at bipolar symptoms in the pediatric (under eighteen) age range, nearly a third of the patients were younger than twelve, and the average age of onset for these young bipolar patients was eight and a half.[1] This same research is also shedding light on why psychiatrists used to think

TABLE 13-1 Comparison of Adult and Pediatric Bipolar Disorder

	Pediatric	Adult
Initial episode:	Major depression	Mania
Episode type:	Rapid cycling, mixed	Discrete episodes
Duration:	Chronic, continuous	Weeks
Functioning between episodes:	Poor (continuous cycling)	Improved

pediatric bipolar disorder was a rare diagnosis: bipolar disorder in children doesn't look the same as bipolar disorder in adults (see table 13-1). If you look for adult symptom patterns in young children, you won't find them very often.

It appears that when bipolar disorder occurs in young children (before puberty), it is a more severe form of the illness. Perhaps this is because children who develop symptoms of bipolar disorder at so young an age seem to have a heavier genetic "loading" for mood disorders than do people with older-adolescent- and adult-onset bipolar disorder. Bipolar children often have more individuals with mood disorders in their families than adult-diagnosis bipolar patients; many of these children have individuals with mood disorders on both sides of the family.[2] Another difference between childhood- and adult-onset bipolar disorder is that rather than mania or hypomania, a major depression is frequently the first sign of the disorder in children. Several studies indicate that 20 to 30 percent of young people with major depressions go on to develop manic symptoms later in life.[3]

But the most striking difference between childhood-onset and later-onset bipolar disorder is the course of the illness. Pediatric bipolar disorder is a much more continuous illness than adult bipolar disorder. In most adults the illness usually appears in discrete episodes of depression or mania, and the symptoms go into remission for months or years at a time. Children, on the other hand, often have long periods of continuous rapid cycling. These children sometimes cycle between depression and mania several times a day, having a laughing fit one moment and talking about wanting to shoot themselves the next.[4] One study of bipolar disorder in the pediatric age range described bipolar children who had over a hundred mini-manias in a year, mood episodes that lasted only a day or two. In this study, none of the research subjects under the age of nine had a single mood episode lasting two weeks or more as his or her only episode. In these children a complex pattern of frequent, short episodes was the rule, not the exception.[5]

Symptoms of Pediatric Bipolar Disorder

Depression is comparatively easy to spot in children: the weepy, listless, and lethargic child is quickly recognized as a sick child. But how do you distinguish hypomanic or manic behavior in a child from the boisterousness and high energy of normal children? An even more difficult task is to differentiate manic symptoms from the hyperactivity and "can't sit still" picture of attention deficit–hyperactivity disorder (ADHD).

The differentiation is possible if close attention is paid to changes in mood. Children with ADHD are hyperactive but don't have the expansive, grandiose mood of mania. The child with ADHD may disrupt a classroom with clowning around and restlessness, but a manic child may tell the teacher that the lessons are being taught incorrectly and try to take over the class. The manic child caught taking things that belong to someone else may say that it's wrong for other people to steal but not for him or her. The manic child may be convinced that he or she is destined for a brilliant career as a doctor or lawyer despite failing nearly every subject in school. The child may believe that he or she is on the verge of becoming a rock star despite being unable to play a musical instrument.

Normal children, of course, will fantasize in similar ways about their future, but they will be able to separate their fantasies from reality and will apply themselves to school work and follow the rules at home. Manic children, on the other hand, convinced of the reality of their grandiose ideas, state and act on the belief that the usual rules and requirements don't apply to them.

Manic children jump from topic to topic in their speech patterns, are difficult to interrupt, and complain that their thoughts are moving too fast. Hypersexuality is a symptom in older children, who may become sexually promiscuous or masturbate excessively; they may suddenly start using sexual profanity or express the belief that a teacher or famous person is in love with them. Spending sprees may take the form of ordering items over the phone using 1-800 and 1-900 numbers.

Very young children may have manic exaggerations of the normal magical thinking of childhood but will act on this thinking instead of using it as a basis for play. Normal children may imagine that they can fly and may run through the back yard "flapping" their arms like the wings of a bird or making airplane noises. Manic children under the influence of the delusion that they've become an angel or a superhero may jump out of a window or off the roof of a house. The symptoms of bipolar disorder in children can be every bit as deadly as they are in adults.

When a young person develops serious depression, how can we tell whether he or she might be having the first episode of what will turn out to be bipolar disorder? Although it's impossible to know for sure, there are some indicators that seem to be fairly reliable. In one study, researchers investigated a group of sixty adolescents, aged thirteen to sixteen years, who had been hospitalized for major depression over the course of three to four years; the purpose was to see whether any particular clinical variables might predict which of them would eventually develop a bipolar course of illness (20% of the group eventually did). Statistical analyses showed that bipolarity was predicted by a depressive symptom cluster that included rapid symptom onset, a slowed down, "retarded" type of depression, and psychotic features (hallucinations or delusions). A family history of mood disorders (bipolar disorder or major depression) in many family members and through successive generations was also a predictor, as was a history of the adolescent developing hypomanic symptoms when he or she took antidepressant medications—a clinical indicator that turned out to be 100 percent accurate in predicting bipolar disorder in this group.[6]

Bipolar Disorder and ADHD

Psychiatrists use the term *co-morbidity* to describe two separate conditions or illnesses that frequently occur together in the same patient. There is a high degree of co-morbidity between ADHD and mood disorders, in some studies as high as 75 percent.[7]

Children and young adolescents with bipolar disorder often do not have the discrete periods of elevated, usually euphoric mood seen in older adolescents and adults. Rather, extreme irritability and prolonged aggressive temper tantrums called "affective storms" are common, and the abnormal mood is ongoing and continuous rather than episodic as in older individuals. Distractibility, impulsivity, hyperactivity, and "mood swings" are symptoms of both ADHD and mania. For these reasons, the diagnosis of both mood disorders and ADHD is difficult in young people, and the relationships between the two diagnoses are, at this point, poorly understood.

It is possible to differentiate between the symptoms of ADHD and bipolar disorder in many young people, but there are some individuals who seem to have both disorders simultaneously. In one study of children who had already been diagnosed with ADHD, 21 percent were also found to meet the diagnostic criteria for bipolar disorder by age fifteen—that is, they seemed to have both disorders. This suggests that, in some youngsters at least, ADHD symptoms may in fact be early signs of bipolar disorder. The ADHD children who eventually developed bipolar symptoms had more severe symptoms and more disturbed behaviors than those who did not. Even more of these ADHD children with more severe symptoms met the criteria for a diagnosis of major depression: by age eleven, 29 percent had major depression; and by age fifteen, 45 percent—nearly half—had been diagnosed with major depressive disorder.[8]

How do we understand the children whose ADHD seems to develop into bipolar disorder? Did they really have ADHD symptoms in the first place, or does very-early-onset bipolar disorder mimic ADHD in its early stages? Are ADHD and early-onset bipolar disorder two separate illnesses that share similar symptom pictures but have different causes? Can ADHD develop into bipolar disorder? If so, how? And what do we make of the extremely high comorbidity between ADHD and mood disorder? These questions are, as yet, unanswered, and the nature of the connection between ADHD and pediatric mood disorders is unclear.

It has been suggested that the link may be genetic. When family members of ADHD children are studied, they are found to have high rates of mood disorders. Children of parents with mood disorders have high rates of ADHD. The researchers studying the group of young people with ADHD described above investigated the prevalence of mood disorders in family members. They found that relatives of children with both ADHD and bipolar disorder were five times as likely to have bipolar disorder themselves as family members of children with only ADHD. They also found high rates of major depression among the relatives of the children with ADHD and bipolar disorder. The researchers speculate that ADHD with bipolar disorder is a particular subtype of the illness.[9] Or perhaps these are two separate illnesses that happen to be inherited together frequently because the genes that cause them are located near one another on the chromosome and thus are usually inherited together. The only thing about this mysterious connection that we are really sure of is that much research in the area remains to be done.

Treatment and Prognosis

The treatment of pediatric bipolar disorder is still evolving. As you might expect, most of our treatment experience has been with lithium. Several studies indicate that lithium is effective in children, but there is also some evidence that it is not as effective in children as in adults. If complicated rapid-cycling bipolar disorder is indeed the rule in early-onset bipolar disorder, then lithium resistance should not be a big surprise: similar types of bipolar symptoms seem relatively lithium-resistant in adults, too. Pediatric lithium doses are, of course, lower than adult doses, but the effective therapeutic range for lithium in the bloodstream when it does work seems to be about the same in children as in adults. (Remember that the therapeutic range in the bloodstream is a measure of lithium concentration. Because children have a smaller total blood volume than adults, a lower dose of lithium for a child will result in the same concentration in the bloodstream.)

Getting regular blood tests done is, of course, more challenging with children than with adults, but given the toxicity of lithium, blood levels are if anything even more important in children. Several studies have been done using methods that avoid the needles, taking lithium levels from saliva rather than from blood, but the results have been disappointing, and so for now these little patients must, unfortunately, have blood tests.

The efficacy in children of other adult treatments for bipolar disorder—anticonvulsants, antipsychotic medications, and so forth—has been reported on here and there, but not enough research has been done to provide definitive recommendations regarding first-line treatment for children. Improvisation is, unfortunately, still necessary to some extent. Much work remains to be done to determine the optimum treatment approach for childhood bipolar disorder.[10]

The combination of ADHD and bipolar disorder seems to be especially difficult to treat, and combinations of medications are often necessary. In a study of adolescents being treated with lithium for a manic episode, a comparison was made between the treatment response in adolescents with and without a history of childhood-onset of ADHD. The adolescents with the ADHD history took significantly longer to get better on lithium than the adolescents with no history of ADHD symptoms. This seems to be further evidence that the combination of ADHD and bipolar disorder may be a subtype of illness and that it is especially challenging to treat.[11]

Many clinicians recommend avoiding stimulant medications completely in young persons with bipolar disorders. The same goes for some other treatments for ADHD, most notably antidepressants. The problem here is the same as with stimulant medications: the possibility of precipitating mania in a predisposed youngster. Another medication used to treat ADHD, atomoxetine (Strattera), has also been reported to precipitate mania. When it was given to an eleven-year-old boy who had been diagnosed with ADHD, had a family history suggestive of bipolar disorder, and had experienced manic-type symptoms from antidepressants, he developed severe manic symptoms.[12]

Clonidine (Catapres) and guanfacine (Tenex), medications used to treat high blood pressure in adults, have been found to be helpful in ADHD. Whereas stimulant medications help with inattention but are not very helpful for impulsivity and hyperactivity, clonidine and guanfacine seem to be effective in reducing these symptoms. There is also very preliminary evidence that medications that affect the neurotransmitter acetylcholine may be helpful for the symptoms of ADHD. Tacrine (Cognex) and donepezil (Aricept), two medications with this therapeutic mechanism that are used to treat Alzheimer's disease in the elderly, have been reported to be helpful for the treatment of ADHD.[13] These alternatives may be safer for youngsters with bipolar disorder who need additional treatment for ADHD.

How is normal psychological development in children affected by bipolar disorder? Relationships with family members are often strained for these patients, as are relationships with peers. Their educational development inevitably suffers as well. Clearly, attention to the psychological needs and the special educational requirements of these children is vitally important to minimize the effects of the illness on their psychological development. Thus, perhaps even more than in adults, counseling and therapy must be a high priority when developing treatment plans for children with bipolar disorder.

Does earlier onset of bipolar symptoms predict a stormier course of illness later on? As noted previously, children frequently have continuous rapid cycling and mixed symptoms. Does the illness take on the more usual adult pattern of discrete episodes as these children age? If so, are the episodes more frequent than in persons with later-onset illness? The jury is still out on this question, and research results are lacking. But at least one small study shows that bipolar disorder in young persons can indeed be a difficult illness to manage. In this study, fifty-four adolescents who were admitted to a university hospital with a diagnosis of bipolar I disorder were followed for five years.[14] Of these youngsters, nearly half had a relapse, and about half of these had two or more episodes during the five years of the study. This study was done on patients who needed to be admitted to the hospital, and so it is biased toward looking at sicker patients. This type of research problem is called *ascertainment bias:* the results of the study may be skewed because of the method used to gather patients for the study. In this case, since patients who were not ill enough to need hospitalization would not have made it into the study, the study group may not be representative of all pediatric bipolar I patients. Nevertheless, these results would seem to indicate that at least some of these young patients are especially prone to relapse and so need careful monitoring.

But as to the longer course of bipolar disorder that begins in childhood, there is practically no information. Is the course of illness different at age thirty or forty depending on whether it started at the age of ten or at twenty? There are no definitive answers to this sort of question for now.

Several tasks lie ahead for those researching bipolar disorder in children. First will be to improve upon the diagnostic process and find out how to better separate bipolar (especially manic) symptoms from other similar diagnostic pictures—especially attention deficit–hyperactivity disorder. Clarifying the relationship between bipolar disorder and ADHD will be a very instructive area of research for other reasons as well and will surely lead to better understanding of and treatments for both disorders. More research to determine which of the available treatments for bipolar disorder work best for children and adolescents is also needed, as are long-term follow-up studies to see if pediatric-onset bipolar disorder looks different from late-adolescent-onset bipolar disorder as the patient grows to adulthood.

CHAPTER 14

Women with Bipolar Disorder: Special Considerations

ALTHOUGH WOMEN ARE NO MORE LIKELY THAN MEN TO SUFFER FROM bipolar disorder, the hormonal changes that accompany menstruation and pregnancy affect the course of bipolar disorder in women and deserve special attention, as do some patterns of symptoms more often experienced by women than men with bipolar disorder. Finally, medication use during pregnancy and while breast-feeding requires careful consideration.

Premenstrual Syndromes

There has been intense interest for many years in the mood symptoms that many women experience for several days before the monthly onset of menstruation. The *DSM IV* contains a description of *premenstrual dysphoric disorder,* with diagnostic criteria that include depressed mood, change in energy level and appetite, and physical symptoms like bloating and breast tenderness. (Premenstrual dysphoric disorder is not in the main part of the *DSM* but rather in an appendix called "Criteria Sets and Axes Provided for Further Study." This means that the diagnosis is not well enough understood and characterized for the experts to agree on what should constitute diagnostic criteria.) The most common designation for mood symptoms that cycle with menstruation continues to be *premenstrual syndrome,* or *PMS.* Is PMS a separate disorder, or is it an "ordinary" mood disorder whose symptoms simply fluctuate with the hormonal changes of the menstrual cycle? This is the big unanswered question about PMS, and one of the reasons why

PMS is not in the *DSM* as an "official" diagnosis. Investigations into things like hormone levels in patients with PMS have not, for the most part, found anything abnormal. Moreover, the best relief from the symptoms of PMS seems to come from the usual treatments for mood disorders, rather than hormonal treatments. Another confusing factor in the study of PMS is the finding that many, perhaps even most, women experience some unpleasant physical and psychological symptoms for a few days prior to the onset of menstrual flow. Finding a group of women with "PMS" whose symptoms can be clearly distinguished from those of women with "normal" premenstrual symptoms and whose timing and profile of symptoms clearly separate them from women with other mood disorders is a clinical research challenge still unmet.

The situation with bipolar disorder is just as murky: some studies indicate that the timing of bipolar symptoms relates to the menstrual cycle, and others have not found any such relationship. In a study wherein women with bipolar disorder were given questionnaires asking about premenstrual symptoms, 60 percent reported a worsening of symptoms premenstrually. But since this is a *retrospective* study—patients were asked to remember something that had happened in the past—the results are highly questionable. Retrospective studies, especially questionnaire studies, are handicapped by the known tendency of people to connect their symptoms to events in their past and try to make sense of them in this way; people tend to overstate their symptoms in questionnaires and make connections where there aren't any. In another study of bipolar disorder and the menstrual cycle, the research subjects rated their moods every day, making it a *prospective* study— usually considered to be a better research technique. In this study *no association* between mood symptoms and menstrual cycles was found in a group of women with rapid-cycling bipolar disorder. But in a study looking at hospitalization, it was found that women with bipolar disorder were more likely to be hospitalized during the premenstrual and menstrual phases of the menstrual cycle than at other times.[1]

So the relationship between bipolar symptoms and the menstrual cycle is still unclear. There may be a group of women with bipolar disorder who are at higher risk for developing symptoms premenstrually, but how this should affect their treatment is unknown.

I can't leave behind the subject of premenstrual mood symptoms without mentioning an intriguing study published in the *American Journal of Psychiatry* in 1997.[2] The researchers had noticed that there is a significant overlap between PMS symptoms and the symptoms of seasonal affective disorder (SAD). In both syndromes depressed mood is accompanied by low energy, a tendency to sleep too much rather than too little, and an increase in appetite with carbohydrate craving. (We'll go into the details of the symptoms of SAD in chapter 16.) When the researchers asked patients referred to a PMS clinic if their PMS was worse during the winter, about two-thirds said that it was. Thirty-eight percent of the original group met diagnostic criteria for full-blown seasonal affective disorder. These women, then, had a mood disorder that cycled in at least *two* ways: with the monthly menstrual cycle, and with the twelve-month cycle of the seasons. This study shows us once more that there are intricate and complex relationships between mood and bodily rhythms and cycles, and that mood disorders are affected by many different factors in ways we are only beginning to understand.

Symptom Differences in Women

Of the various differences between the genders in the course of illness and symptoms of bipolar disorder, the greater incidence of rapid cycling in women is the best documented. A review article on bipolar disorder in women looked at ten studies involving several hundred persons with rapid-cycling bipolar disorder and found that 74 percent of the rapid-cycling patients were female.[3] Thus, the ratio of women to men with rapid-cycling disorder is 3:1.

Several reasons have been proposed for this difference. Since thyroid problems have been associated with rapid cycling in bipolar disorder, and since women are more likely than men to have certain types of thyroid problems, it was thought that a higher incidence of thyroid disease among women might explain the difference. But when women with rapid-cycling bipolar disorder were tested for thyroid problems, no greater incidence of thyroid disease was found. Theories implicating female hormones have also been suggested, but so far they are mostly speculative, and no research data exist clearly proving that hormonal differences between men and women explain this difference.

Another intriguing idea about the increased incidence of rapid-cycling bipolar disorder in women is related to the finding that women with bipolar disorder have a slightly greater ratio of depressive to manic episodes than men have. Several studies have found that women with bipolar disorder tend to have more episodes of depression during the course of their illness than men have.[4] This being the case, it may be that women with bipolar disorder are more likely to be treated with antidepressants that can cause them to enter a rapid-cycling phase of the disorder. The types of clinical studies that would prove this theory have yet to be carried out.

The finding that women with bipolar disorder have more depressive episodes than their male counterparts seems to fit with the finding that women are more likely than men to suffer from nonbipolar depression. No one understands this greater tendency of women to suffer from depressive illnesses. As I noted above, research on the levels of the female reproductive hormones in depressed women has generally been unrevealing.

It is now known that there are many differences in brain organization between women and men, differences that have little to do with sex and reproduction. Psychological testing profiles indicate that women are superior to men in their performance on certain tests of language and memory, and men perform better on certain specialized tests of three-dimensional visualization. It is thought that there are subtle differences in the way the brains of men and women are "wired" during prenatal development, probably under the influence of hormones in the womb, especially testosterone. The differences between men and women in the incidence and symptom profile of mood disorders may be due to these differences in "wiring." Explaining the significantly higher incidence of serious depression, including bipolar depression, in women is perhaps the most important unanswered question before us in the field of women's mental health.

Postpartum Mood Disorders and Family Planning

Emil Kraepelin noticed that women often had episodes of mania after giving birth, and for many years the term *postpartum psychosis* was a familiar one in medicine. With the reawakening of interest in careful diagnosis in psychiatry, however, it has become clear that most of these episodes of "psychosis" are episodes of bipolar disorder. Many clinical studies indicate that women with bipolar disorder are at very high risk for an episode of illness in the period after giving birth. One review article on bipolar disorder in women put it this way: "There is no other time in the life of a male or female bipolar patient when the risk of an episode is higher than it is for a female bipolar patient in the post-partum period."[5] One can speculate on the reasons for this: the emotional and physical stress of labor and delivery with the inevitable sleep deprivation, periods of physical pain, and dramatic changes in the levels of reproductive and stress hormones that attend childbirth. But the exact reasons for this very striking finding remain unknown.

Women with bipolar disorder who want to have a child are thus faced with a challenging dilemma. On the one hand, physicians usually recommend that a woman not take any medications during pregnancy, in order to protect the unborn child from prenatal exposure to pharmaceuticals. On the other hand, it is clear that a woman with bipolar disorder is at high risk for relapse after giving birth and perhaps needs medication late in her pregnancy more than at any other time in her life. Another problem is that the most commonly used mood-stabilizing medications—lithium, valproate, and carbamazepine—all have been associated with birth defects.

There are no easy solutions to these problems, but a few facts suggest some ways out. Most embryonic development has been completed by the final months of pregnancy, and lithium may be safer during pregnancy than originally thought. Current recommendations include avoiding most medications, especially the ones most closely linked to birth defects, during the early months of pregnancy and restarting treatment as soon as possible after delivery, possibly even in the latter stages of pregnancy.

But this much is very clear: simply stopping all medications while trying to get pregnant and for the duration of the pregnancy in order to eliminate all risk to the fetus is *very* risky for the mother. Some women will, of course, be willing to take this risk, and there are many arguments to support this approach. On the other hand, the first weeks and months—and some say the first few moments—of mother-child contact are very important for mother-child bonding, and this process may be disrupted if the mother is depressed or hospitalized with bipolar symptoms.

Many women with bipolar disorder have healthy babies and remain well in the weeks and months following delivery. Careful planning, conscientious symptom monitoring, and timely resumption of treatment will probably increase the chances of this happening. The woman with bipolar disorder owes it to herself and to her child to think and plan carefully about pregnancy. She should find an obstetrician and a psychiatrist who will support her decision to become pregnant and work closely with her and with each other toward the healthiest possible outcome for both mother and baby.

Is it safe to breast-feed while taking medication? Many medications are secreted in breast milk, but there is little research about the effects of these medications on infants. Although the Food and Drug Administration has not approved any psychiatric medication for use during breast-feeding, a few clinics provide careful monitoring for infant exposure to pharmaceuticals by testing breast milk and the baby's blood and urine, thus making it possible for some of their patients to breast-feed more safely while taking medications.[6]

CHAPTER 15

Alcoholism and Drug Abuse

Of all the statistics associated with bipolar disorder, here is one of the most significant and most disturbing: according to one very important study, more than 60 percent of persons with bipolar disorder also suffer from alcoholism or drug-abuse problems.[1]

Does having bipolar disorder make individuals more likely to use and abuse drugs and alcohol? Can alcoholism or drug abuse trigger the development of bipolar disorder in someone who is genetically vulnerable? Do bipolar disorder and substance-abuse disorders have a common biochemical or genetic cause? There is evidence to support an answer of yes to all of these questions.

Bipolar Binges

Perhaps the easiest-to-understand model for the observed link between bipolar disorder and alcoholism and drug abuse is the idea that the mood changes of bipolar disorder propel people into situations they would otherwise be able to avoid and cause them to do things they otherwise wouldn't do.

Brad was a forty-two-year-old writer. He had a day job as a copywriter for a small advertising firm, but his creative juices really started flowing late at night when he worked on his "stories." In college Brad had won a writing contest and had seen his very first attempt at writing a short story published in a prestigious national publication. Since then he had published one or two stories a year, sometimes in little literary journals that paid him practically nothing, once in *Atlantic Monthly*, most often in something in between.

I first met Brad when he was starting to get treatment for alcoholism at the substance-abuse treatment facility affiliated with the hospital where I worked. A psychiatric consultation had been requested because Brad had told the staff he had been troubled by depression and thought it made his drinking problems worse.

"I know what you're thinking: another alcoholic writer. But I'm not."

"Slow down, Brad," I said. "I didn't even know you were a writer until you told me just now." He was a serious and intense man with dark, deep-set eyes. I had to admit he looked the part of the troubled writer. "But I'm interested in hearing your ideas about your drinking problem."

"Sorry, I shouldn't jump to conclusions. But people always think of writers as alcoholics. You know, Hemingway, Tennessee Williams, sitting at their typewriters with a glass of Scotch. Well, I don't drink when I write, I drink when I can't write."

This was beginning to sound interesting. "What do you mean?" I asked.

Brad drank when he couldn't write because it made him feel better. And it gradually became clear to me that when he couldn't write, it was because he was depressed. "My mind just goes blank for days at a time. I get behind at work, I sleep too much, and I don't even bother turning the computer on at home. I can get the car-wax and potato-chip commercials written at work, but I couldn't be really creative if my life depended on it. This 'what's the use?' feeling comes over me, and I find myself bringing home a fifth of vodka two or three times a week and just sipping the nights away."

"Have you ever used any other drugs? Marijuana? Cocaine?" I asked.

"Oh, yes," Brad said with a deep sigh. "About three years ago I drained my bank account over a summer—blew it all on cocaine. If I hadn't ended up in the hospital, I might never have stopped."

"What happened?"

"Well, this is really embarrassing. I don't know what got into me, but I got this inspiration to try writing for TV. I had never tried scriptwriting before, but I was sure I could do it. I got an idea for a script about a guy who falls in love with a woman with a cocaine problem. I thought I needed to do some research—you know, where you go to buy the stuff, what those areas of town are like, the people involved."

"Maybe you should have tried the library first."

Brad turned, looking at me intently. At first I thought I had offended him with my little attempt at humor. But I hadn't. "That's just it," he said. "That what I usually *would* have done." He looked away again. "I'm not a particularly brave person, and certainly not a fool. But I was . . . I don't know quite how to put it . . . uninhibited, confident. I found myself walking down streets at midnight that I would have been nervous walking down in broad daylight. I bought the stuff and had no qualms about using it. And I was hooked in no time at all. I would get off work, go home, and write until it got dark. Then I'd make a run for the cocaine, kind of cruise around for a while, then come home and snort it. I'd get back to the writing and go at it until the sun came up."

"When did you sleep?" I asked.

"I didn't, not for days at a time. I didn't need to. I felt energized all the time."

"All the time?"

"Yes, I think cocaine must affect me differently than it does most people. I was feeling high even hours and hours after I had used. Once the high lasted three days."

This was sounding like more than just a drug and alcohol problem. People don't feel high from cocaine for three days. Something else had energized Brad that summer. His mood and behavioral changes had all the hallmarks of hypomania.

"So how did you end up in the hospital?"

"One morning my heart started beating real fast and my chest started to hurt. I left the office and got myself to the emergency room. They wanted to admit me right away, but I wouldn't let them."

"Why not?"

"It didn't seem necessary to me. I thought my heart was fine; I just wanted something for the pain. I know that sounds crazy now, but I think I *was* a little crazy by then. I don't remember much about what happened next, but they told me I started shouting and fighting. All I know is I got two shots in the butt and didn't wake up until eleven hours later."

Fortunately Brad's heart *was* fine, but he was discharged with a prescription for Risperdal to take for a few days for what was called a "cocaine-induced psychosis." His sleep patterns and energy level got back to normal.

"It's funny," he added, "I haven't had even the slightest temptation to use cocaine again. I didn't drink either for the whole next year. But then I found myself slipping into the pit again, and I didn't have the energy to say no anymore. But this time I knew I needed help. I think memories of that cocaine summer made me realize that the drinking might lead to something else again if I didn't get some serious treatment. That's why I checked in here."

I couldn't help asking one more question before telling Brad I thought he probably had bipolar disorder: "Did you finish the script?"

"Yes, I did. It turned out great. I've sent it to a producer, and she's interested. You know, I might even make back the money I spent on my, uh . . . research."

Not all stories like Brad's have such a happy ending. Some persons with bipolar disorder can indeed pull out of substance abuse when their mood episodes come to an end, either spontaneously or with treatment, but for others the substance-abuse problem takes on a life of its own. In the worst-case scenario, the mood disorder and the substance-abuse disorder start feeding on each other, and a vicious cycle of mood symptoms, increased substance abuse, and even more severe mood fluctuations takes over until it's impossible to separate one problem from the other.

Psychiatrists used to talk a great deal about "self-medication" in discussing the relationship between bipolar disorder and substance abuse. The idea was that bipolar patients sometimes started down the road to a full-blown substance-abuse problem by attempting to "treat" their mood symptoms with alcohol or drugs of abuse. Although this certainly occurs in some patients, it doesn't seem to be the most common scenario. Although some patients, like Brad, find themselves drinking while depressed because it deadens the psychic pain of depression, bipolar patients seem at greater risk for alcohol and drug abuse when they are hypomanic or manic. Brad's cocaine binge is actually the more typical story. The "self-medication" hypothesis might predict that bipolar patients would use stimulants like cocaine to alleviate their depressions. But studies show that, like Brad, bipolar patients are more likely to use cocaine—and to a lesser extent alcohol—to intensify and prolong their hypomanic and manic states.[2]

The link between mania and cocaine abuse has convinced many researchers that it is manic disinhibition and loss of judgment rather than a tendency to "self-medicate" that puts bipolar patients at such high risk for substance abuse.

Effect, Cause, or Association?

Another possible relationship between bipolar disorder and substance abuse works in the other direction—that is, alcohol and drug abuse may bring on episodes of abnormal mood in bipolar-disorder patients, perhaps by triggering episodes in persons who are vulnerable to the disorder because of genetic factors. Several studies have shown that bipolar patients who have a substance-abuse disorder have a stormier course to their mood disorder than patients who do not abuse alcohol or drugs. "Dual-diagnosis" patients, on average, first develop symptoms of their bipolar disorder at a younger age, and in some studies they have been shown to have more frequent hospitalizations. This has been interpreted to indicate that substance abuse may worsen the course of bipolar disorder, perhaps because of some direct effect on the brain of repeated use of drugs and alcohol.[3]

Finally, it may be that, like bipolar disorder, a vulnerability to addiction has a strong genetic component, and the two problems tend to occur together simply because the genes for both are located close to one another on the chromosomes and tend to be inherited together. I, for one, have seen too many patients like Brad—patients whose bipolar-disorder symptoms and substance abuse seem to trigger and reinforce each other—to believe that these so often tightly intertwined problems are randomly associated.

Use or Abuse?

At what point does substance use become "abuse" (see table 15-1)? It would be easy for me to launch into a long and complex discussion of diagnostic criteria for substance abuse and chemical dependency, but that probably wouldn't be very helpful. I think the issue is quite clear for individuals with a mood disorder: with the possible exception of occasional alcohol use, I advise persons with a mood disorder to *scrupulously avoid any and all intoxicating substances in any quantity whatsoever.*

TABLE 15-1 Signs of Alcoholism

Many medical and professional organizations endorse the **CAGE** questionnaire to identify problem drinking:
1. Have you ever felt you should **C**ut down on your drinking?
2. Have people **A**nnoyed you by criticizing your drinking?
3. Have you ever felt bad or **G**uilty about your drinking?
4. Have you ever had a drink first thing in the morning to steady your nerves or get rid of a hangover (an **E**ye opener)?

One *yes* suggests a possible alcohol problem. More than one *yes* means that an alcohol problem is highly likely.

Source: National Institute on Alcohol Abuse and Alcoholism, *Alcoholism: Getting the Facts,* 1996.

All abused substances appear to work by stimulating "reward" centers in the brain. You have probably heard that laboratory animals will push a lever that delivers an electrical stimulus to certain brain regions rather than another one that delivers food to their cage, and will continue doing so until they're practically dead from hunger. When a similar lever device is used to deliver an intravenous dose of alcohol or another drug to laboratory animals, the substances that animals will willingly and persistently self-administer in this way are almost exactly the same ones that humans use to get intoxicated: narcotics, cocaine, and certain stimulants and tranquilizers. These are the same substances that humans abuse and become addicted to. Some drugs, like cocaine, affect these centers quickly and powerfully; others, like marijuana, work more slowly, but they all work the same way: by disrupting the normal operation of the brain's "feel-good" circuitry.

Now, you don't need to be a psychiatrist to realize that persons with bipolar disorder already have enough problems with the "feel-good" circuits of the brain, and that mucking things up further with "recreational" drugs is a *very* bad idea. There is some evidence to suggest that intoxicating substances actively interfere with the therapeutic effects of the medications used to treat mood disorders. It seems to me that *any* use of intoxicating substances by persons with bipolar disorder is unhealthy and extremely risky and for those reasons amounts to substance abuse.

The question that usually comes next is, Can't I even have an occasional glass of wine with dinner? Although I'm hard-pressed to forbid my patients ever to drink, it's clear that when it comes to alcohol, less is better. Given the known high risk of bipolar patients for serious substance-abuse problems, the best course is probably no alcohol at all.

A Deadly Combination

There is one well-established research finding that is much more significant than all the speculation about the nature of the association between bipolar disorder and substance abuse and even more disturbing than the extremely high rate of substance abuse among people with bipolar disorder. This is the finding that persons who have mood disorders and also abuse alcohol or drugs have a greatly increased risk of completed suicide. Severe depression complicated by alcoholism or drug abuse has been found to be one of the most frequent diagnostic pictures in study after study of the psychiatric diagnoses of suicide victims. In a 1993 study attempting to make psychiatric diagnoses on suicide victims, clinicians reviewed the medical records and interviewed the relatives of almost fourteen hundred persons who had committed suicide. This study, which found that most of the suicide victims had suffered from a mood disorder, also found that *nearly half* (48 percent) had suffered from alcoholism or drug abuse.[4]

Another point to emphasize here is that when bipolar disorder and a substance-abuse problem coexist, they *both* need treatment. Getting proper treatment for the mood disorder will certainly make the substance-abuse problem easier to treat, but it cannot be assumed that a substance-abuse problem will simply go away when a coexisting mood disorder is treated. An active substance-abuse problem will in fact make the mood disorder difficult to diagnose, let alone treat.

Psychiatrists and other mental-health professionals are well versed in the available treatment resources in their community for chemical-dependency problems. But perhaps more than most other types of mental-health problems, the treatment of alcohol- and drug-abuse problems requires a wide range of specialized services and support groups. Mental-health professionals will usually refer a patient to a chemical-dependency center or organization for evaluation and treatment of a chemical dependency. Treatment options might include in-patient rehabilitation, out-patient treatment, or a new type of treatment program wherein patients spend the day at the program and return home at night. There are even evening programs that allow people to return to work during the day.

The first step is admitting that there might be a problem. This is often the most difficult step. When in doubt, talking about these concerns with the psychiatrist or therapist is not just important, it can be literally lifesaving.

CHAPTER 16

Seasonal Affective Disorder and Chronobiology

CHRONOBIOLOGY (FROM *KHRONOS*, THE GREEK WORD FOR "TIME") IS the science of bodily rhythms and biological clocks. Nearly every organism on the planet lives in rhythm with the astronomical cycles of the earth, sun, and moon. The activities of animals and the growth cycles of plants harmonize with the daily rising and setting of the sun, the monthly ebb and flow of ocean tides, the annual cycle of the changing seasons.

Ancient peoples erected immense astronomical calculators and observatories like Stonehenge in England and the monuments at Carnac in France, where rows of more than a thousand stones stretch across the countryside. At these sacred places and at others, like the pyramids of the Mayans and Incas, ancient astronomers determined the dates and times of solstices, equinoxes, and eclipses. In festivals like the Roman Saturnalia our forebears celebrated the lengthening of the daylight hours that heralds the arrival of spring and the return of the sun. Our modern midwinter holidays, Christmas and Hanukkah, recall these sentiments with traditions centered around candles, lights, and greenery.

Once we humans learned how to predict eclipses, we were no longer terrified by them. As we learned how to extend the daylight hours with fire and gaslight and electricity, we depended less on the cycles of the sun to structure our activities and felt more in control of time. We learned to warm ourselves in winter and cool ourselves in summer. The changes of seasons were still lovely to watch and interesting in the way they affected the plants and animals around us, but they didn't really affect us very much anymore—or so we thought.

But the changes of the seasons certainly *do* affect other creatures: the migration of birds, salmon, and whales, Arctic rabbits that change color in winter, the astonishing changes in plant life that occur from fall to winter to spring, and, of course, those hibernating bears. But humans have evolved beyond all that, haven't we? Our cycles of activity, like our sleeping at night and being awake during the day, are just conventions set by our culture rather than expressions of our biology. We humans have severed our connections with the rhythms of the celestial bodies. Haven't we?

That's what many of us thought—until 1982, when a paper by researchers from the National Institutes of Mental Health appeared in the *American Journal of Psychiatry*.[1] This paper, called "Bright Artificial Light Treatment of a Manic-Depressive Patient with a Seasonal Mood Cycle," described a patient with bipolar disorder whose symptoms occurred in a pattern related to the seasons: depression in winter and mood elevation during the summer.

Seasonal patterns in bipolar disorder had been described previously by a number of astute clinicians, including (as you might expect) Emil Kraepelin, who observed, "Repeatedly in these cases, I saw moodiness set in in autumn and pass over in spring 'when the sap shoots in the trees,' to excitement."[2] But there had been little organized research activity into the relationship between mood and the seasons. Then in the late 1970s a group of researchers were drawn together at NIMH by a mutual interest in seasonal mood changes, and they started to look at these relationships. One of them, Norman Rosenthal, had noticed his own seasonal shifts of mood for a number of years in his native South Africa, and had seen these mood swings worsen when his psychiatric training brought him to New York—a city located much farther from the equator than his native Johannesburg had been. In New York the summer days are much longer and the winter days much shorter than in South Africa. Rosenthal recalled his first autumn in New York this way:

> Daylight-saving time was over and the clocks were put back an hour.
> I left that first Monday after the time change and found the world in
> darkness. A cold wind blowing off the Hudson River filled me with
> foreboding. Winter came. My energy declined, and I wondered how
> I could have undertaken so many tasks the previous summer. Had I
> been crazy? Now there seemed to be no alternative but to hang in and
> try to keep everything afloat . . . Finally, spring arrived. My energy level
> surged again, and I wondered why I had worried so over my
> workload.[3]

A number of mood-disorder patients with seasonal mood changes found out about the NIMH group and sought out Rosenthal and the other scientists working on seasonal mood disorders. One was a woman who experienced regular winter depressions characterized by low mood and the development of an intense craving for sweets and starches. She had made an important observation during the two winters before she came to NIMH: during both these winters, she had taken vacations in the Virgin Islands. On both occasions traveling south toward the equator—to a latitude where the winter days were significantly *longer*—resulted in a dramatic improvement in her mood. Further, the improvement vanished abruptly when she returned to her colder—and darker—home up north. It was becoming obvious to the NIMH team that the crucial factor in seasonal mood changes was *light*.

The word *photoperiod* refers to the length of daylight hours in the twenty-four-hour day. It has been known for many years that photoperiod has a profound effect on many living things. If you've ever put a poinsettia plant or Christmas cactus in a dark closet to coax it into bloom for the holidays, you've used photoperiod manipulation to influence the plant's physiology. The shortened photoperiod causes the plant to produce hormones that cause flower buds to be set.

One member of the NIMH team suggested trying to treat winter depressions by artificially lengthening the photoperiod. Several patients volunteered to sit in front of bright lights for several hours before dawn and several more after sunset. Within three days the first patient began to feel better. "The change was dramatic and unmistakable," Rosenthal later wrote.[4] Phototherapy had been born.

Biological Clocks

In the 1920s the great psychobiologist Curt P. Richter—whom some consider to be the father of chronobiology—started investigating "biological timing devices" in laboratory rats.[5] (He was still pursuing this area of research in the 1980s as a small, stooped but bright-eyed man of ninety-something whom I would see walking through the halls of Johns Hopkins' Phipps Psychiatric Clinic with his battered leather briefcase in hand.)

Dr. Richter recorded the daily activity levels of his rats by putting them in individual cages with revolving drums similar to the wheels you see in pet hamster cages. Each rat's drum was connected to a device that continuously recorded its turnings, providing extremely accurate and totally objective measurements of each rat's activity level on a twenty-four-hour-a-day basis for as long as Richter cared to continue the observations. Each day the windowless laboratory's lights were switched on at 6 A.M. and off at 6 P.M. Richter noticed that his rats, as rats are wont to do, became active and started their exercise wheels spinning shortly after the lights went out, slowed down shortly before their artificial "morning" began at 6 A.M., and slept during most of the day. But his cleverly designed measuring devices were so accurate that they allowed Richter to make another very interesting observation: each rat's activity schedule was almost *precisely* the same night after night (see figure 16-1). One rat might start his nightly exercises minutes after "lights out" and continue until 4 A.M. while another didn't get going until, say, an hour after "nightfall" and then continued until 5:30. But whatever an individual rat's schedule was, he stuck to it night after night, often not varying by more than a few minutes. Now, since Dr. Richter had not equipped his rats' cages with tiny wall clocks, he concluded that each rat must have his own *internal* clock—one that kept very good time.

But what if the light/dark cues were eliminated? Would the internal clocks still run properly? At first Richter tried keeping the rats in total darkness by darkening the lab all the time. This proved increasingly impractical: a technician or janitor switching the lights on at the wrong time might ruin weeks or even months of work. To eliminate this or any other possibility of light contamination, the rats were surgically blinded. What happened next was remarkable: "The rats continued for some days or weeks to start running at exactly the same time each day, just as if they could still see, [but] sooner or later [they] started running either earlier or later day after day *by strikingly constant intervals.*"[6]

Each rat's internal clock continued to keep excellent time; the trouble was, it wasn't exactly a twenty-four-hour clock. A particular rat's internal clock might have, say, a cycle of twenty-three hours and fifty-five minutes. This particular rat would start waking up five minutes earlier every night, and the rat's sleep/wake cycle would shift in relation to the twenty-four-hour cycle by five minutes a day. As Richter discovered, each blinded rat's internal clock kept to a twenty-four-hour cycle for a while, but then the rat's *internal* clock started keeping to its own particular variation on the twenty-four-hour theme, and the rat's activity schedule started shifting (see figure 16-2).

Since the internal clock of the rat didn't quite keep a twenty-four-hour cycle, the internal clocks of the normal rats (the rats that could see normally) must have been "set" every once in a while in order for them to be accurately synchronized within a twenty-four-hour day. Obviously the "setting" mechanism was exposure to light. That burst of bright light at 6 A.M. every day when the laboratory lights went on accurately tuned the normal rat's clock to a twenty-four-hour day.

The blinded rat's internal clock no longer kept to a twenty-four-hour schedule because it had lost what we now call its *zeitgeber*, a German word that means "time giver." The blinded rat's internal clock could no longer be *entrained* (brought onto schedule, or reset) by its external "setting" signal: light.

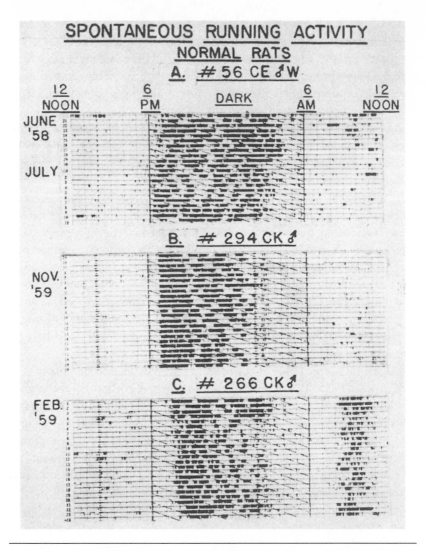

FIGURE 16-1 Original records from three of Dr. Richter's rats. Each line in the records represents one day, the lines becoming thicker when the rat becomes active. Rat A starts running in his cage at exactly 6 P.M. every evening, rat B starts about an hour later, and rat C a bit later still. The records illustrate the remarkable consistency of each animal's internal clock and activity schedule.

Source: Curt Paul Richter, *Biological Clocks in Medicine and Psychiatry* (Springfield, Ill.: Charles C Thomas, 1965). Courtesy of Charles C Thomas, Publisher, Ltd., Springfield, Illinois.

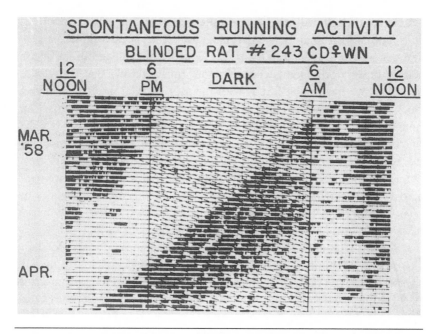

FIGURE 16-2 Activity record for a blinded rat. Each line again represents a twenty-four-hour period. This rat's activity period is shifting by almost exactly thirty minutes every day: the dark line indicating activity starts a little further to the left (earlier) every day.

Source: Richter, *Biological Clocks in Medicine and Psychiatry.* Courtesy of Charles C Thomas, Publisher, Ltd., Springfield, Illinois.

Now fast-forward to Manchester, England, in the mid-1990s. Fourteen healthy young men and women have volunteered for a biological-clock experiment. The vocabulary of chronobiology had changed a bit, the "internal timing device" now being called an "endogenous circadian pacemaker." (*Endogenous* means "inner" or "internal," and *circadian* is a word that refers to a twenty-four-hour cycle.) Two or three at a time, the volunteers enter experimental living quarters where, for about a month, instead of a twenty-four-hour day they live on a thirty-hour day: twenty hours of wakefulness, ten hours of sleep. Every couple of hours while awake they take a ten-minute battery of psychological tests and rate their mood. What did the mood ratings show?

Here's a hint: like rats, humans also have a close-to-twenty-four-hour internal clock. Although it might be possible to investigate this pacemaker by asking volunteers to live for a month or so like Dr. Richter's rats (in a little room with a cot and an exercise bike hooked up to a recording device), the human endogenous circadian pacemaker can be demonstrated with much simpler equipment. All you need is a thermometer. Our body temperature rises and falls throughout the day, like—well, like clockwork. It is highest at 6 P.M. and lowest at about 6 A.M. Under experimental conditions of constant darkness or dim light, when this clock runs at its own pace, our cycle is about twenty-five hours. But as with the rat's internal timer, our internal clock is entrained by environmental cues, primarily light, to a twenty-four-hour cycle.

Here's another hint: our internal clock can shift only about one or two hours per day. When we reset our watches for daylight-saving time or travel to an adjacent time zone, we hardly notice the change. But when we travel across several time zones, it takes several days for our internal clock to become entrained to the new time. The farther we've traveled, the longer it takes: about one day for each hour of time change.

So what happened to our English volunteers? Since they were forced to live on a thirty-hour cycle, their internal clocks could *never* catch up with their sleep/wake cycle. Their internal clocks started running as quickly as possible but inevitably went in and out of synchronization with their artificially prolonged sleep/wake cycle. The researchers found that the more out of synchronization the volunteers became, the worse their mood became. In fact, it was the *interaction* of the two cycles that seemed to make the most difference in their mood. They felt worst when their internal temperature clock was telling them it wasn't time to get up yet and their sleep/wake cycle was telling them it was time to start winding down from a long day. The researchers proposed that "temporal alignment between the sleep-wake cycle and the endogenous circadian rhythms affects self-assessment of mood in healthy subjects."[7] Put more simply: when our sleep/wake cycle and our internal clock are out of synchronization, it has a very *negative* effect on our mood.

Seasonal Affective Disorder

So let's get back to the patients with winter depressions and summer mood elevations (see table 16-1). What can all these findings in chronobiology tell us about the causes of this illness? Do seasonal affective disorder (SAD) patients, with a mood control system abnormally sensitive to light, have some kind of problem with their internal clock? Perhaps a chronic dyssynchrony between various circadian cycles and rhythms?

Several theories for SAD involving circadian rhythms have been put forward, but none fits the experimental findings very well. It had been proposed that people with SAD might have an abnormal delay in circadian rhythms. Early-morning bright light would be expected to correct this problem by advancing the cycle. Evening phototherapy would be expected to have the op-

TABLE 16-1 Symptoms of Seasonal Affective Disorder

Winter depressions
Mania, hypomania, or normal mood in summer
Carbohydrate craving during depressions
Low energy, sleeping too much during depressions
Reverse diurnal variation of mood (afternoon or evening "slump")

posite effect and make things even worse. But research clearly shows that morning and evening phototherapy are equally helpful for SAD. It has also been suggested that SAD patients have lazy circadian rhythms, and even that they are abnormally sensitive to light. But tests of these various hypotheses have led to more confusion than clarity, and no one has come up with a theory that ties SAD to a particular circadian rhythm disturbance.

A research group from Columbia University attempted to discover the factors that predicted who would have a good response to photoperiod manipulation. They gave a course of phototherapy to 103 people who reported seasonal mood changes. Some of these individuals met diagnostic criteria for bipolar I, some for bipolar II, and some had unipolar depressions—that is, they had never been manic or hypomanic.

The researchers found that it was not diagnosis (as bipolar I or II or non-bipolar depression) but a particular *pattern* of depressive symptoms that predicted a good response to phototherapy. The people helped by phototherapy tended to sleep more rather than less when they were depressed (hypersomnia) and to complain of low energy and fatigue. They noticed increased appetite during depressions, especially for sweets and starches ("carbohydrate craving"), and an accompanying weight gain. Finally, they had a striking diurnal variation in mood (a consistent pattern of change in mood through the day), but in a pattern that was the opposite of that usually seen in severe depression: instead of waking up early in the morning with the worst mood of the day and then feeling better as the day went on, these people felt better in the early part of the day but had an afternoon or evening "slump," a pattern called *reverse diurnal variation.*[8]

Let's recap some of the symptoms that predicted a good response to phototherapy in this study: a seasonal pattern of symptoms (fall/winter onset with remission in spring), low energy, carbohydrate craving, and hypersomnia. In other words, as winter approaches, these people begin feeling increasingly sluggish mentally and physically, find that they crave carbohydrates, and sleep a lot more than usual. When spring arrives, the symptoms subside. Sound familiar? The similarity to the hibernation behavior of bears is certainly striking.

The serotonin level in an area of the brain called the *hypothalamus* shows a seasonal (twelve-month) rhythm, with the lowest levels of serotonin found in December and January.[9] It is thought that the hypothalamus is the location of our biological clock, and this part of the brain is also thought to be important in the development of SAD.

We also know that serotonin levels in the brain increase after a meal high in carbohydrates. High carbohydrate intake shifts the balance of certain amino acids in the bloodstream and makes some of them, including *tryptophan,* a serotonin precursor, move into brain tissue more easily.

Together these facts suggest that SAD may be triggered by low serotonin levels in the hypothalamus, perhaps related to the short photoperiod of winter days. SAD patients discover that they feel a little better after they have a carbohydrate meal—because such a meal boosts brain levels of serotonin—and they tend to binge on sweets and starches. The fact that the serotonin-boosting SSRI antidepressants are very effective in SAD lends support to this line of reasoning.

But this is in all probability only a crude outline of some of the facts about SAD, and it leaves much unexplained. I've been talking about SAD as if it were a diagnostic category of its own, but it's not. SAD can refer to a bipolar I, bipolar II, or nonbipolar depressive illness that shows a seasonal pattern to symptoms. But a lot of what we know about mood disorders suggests that bipolar I, bipolar II, and nonbipolar depressive illnesses are very *different* illnesses in course and causation. What does it mean that *each* can have a seasonal pattern? The study I described earlier showed that it was not diagnosis but rather symptom pattern that predicted who gets better with light therapy. Does this mean that our whole diagnostic classification system is called into question?

Don't throw out your *DSM* just yet. The "bipolar/nonbipolar" and "bipolar I/bipolar II" diagnostic divisions are still very useful in picking treatments, and so is the "with seasonal pattern/without seasonal pattern" designation. It may just be a few more years before we figure out how all the classifications fit together.

In the meantime, patients with bipolar symptoms who notice a seasonal pattern should talk with their physician about phototherapy, especially if they have the typical SAD depressive symptom pattern: low energy, hypersomnia, carbohydrate craving, weight gain, and reverse diurnal variation of mood (afternoon or evening "slump").

In phototherapy, the person is exposed to bright light in either the morning or the evening, normally using a light-box (similar to the one depicted in figure 16-3). The therapeutic effect is sometimes evident within days, but as with antidepressants, several weeks of therapy are sometimes needed to obtain good remission of symptoms. Side effects are generally minor: head-

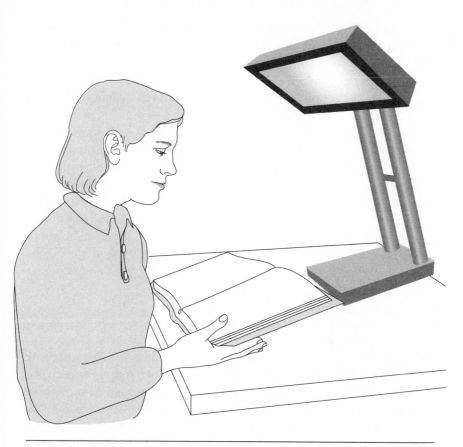

FIGURE 16-3 Phototherapy

aches and eyestrain, for example.[10] The heat generated by the lights can cause dryness of the eyes or nasal passages. Too much light exposure can sometimes precipitate hypomanic symptoms: irritability, insomnia, feeling "hyper." Fortunately this problem seems to respond quickly to decreased light exposure, and phototherapy doesn't seem to have the risks of mood destabilization that taking antidepressant medication does.

The details of the optimum intensity and duration of light exposure are still being investigated, but several studies suggest that if the light is bright enough, exposure for an hour or even less may be sufficient. The main light-gathering organs of our bodies are, of course, our eyes, and it had been assumed that light falling upon the retinas sends the signal to the brain that resets our internal clock. Some research, however, suggests that the eyes are not the only, or even the most important, means of transmitting light signals to the body's internal clock. A study published in 1998 reported that the circadian rhythms of volunteer subjects could be shifted by delivering a three-hour pulse of light to the back of the knee joints.[11] As with the English study, body temperature was measured to track circadian rhythm. This finding might seem strange indeed at first, but is it really so unexpected to find that exposing the surface of the body, rather than the eyes, to light might affect our internal clock? After all, poinsettia plants don't have eyes, and they can sense a change in photoperiod quite well! It is thought that hemoglobin and other blood pigments may somehow be activated by exposure to light through the skin, in much the same way that chlorophyll, the green pigment in the leaves of plants, is activated by light. This would suggest that the light's signal is carried to the brain by the blood, with an activated blood pigment acting as a kind of "light hormone."[12] Perhaps someday instead of sitting in front of lights during the day, phototherapy patients will strap on fiberoptic cables that deliver light to the backs of their knees while they sleep.[13]

The Sleep Cycle and Bipolar Disorder

We're not finished with circadian rhythms yet. Even if they haven't turned out to explain very much about SAD, circadian rhythms, especially the sleep/wake cycle, are very significant in bipolar disorder. The study with our English volunteers demonstrated how important the sleep/wake cycle is in the regulation of mood in persons who do *not* have mood disorders. So it should come as no surprise that sleep/wake cycle manipulation has dramatic effects on persons with bipolar disorder. Clinical observations confirm this: sleep deprivation can be used therapeutically to treat the symptoms of depression, and it can also cause a switch into the manic state. To understand these observations, we need to take a closer look at normal sleep.

For quite a long time sleep wasn't of very much interest to experimental psychologists and psychiatrists. This may seem odd, especially considering Freud's and others' intense interest in dreams. Possibly because of a lack of investigative tools, interest in dreams never extended to interest in the process of dreaming, and so the physiology of sleep was a neglected area of research for many decades.

This changed in 1953, when a group of researchers used an electroencephalogram (EEG) machine on sleeping volunteers in a clinical laboratory to investigate the longstanding observation that people move their eyes beneath closed lids during some periods of sleep. When the researchers awakened the subjects during what came to be called *rapid eye movement sleep* (REM sleep), 90 percent of them reported that they had been dreaming. Further studies revealed that sleep is a complex process, with several different stages and rhythms of activity that together are now called *sleep architecture.*

As figure 16-4 indicates, after falling asleep a person passes through

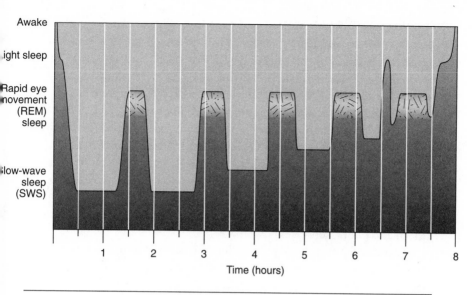

FIGURE 16-4 Normal sleep architecture

lighter and then progressively deeper stages of sleep. Brain activity slows, and the heartbeat and blood pressure drop to the lowest levels of the twenty-four-hour day. The process is like a submarine descending into darker, quieter, deeper water. The very deepest stage is called *slow-wave sleep* (SWS) because the EEG shows slow synchronized rhythms in the electrical activity of the brain. SWS is thought to be the physically restorative part of sleep; experimental subjects who are awakened whenever they enter SWS but are allowed to experience the other stages complain of muscle aches and other symptoms of physical discomfort.

About ninety minutes after a person falls asleep, the sleep "submarine" begins to rise again. The EEG indicates a brain activity pattern not very different from that seen in awake individuals. The EEG electrodes that track eye movements measure intense activity, and individuals awakened during this stage report dreaming: the sleeper has entered a period of REM sleep. After fifteen to twenty minutes of REM sleep, eye movement ceases, and the sleeper drifts back down into the deeper stages again and has another period of SWS, which predominates during the first part of the night. As the night progresses, the sleeper spends more time in REM sleep and less in SWS. Toward dawn, sleep becomes lighter and REM periods become longer until finally the person wakes up. It is thought that REM sleep and body temperature are both tightly linked to the body's main circadian clock (often called the *strong oscillator*) because the lowest point of the body's temperature cycle coincides with the most intensive period of REM sleep.

When we look at EEG sleep studies done on depressed persons, the REM cycle seems to have shifted. Depressed individuals go into REM almost immediately after falling asleep, a phenomenon called *decreased REM latency.* Some slow-wave sleep still occurs in the later part of the night, but the overall amount of SWS is reduced. Some researchers have interpreted these findings as indicating that depressed individuals suffer from a *phase advance* of the REM cycle, and that the rhythm of the strong oscillator has gotten out of phase with other bodily rhythms. We saw from the study on the English volunteers that when the strong oscillator (as measured by their temperature cycle) is out of synchronization with the sleep/wake cycle, dips in mood occur. In the few patients with bipolar disorder who have been studied, striking shifts of the REM and temperature cycles were observed as the patients cycled in and out of depression and mania.[14]

These findings bring together a lot of what we know about the symptoms of depression and about circadian rhythms. The decreased amounts of SWS may explain the fatigue and bodily discomfort typical of depression. The shifting of the usual period of REM from the early-morning hours to the early part of the sleep cycle may explain the early-morning awakening typically seen in depression.

These findings may also explain the therapeutic effects of sleep deprivation on symptoms of depression. Patients with the typical diurnal variation of mood seen in depression often report that they have their best mood of the day during the late evening, before they go to sleep, and feel their worst in the morning after they've slept. This and other observations led some researchers in the 1950s to experiment with sleep deprivation as a therapeutic technique for the treatment of depression. With the introduction of antidepressant medications, interest in sleep deprivation faded, but recently it has been growing again. This work shows that if patients are totally deprived of sleep—kept up all night—about 60 percent of them report a sometimes dramatic improvement in their mood. Unfortunately the effect is temporary; in most patients the benefits disappear after even a brief nap, making this interesting technique a not terribly useful one. But experiments with partial sleep deprivation indicate that waking patients up at about 2 A.M. and making sure that they do not sleep during the second half of the night is nearly as effective as total sleep deprivation. Advancing the sleep cycle by six hours, so that patients go to sleep at 6 P.M. and get up at 2 A.M., has also been found to have antidepressant effects.

Although the technique has not caught on in the United States, sleep deprivation and phase advance are popular in Europe as adjuncts to medication in the treatment of bipolar and nonbipolar depression. An Italian study published in 1997 compared the recovery time from depression in ten bipolar patients. All of them were treated with fluoxetine (Prozac), but five were also given several cycles of total sleep deprivation. The patients who had sleep deprivation got better faster on the medication than those who did not.[15]

The other relevant clinical observation about sleep in persons with bipolar disorder is that sleep deprivation can precipitate mania. This is a very well documented finding, and for this reason my discussion of sleep deprivation as a treatment for depression comes with a "don't try this at home" warning: even one night of sleep deprivation can precipitate mania. There have been numerous reports of individuals with bipolar disorder becoming manic after transatlantic flights or after sleep deprivation caused by medical emergencies or family crises. Emotional upsets can, of course, lead to insomnia and poor sleep due to anxiety. It has been proposed that lack of sleep for *any* reason may be what tips the balance for many bipolar patients and brings on an episode of mania.[16]

All of the work on chronobiology and biological clocks indicates that there are important links between bodily rhythms and mood, and we've barely scratched the surface of this fascinating area of study. But so far we have only tantalizing hints about these links rather than clearly understood mechanisms and relationships. Nevertheless, studies of sleep and SAD point the way toward new and safer treatments for certain mood disorders—techniques like phototherapy and sleep phase advance. This work also indicates the importance of lifestyle regularity in controlling the symptoms of bipolar disorder, a topic we'll explore in more detail in chapter 20.

The Genetics of Bipolar Disorder

IT HAS LONG BEEN RECOGNIZED THAT BIPOLAR DISORDER EXISTS IN clusters within families and seems to be inherited in some individuals. In *Manic-Depressive Insanity,* Emil Kraepelin wrote of one family in which "of the ten children of the same parents who were both probably manic-depressive by predisposition, no fewer than seven fell ill the same way; of the five descendants of the second generation, four have already fallen ill."[1]

For many years research on the genetics of bipolar disorder was hampered by foggy diagnostic criteria and a lack of laboratory methods to identify genes. But this is changing. Not only have psychiatrists become more skilled in the diagnosis of bipolar disorder, but the biochemical methods available to locate and identify genes on the human chromosome have become tremendously more sophisticated. These developments will, sooner or later, lead to a better understanding of the genetic mechanisms of bipolar disorder, which will in turn lead to better diagnosis and treatment of the disorder.

Genes, Chromosomes, and DNA

A brief discussion of the principles of genetics, the scientific study of the inheritance of biological attributes, will lead us into our discussion of the heredity of bipolar disorder.

The patterns and rules of inheritance in living things were first described by Gregor Mendel, an Austrian monk who over many years performed elegantly planned and executed experiments with plants, mostly garden peas, in his monastery garden. Prior to Mendel's work in the latter half of the nineteenth century, it was thought that the traits of one parent were simply blended with those of the other parent in their offspring, who were thought to have traits that were intermediate between the two parents. Mendel discovered that this was not always or even usually true. He found, for example, that crossing a pea plant that produced green peas with a pea plant that produced yellow ones did not produce plants with yellow-green peas (that is, an intermediate form). Instead Mendel discovered that *all* the seeds formed by the cross grew green peas. When he went on to cross these offspring seeds, he found that exactly *three-quarters* of the second-generation seeds produced green peas and *one-quarter* produced yellow ones. There were no intermediate forms and no blending of traits. The offspring seeds got either a "green" inheritance or a "yellow" one; there were no "in-betweens." Mendel concluded that each parent contributed something that determined pea color, and these "somethings" were distributed to the offspring—in this case, seeds—to determine the trait. These "somethings" are now called *genes*, the units of inheritance.

We now understand that genes are sets of instructions for building proteins. All plants and animals from seaweed to snapdragons and from earthworms to elephants are constructed of and operate by means of proteins. Myosin (muscle protein), hemoglobin (the oxygen-carrying protein of red blood cells), and collagen (the structural protein of skin and cartilage) are just a few examples. Even the nonprotein structural materials of the body, like the calcium salts in our bones, depend on proteins. Proteins called enzymes direct the manufacture of bone from calcium salts by expediting certain chemical reactions. Many hormones are proteins (insulin, for example), and those that are not (like testosterone and cortisol) are manufactured by protein enzymes. I've already mentioned some members of the protein family that are of enormous interest to those studying bipolar disorder: *G proteins* and the receptor molecules for the neurotransmitters are proteins. All proteins are built according to specifications contained in genes.

For many years it was believed that genes were proteins also—that is, that genetic information was somehow encoded in protein molecules. But by the mid-1940s experiments with bacteria had proven that a far simpler family of biochemical compounds, called *nucleic acids,* contained genetic information. In 1953 James Watson and Francis Crick published a paper in the British scientific journal *Nature* describing the structure of the most important of these compounds, deoxyribonucleic acid (DNA), and the modern age of genetics had begun.

DNA molecules are long spiral chains whose links consist of four simpler compounds called nucleotides. The four DNA nucleotides, adenine, cytosine, guanine, and thymine (usually abbreviated as A, C, G, and T), are the elements of an elegantly simple code used to write out instructions for the manufacture of proteins. Just as you can write out a Morse code version of *Hamlet* using only dots and dashes, you can write out instructions for building hemoglobin, myosin, collagen, or any other protein using A's, C's, G's, and T's. That's what DNA does. You can think of the physical structure of a gene as the section on the DNA molecule that codes for one protein.

When the DNA molecule is doing its work in the cell, it is unraveled and stretched out, surrounded by a whole retinue of ultramicroscopic attendants busily reading the coded instructions and making proteins. When it's time for the cell to divide, another set of attendants carefully coil the DNA molecule into a compact cylinder and surround it with protective proteins to form the threadlike structures you may have looked at under the microscope in high school biology: the chromosomes.

Genetic Diseases

For some disorders, the links from a certain gene to a certain protein to a certain trait or disease are easy to follow. Sickle-cell anemia is one such disease. When the blood of sickle-cell patients is examined under the microscope, instead of seeing the normal saucer- or disk-shaped red blood cells, one sees abnormal crescent- or sickle-shaped cells. Once scientists had the biochemical methods that allowed them to look at the components of blood cells, they discovered that sickle-cell patients had an abnormally shaped hemoglobin molecule (hemoglobin is the protein in red blood cells that transports oxygen). This abnormal hemoglobin tends to form abnormal chains within the cell, stretching the normally disk-shaped cells into the sickle shape characteristic of the disease.

Because hemoglobin is easily purified, it was one of the first proteins whose structure was completely described (a feat that earned Cambridge University biochemist Max Ferdinand Perutz the Nobel Prize in 1962). Researchers discovered that sickle-cell hemoglobin (now called hemoglobin S) differs from normal hemoglobin by only a few atoms, the equivalent of a single substitution in the hemoglobin gene on the DNA molecule. Because of several biochemical factors that made the hemoglobin gene especially accessible and easy to work with, it was possible to pinpoint its location early on in the search for genes that cause human diseases. We now know that at one particular spot on the DNA molecule of persons with sickle-cell anemia, there is an A instead of a T in the set of instructions. An abnormal hemoglobin molecule results from the reading of these incorrect instructions, and the abnormal hemoglobin molecules cause the abnormally shaped red blood cells, which block blood vessels and result in the symptoms of the disease.

The pathway from abnormal gene to abnormal protein to abnormal cells to symptoms has been completely described.

Genes have been identified and located in several other human diseases whose inheritance pattern indicates that they are single-gene illnesses (this "single-gene inheritance" is also known as Mendelian inheritance). In some cases this has been possible even though the identity or function of the protein the abnormal gene codes for is unknown. Huntington's disease (or Huntington's chorea), the degenerative brain disease that afflicted folksinger Woody Guthrie, is one example.

One type of genetic search uses *linkage studies* to locate and identify genes. These studies take advantage of the fact that genes that are located close to one another on the chromosome tend to stay together when the chromosomes are packaged into egg or sperm cells. Geneticists then use gene maps that show the location of *marker genes.* In a linkage study, DNA tests are performed on a blood sample of persons with the condition being investigated as well as samples from unaffected family members. Sophisticated mathematical analysis of the marker genes generates a kind of genetic signal along the chromosomes being studied, and if the signal is strong enough, it indicates that a gene for the illness must be nearby. The next step is to take a closer look at the area marked by the signal, searching for stretches of DNA where a gene might be hiding. This method has been highly successful in locating the genes for several other single-gene diseases, including cystic fibrosis and Duchenne's muscular dystrophy.

Another type of search starts with an idea that a particular gene (called a *candidate gene*) might be involved in causing an illness. In bipolar disorder, genes involved with serotonin signaling have been candidate genes for these kinds of studies. Blood is collected from individuals who have and others who don't have the illness being investigated, and then DNA analysis is done to see whether individuals who have the illness share a particular copy (called an *allele*) of the gene. If a particular copy of the candidate gene is consistently found in individuals who have the illness, but not in those who don't, this suggests that the candidate gene is indeed important in causing the illness. This type of study is called an *association study* because the researcher is looking for an association between a particular gene and the illness.

These kinds of studies are very useful when one gene is primarily responsible for the illness (as in sickle-cell anemia), but if several genes are involved, the problem of gene identification becomes tremendously more complicated. If the illness being investigated takes several forms or is difficult to diagnose, the task becomes monumental. Unfortunately, all of these things are true for bipolar disorder: it is fairly certain that many genes are involved and that they probably act together to cause an illness that can take many different forms and is often difficult to diagnose.

Nevertheless, in the late 1980s several reports appeared that purported to link bipolar disorder to specific regions of chromosomes. The most significant report was of an Amish family that seemed to carry a bipolar-disorder gene located on one end of chromosome 11. In this study the researchers thought they had overcome at least one of the usual hurdles to finding a bipolar gene. This particular family pedigree seemed to indicate Mendelian inheritance at work. Even if there were several possible genes that could cause bipolar disorder, this particular family seemed to pass on the disorder through only one. Mathematical analysis of previously identified DNA markers pointed to chromosome 11, and the statistical significance of the findings appeared solid. Zeroing in on a bipolar gene seemed within reach. Within only months, however, these results were called into question when another team of scientists took another look at the mathematical analysis. But it was the issue of diagnosis that ultimately scuttled this ambitious study. Several of the individuals who had been classified as unaffected when the data were originally collected developed symptoms of bipolar disorder later on. When the new numbers were "crunched," the results fell apart completely.[2]

Linkage studies have pointed to a number of different locations on different chromosomes as possible sites for bipolar genes, but the results are still preliminary, and sometimes, as with the Amish study, repeat testing has cast doubt on the conclusions. Association studies have been similarly disappointing. A team of researchers looked for an association between a particular copy of the gene for a particular G protein in persons with bipolar disorder, but did not find one.[3]

What We Know

In the absence of specific identified genes or any knowledge about what proteins these genes code for, we can talk about the inheritance of bipolar disorder in only a very general way. Children of individuals with bipolar disorder have an increased risk of developing bipolar disorder. Assigning a number to that risk is very difficult, for some of the same reasons that the search for a bipolar gene has been so difficult, especially problems of diagnosis. But the risk seems to be several times that of the general population, on the order of 10 percent. However, children of persons with bipolar disorder are also at a higher risk for unipolar (depression-only) illness, and when you add in this risk, the percentages go up into the high twenties. This means that the children of persons with bipolar disorder have about a one in four chance of developing some kind of mood disorder and about a one in ten chance of developing bipolar disorder.[4]

Individuals with bipolar disorder need to be alert to signs and symptoms of mood disorders in their children and to get them into treatment if such symptoms occur. Although we may be uncertain about the details of the inheritance of bipolar disorder, we are not at all uncertain about the importance of early diagnosis and treatment.

The Search Continues

Several factors make scientists optimistic about eventually discovering genes for bipolar disorder. First, the number of identified genetic markers continues to rise. These markers, like signposts along the length of the chromosome, mark particular locations in the DNA molecule. Imagine that your car breaks down along a barren desert highway that has markers every hundred miles. Imagine yourself on your cellular phone, calling the highway patrol and telling them you remember passing the 100-mile marker, but you're not sure how far back it was. That means you are somewhere between the 100- and the 200-mile markers. Let's hope you brought some water with you because it may be a while before you get picked up! Now imagine that the markers are located every *ten* miles. If the last marker you remember passing was the 100-mile sign, you're somewhere between mile 100 and 110. Obviously, the highway patrol will find you much more quickly.

The same principle applies in the search for the bipolar gene: the more genetic signposts there are, the easier it will be to find a particular gene. More precise diagnoses will also help, as will the study of larger family pedigrees as well as advances in technology—both biochemical methods and more powerful computers and software to do the mathematical analysis.

Even when genes are identified, however, and tests are developed that can look for these genes in individuals, predictions about who will develop symptoms will still be imprecise. This is because several genes are likely involved and also because genetics is almost certainly not the whole story in bipolar disorder. Environmental factors are undoubtedly important (perhaps equally important) in determining who will and will not be affected; psychological and perhaps physical stresses and traumas are probably very important. So even when a gene or genes are identified and can be tested for, finding that a person has a bipolar gene will probably mean that he or she has a higher chance of developing symptoms than someone who does not have the gene—but not a 100 percent chance. This will raise a lot of questions about who should and should not be tested and who is entitled to know genetic test results.

But finding responsible genes may lead to new treatment approaches that will benefit everyone with mood disorders. Gene identification, as well as identification of the function of these genes or the gene products, will undoubtedly shed light on the biochemical basis of bipolar disorder. It may then be possible to design medications or other treatments based on knowledge about the causes of bipolar symptoms on a cellular or biochemical level—rather than stumbling upon treatments by accident, as has been the case so far. Genetics research is one of the most challenging but most promising areas of investigation of bipolar disorder, and it holds the promise of truly revolutionizing the treatment of this disease.

CHAPTER 18

Bipolar Biology

IN THIS CHAPTER I DISCUSS SEVERAL CONNECTIONS BETWEEN BIPO-
lar disorder and other aspects of the biology of the brain and nervous system.

"Medical" Mood Disorders

It has been known for many years that symptoms of mood disorders can
develop during certain medical illnesses. By taking a close look at these illnesses and trying to see what they have in common, we have learned a great
deal about the possible causes of bipolar disorder and other psychiatric illnesses that affect mood.

Psychiatrists used to use the term *organic* to describe mental symptoms
that were caused by medical (as opposed to psychiatric) illnesses. Whereas
symptoms like hallucinations or mood changes can be caused by psychiatric
illnesses like schizophrenia or bipolar disorder, they can also be caused by reactions to pharmaceuticals or by medical problems like epilepsy, hormone
imbalances, or brain tumors. When a mental symptom was caused by this latter type of problem—one that could be diagnosed with blood tests or x-
rays—psychiatrists designated it an "organic" symptom or syndrome. The
implication of this diagnostic system was that "organic" symptoms were not
really psychiatric but rather "physical" problems. The other implication was
that illnesses like bipolar disorder and schizophrenia—for which, remember,
no one could find a physical basis in the brain or nervous system—weren't
brain diseases after all but mysterious psychological maladjustments instead.

Now, of course, we realize that illnesses like major depression and bipolar disorder are "real" medical illnesses too and are caused by disturbances in brain physiology. We just aren't yet able to test for and measure the underlying physiological disturbances that we know must be there. Therefore the word *organic* has been dropped from the psychiatric vocabulary. We have new terminology to talk about patients who have psychiatric symptoms that are clearly related to nonpsychiatric illnesses. Instead of referring to "organic" problems, we now say that the patient has, for example, a *mood disorder due to a general medical condition* (the proper *DSM* terminology). Confused? A case study will help explain.

Bea was a sixty-year-old woman who had suffered a stroke about six months before I first saw her in the clinic. She had worked hard all her life as a nurse—in fact had started out as a nursing aide as a teenager, then got an L.P.N. degree in her twenties and an R.N. degree in her thirties. She had simultaneously raised two daughters, one of whom was now an attorney. Bea had been a few years away from a well-deserved retirement when she had the stroke. She lost her speech and the use of her right arm and leg for several weeks. She had been in a rehabilitation center for several months and had made a substantial recovery. But she continued to be very depressed. I had been asked to find out why.

"Mrs. Washington?" I called from the side of the waiting room. A handsome woman with close-cropped gray hair rose slowly from a chair. A smartly dressed younger woman sitting next to her got up too, though much more quickly, and turned to her. "Mama, do you want me to come with you?" Bea looked at me, then at her daughter, then down at the floor, obviously perplexed. "Why don't you both come into the office," I offered. "I'm sure your daughter will be very helpful and will make you feel more comfortable, right?" An apprehensive look came over Bea's face, then she nodded slightly.

I noticed that she walked with a very slight limp on the right and held her right arm stiffly, but she certainly didn't seem to have much weakness remaining from the stroke. Nevertheless, she walked very slowly and seemed to be clutching her daughter's arm as if she might topple over at any moment. Her slowness and obvious fear of falling seemed out of proportion to her physical impairment—and anything about a person's behavior that's "out of proportion" is always of great interest to a psychiatrist.

Post-stroke Mood Disorders

I should pause here for a moment and talk about what a stroke is. The name is well deserved. It is a sometimes catastrophic medical condition that can come upon a person like a bolt of lightning, striking him or her down suddenly, sometimes fatally. The medical term for what is commonly called stroke is *cerebrovascular accident,* or *CVA.* A stroke is caused by a blockage of one of the major blood vessels of the brain (the *cerebral vasculature*). Deprived of the oxygen and nutrients that are carried in the bloodstream, the sensitive brain tissues swell, various toxic reactions set in, and normal brain function abruptly ceases. If the blockage is complete, tissue death can occur. More frequently, blood flow is not completely blocked, or blood gets to the affected area by way of other, unaffected, tributary vessels; in these cases cell damage, rather than cell death, occurs. We don't really understand how and why some people slowly regain the function of the damaged areas and others do not. Bea had evidently suffered a blockage of the left middle cerebral artery, affecting the speech area of the brain and most of the right side of the body. (Each half of the brain controls functions on the *opposite* side of the body.) Bea had made a substantial recovery, better than most people with similar strokes.

"You seem to have made a lot of progress, Mrs. Washington," I continued. "You must have worked very hard at the rehab center."

"Mama works very hard at everything she does. Don't you, Mama?" her daughter said encouragingly.

"It hasn't done me any good," Bea said with a deep sigh. "Not any good at all. I just wish the good Lord would take me," she said bleakly, with a soft voice and dry eyes.

The younger woman's eyes, on the other hand, were now overflowing. "This is not the way my mother talks, Doctor. This is not the way my mother is. This is why we're here. We want her back."

I leaned over toward Bea a bit and touched her hands. "Mrs. Washington, I want you to squeeze my fingers in your hands. This is a strength test, so I want you to squeeze as hard as you can." I felt a feeble grasp from both her hands. "I know you can do better than that," I said. "Squeeze hard." Her grasp tightened a bit. "Squeeze harder, *squeeze!*" For just a moment her grasp tightened so that my finger joints smarted with pain. Her strength was excellent in both hands— once she put some effort into it. "That's great," I said. "I'm not a neurologist, but I didn't notice much weakness at all in your right hand. It seems, though, that it's hard for you to get going."

"Now that I'm crippled, I just can't do for myself the way I used to."

"Mama, you're not crippled," her daughter said decisively. "The physical therapist said you've done the best of any patient he's seen in a long time. And Dr. Lee said—"

"They say that to be kind, but I'll never be the same."

"It sounds like you've given up hope, Mrs. Washington," I said quietly. Bea looked at her daughter, who reached over and held her mother's hand. Then she looked down at the floor. Silence hung in the room for a moment like a fog. I leaned over toward her again. "And I gather it's not like you to give up." Bea was motionless, silent; another tear trickled quietly down her daughter's cheek.

"Well, I have just a few more questions," I said, straightening up and reaching for a notepad. "But I think we can help you with this problem."

The "few more questions" brought out all the other symptoms of major depression: restlessness and insomnia, loss of appetite, feelings of helplessness and hopelessness. But the most striking symptoms were the frequent complaints of "I can't." Before the stroke this lady's favorite words, it seemed, had always been "I can." There was no family history of mood disorders, and Bea had never suffered from depression before. Clearly this depression was related to her stroke.

But, you might ask, who wouldn't be depressed? After all, this proud and independent-minded woman had suffered a catastrophic illness that had forced her into an early retirement and had left her with a limp. Isn't her depression perfectly understandable?

This view of the matter is the one most people took in the late 1970s, when Dr. Robert Robinson began studying depressive symptoms in stroke patients. Why, people wondered, was this bright young clinical scientist spending his time doing research on something so obvious? As is often the case in science, however, taking a close look with an open mind at what seems obvious sometimes leads to unexpected discoveries. This was certainly the case in Robinson's research on the connection between stroke and mood disorders.

The first indication that the obvious explanation for depression in stroke patients—that their disabilities made them depressed—might not be the whole story had come a few years earlier, when a study appeared showing that stroke patients had more problems with depression than other patients with comparable disabilities.[1] These researchers studied twenty stroke patients and ten patients who had suffered other kinds of injuries, like a broken back or neck, that had caused the same level of impairment as in the stroke patients but without injury to the brain itself. A higher percentage of the stroke patients were depressed. When Robinson and his colleagues studied stroke pa-

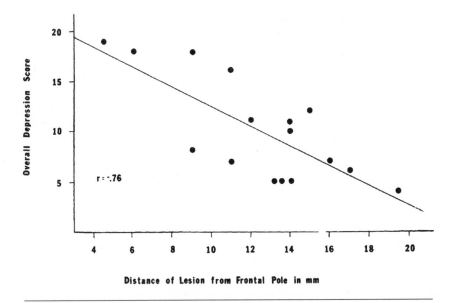

FIGURE 18-1 This graph illustrates the relationship between the severity of depressive symptoms in stroke patients and the location of the stroke within the brain. The closer the stroke was to the front of the brain (the further toward the left on the scale), the more severe the depression.

Source: R. Robinson and B. Szeta, "Mood Change Following Left Hemisphere Injury," *Annals of Neurology* 9 (1981): 450. Reproduced with the permission of Lippincott-Raven Publishers.

tients, they discovered that a surprising number of them developed a full-blown major depression eight to nine months after their stroke: 67 percent, in Robinson's original study.[2] There were other intriguing findings: patients who had suffered an injury to the *left* side of the brain were more likely to become depressed than patients who had suffered a right-sided stroke. And the most intriguing finding of all: the closer the location of the stroke injury was to the front of the brain, the more severe the depression (see figure 18-1).

These studies helped pinpoint the types and locations of cells and fibers in the brain that we now believe are important in the control of mood. Specifically, they indicated the crucial role of some structure in the forward part of the left side of the brain. This may seem odd if you remember from chapter 5 that the hypothalamus and other structures deep in the lower part of the brain are thought to be the most important centers for mood control. But you may also remember that these centers do their work by way of a bundle of fibers that project throughout the brain. It is thought that this bundle is affected in the stroke patients who suffer depression. The closer the stroke-damaged area is to this bundle, the more likely it is that the patient will be depressed and the more severe the depression will be. These fibers originate in serotonin and norepinephrine neurons, and we know that these neurotransmitters are very important in mood. Just as a single point of damage to a main electrical line can cause a whole section of a city to plunge into darkness, a small stroke in just the right location can affect important bundles of norepinephrine and serotonin fibers extending into large regions of the brain. The result is a change in brain chemistry that causes a major depression. (You might think that medication wouldn't be very helpful for these patients, but fortunately this is not the case. Antidepressant medications are very effective treatments for post-stroke depressions.)

These patients had all the classic symptoms of major depression, and they were caused by the stroke (they therefore had a *mood disorder due to a cerebrovascular accident*). But what about mania? Can a stroke cause a patient to have a manic episode? There have been a number of case reports of people becoming manic after a stroke, but mania occurs much more rarely than depression. For this reason mania hasn't been studied nearly as well as depression in stroke patients. Whereas people who develop depression following a stroke tend to have damage to the left side of the brain, people who develop mania tend to have damage to the right side. They also tend to have damage to one of several linked brain areas collectively called the *limbic system*. Although the functions of the limbic system are very poorly understood, the experience of strong emotions seems to depend on the limbic system being intact. Persons who have large areas of the limbic system damaged by tumors often experience a *loss* of emotional responsiveness, becoming listless and apathetic. It may be that stroke patients who become manic have damage to some small discrete area of the limbic system that usually exerts control over strong emotions in some way. Damage to these "damper" areas thus results in a loss of control over strong emotions: the euphoria and irritability of mania. Patients who become manic after a stroke often have a family history of psychiatric problems and therefore may have a genetic predisposition for mania that the stroke activates in some way.[3]

Mood-disorder symptoms can occur in other brain diseases that involve the limbic system—Parkinson's disease and Huntington's disease, for example. Individuals who have brain injuries from motor vehicle accidents can also have periods of depression. In all these cases, the mood symptoms are thought to be caused by physical damage to brain circuits resulting in chemical malfunctions and changes in neurotransmitter activity levels.

Mood Disorders Due to Hormonal Problems

Another broad category of "medical" mood disorders are those related to various hormone imbalances. By far the most important hormone systems in the regulation of mood are the thyroid hormones and the adrenal hormones.

The thyroid gland is located just below the larynx (the "voice box") at the base of the neck and secretes several hormones into the bloodstream. These hormones are very important in the body's regulation of energy. Thyroid hormones help control the rate of calorie consumption by the body, known as *metabolism,* and the rate at which calories are converted to and stored as fat. If the thyroid gland is secreting too much of its hormones (*hyper*thyroidism), metabolism speeds up; if there's not enough thyroid hormone (*hypo*thyroidism), metabolism slows down. This "speeding up" or "slowing down" affects emotions and behavior as well and can cause symptoms that can be mistaken for those of a mood disorder (see table 18-1).

When a person is suffering from *severe* hyper- or hypothyroidism, the clinical picture is pretty unmistakable. But changes in mood and activity level can be the *only* symptoms of mild thyroid problems. Not only can thyroid disease cause mood symptoms directly, it can also make the symptoms of a preexisting mood disorder more difficult to treat. We have already discussed the link between rapid-cycling bipolar disorder and thyroid disease, and major depression can be very resistant to treatment if there is even the slightest thyroid problem. These are more reasons why it is very important to pay attention to this hormonal system and to test for thyroid hormone levels in persons with mood disorders.

The adrenal glands sit atop the kidneys in the lower back and secrete many hormones, including cortisol and adrenaline, which are also important in the regulation of metabolism. Some adrenal hormones are often referred to as "stress hormones" because they tend to be released during episodes of fright or psychological stress and also after physical injury.

Adrenal hormones have potent anti-inflammatory actions; many phar-

TABLE 18-1 Psychiatric Symptoms of Thyroid Disease

Hyperthyroidism	Hypothyroidism
Irritability	Depressed mood
Insomnia	Drowsiness
Restlessness	Lethargy
Hyperactivity	Poor concentration
Paranoia	Slowed thinking
Poor concentration	Apathy and social withdrawal
Delusional thinking	Hallucinations

maceutical products, such as cortisone, are artificial versions of adrenal hormones. These drugs, usually called *steroids,* are a component in some creams used to treat allergic skin reactions, but steroids are also given orally and intravenously to treat inflammatory conditions such as rheumatoid arthritis, asthma, and inflammatory bowel disease. (Steroid creams do not cause psychiatric symptoms. The creams are formulated so that the medication affects only the tissue it comes into direct contact with. Only minute amounts of the active ingredient are absorbed into the bloodstream.)

Excessive cortisol from adrenal tumors can cause symptoms of agitated depression with suicidal thinking. On the other hand, hypomanic symptoms seem to be more common in patients being treated with artificial steroids for medical conditions. Mood-stabilizing medications are helpful in minimizing the psychiatric side effects of steroid treatment. There have been several case reports of lithium, carbamazepine, and valproate helping to prevent irritability and mood instability in patients taking steroid medication for illnesses like multiple sclerosis.[4]

Unlike thyroid disease, the diseases that cause excessive adrenal hormones are fairly uncommon. Too much cortisol causes many physical symptoms, including a change in fat distribution that causes a distinctive facial appearance, muscle wasting, and changes in skin texture as well as blood-pressure and blood-sugar abnormalities.

As with the study of mood changes in stroke patients, we have learned a lot about the normal regulation of mood by studying these hormonal problems that cause mood symptoms. There are complicated control systems for the regulation of thyroid and adrenal hormone production that also involve areas of the brain. Deep in the brain, the hypothalamus helps to regulate metabolism and our physical responses to stress and illness by means of complex feedback loops of chemical signals to the thyroid and adrenal glands. And you've already heard about how important the hypothalamus is thought to be in mood regulation. These intricate mechanisms linking mind and body are undoubtedly important in the regulation of the complex mental and physical experience we call mood. Better understanding of how hormone problems cause mood symptoms will undoubtedly lead to better understanding of how hormones are involved in the normal regulation of mood and in mood disorders such as bipolar disorder.

Picturing Bipolar Disorder in the Brain

For decades clinical scientists have searched for a way to test for bipolar disorder. As we have developed more sophisticated ways of probing the workings of the brain, we have been able to measure subtle differences in brain functioning in mood-disorder patients, and although none of these observations has yet led to the development of reliable tests, we are nevertheless learning a great deal about the disorder with these techniques.

As we saw in chapter 4, early researchers who dissected the brains of persons with bipolar disorder in pathology labs or examined brain tissues under the microscope found no abnormalities of brain structure and questioned whether bipolar disorder was really a brain disease at all. We now know that it is—but that's because we have learned how to look for and measure abnormalities of brain *chemistry*. Looking at the *structure* of the brain, whether with the naked eye, the microscope, or the x-ray machine, has been unrevealing until quite recently. But now two new imaging techniques are beginning to allow us to picture bipolar disorder in the brain.

The first of these is *magnetic resonance imaging,* or *MRI.* This imaging technique is based on the finding that the atoms of objects placed in a powerful magnetic field absorb energy or "resonate" at characteristic frequencies that can be measured with the proper equipment. In medical MRI scans, the patient lies encircled by a large doughnut-shaped instrument that generates a powerful magnetic field. Sensitive instrumentation measures the different resonances of different tissues: bone, muscle, fat, blood, and so forth, and the signals from each are assembled by computer into a picture. MRI is a very sensitive technique, and even small and subtle tissue differences show up with astonishing clarity.

A number of studies have shown that persons with bipolar disorder have an increased number of unusual MRI findings called T_2 *hyperintensities.* These are small areas of high MRI signal intensity thought to indicate change of water content in brain tissue. Persons with blood-vessel diseases of the brain and several other brain diseases are also found to have T_2 hyperintensities on MRI scans, and T_2 hyperintensities also seem to increase with the normal aging process. But although T_2 hyperintensities are not unique findings in bipolar disorder, they are found in higher numbers in people with bipolar disorder than in control subjects matched for age. In one study, hyperintensities were found 1.6 times more often in bipolar I than in bipolar II patients and twice as often in bipolar I patients as in comparison subjects who did not have bipolar disorder.[5]

It's not clear exactly what these signal differences on the MRI images of persons with bipolar disorder represent. Most of the other conditions in which T_2 hyperintensities are found involve loss of neurons and other brain cells and also the pathological process called demyelination, the loss of the fatty insulating material of nerve fibers. Perhaps T_2 hyperintensities are a result rather than the cause of bipolar disorder; perhaps permanent brain changes occur after many years and many episodes of bipolar disorder symptoms, and T_2 hyperintensities are the tiny "scars" of these episodes. Much work remains to be done to explain the significance of these intriguing findings.

The other new imaging technique that is being used to investigate bipolar disorder is *positron emission tomography,* or *PET.* Positrons are subatomic particles emitted by radioactive materials. The PET scan visualizes tissues where positrons are being emitted. In most brain studies, a radioactive substance similar to glucose—the sugar that is the basic energy source of living things—is injected into the bloodstream, and the PET scanner shows which areas of the brain the glucose travels to. There will be higher levels of glucose where there are high levels of brain activity; brain areas with high metabolic activity thus "light up" on the scan. The PET scan gives a glimpse of the brain at work, a *functional* image of the brain that has been a tremendous advance for researchers. PET scans have been used to discover precisely which areas of the brain are involved in particular language functions, and they have been used to investigate the operation of the brain's visual system. The PET scan is also proving to be a powerful tool for the investigation of psychiatric illnesses.

The most consistent PET scan finding in bipolar disorder is a decrease in metabolic rate in the frontal lobes of the brain during periods of depression.[6] The frontal lobes are thought to be important for complex information processing and integration and are also involved in some aspects of emotional control. People who have damage to the frontal lobes from tumors or injuries have difficulty with complex problem solving and are often emotionally dulled and apathetic, two problems that bear a striking resemblance to depressive symptoms. One unanswered question is whether these PET scan findings are unique to the depression of bipolar disorder. Similar results have been found in patients with unipolar depression; the PET scan may be measuring depression rather than marking bipolar disorder. (A related finding was reported in 1997 in an autopsy study that compared levels of inositol in the frontal cortex of persons with bipolar disorder, suicide victims, and control subjects. Inositol is a molecule involved in the second-messenger system of neurons. This study found that there were decreased levels of inositol in the frontal lobes of both the bipolar patients and the suicide victims compared with the control subjects.[7] This study also seems to suggest that there are changes in frontal lobe functioning in severe depression.)

PET scanning in psychiatric illness is still in its infancy. The metabolic patterns seen in the PET scans of bipolar patients are not different enough from those seen in controls and in patients with other neurological and psychiatric problems to form the basis for a reliable test for bipolar disorder— not yet, at least. But as with the MRI findings, the PET findings show conclusively that bipolar disorder is a brain disease with real physical changes in the function of brain areas that can be visualized and measured with the right equipment.

Viruses and Bipolar Disorder

For many years there has been great interest in the possibility that viruses are in some way connected to the development of psychiatric illnesses. Most of the work in this area has focused on the role of viruses in the causes of schizophrenia, but there is growing interest in the possibility that viral infections may have something to do with the causes of bipolar disorder as well.

Links between viruses and psychiatric illness have been sought in several ways: (1) examining birth records to determine if persons with psychiatric illnesses tend to be born during times when viral infections are more common, (2) doing autopsy studies to look for virus particles in the brains of individuals with psychiatric illnesses, and (3) testing living individuals for immunological evidence of viral infections. All three of these methods have revealed the possibility of a link between bipolar disorder and certain viruses.

It has been known for many years that persons with schizophrenia are somewhat more likely to have been born in the winter and spring months when viral infections are more common. A number of studies also suggest that there is an increased incidence of schizophrenia in children born during times of higher-than-usual rates of influenza, measles, and chicken pox. It has been suggested that viral infection of the developing brain during the third to seventh month of gestation may somehow lead to the development of schizophrenia in some people. Several studies have found that individuals with bipolar disorder are more likely to have been born in winter, suggesting that prenatal viral infections may have some role in the later development of bipolar disorder as well.[8]

Testing for evidence of viral infections by looking for viral DNA and RNA in the brains of individuals with bipolar disorder has become possible with the development of sophisticated biochemical techniques that allow tiny amounts of viral genetic material to be isolated and identified. As you probably know from the news coverage of criminal trials, DNA and RNA are unique molecular "fingerprints" that can identify individuals with great certainty. DNA and RNA can be used to "fingerprint" viruses in the same way. DNA and RNA from certain viruses have been found in the brain tissue of persons with bipolar disorder but have not been found, or have been found in lower concentration, in control subjects. These findings provide additional evidence that viral infection may be involved in some way with the development of bipolar disorder, at least in some individuals.[9]

A third method of investigating the possibility that viral infections are involved in the development of bipolar disorder is to test for antibodies to viruses by means of a blood test. Most blood tests for viral infection, such as tests for HIV and hepatitis viruses, don't actually test for the virus itself but rather for chemical defenders called antibodies that the body produces in response to a viral infection. Each type of antibody is shaped precisely and uniquely to fit the invading organism that prompted its manufacture. The presence of antibodies to a particular virus in the bloodstream indicates that the body has encountered that particular virus before. Researchers using this approach have been investigating possible links between bipolar disorder and an animal virus called the Borna disease virus.

Borna disease, an illness that usually affects horses and sheep, is caused by a virus that invades the brain and meninges (the covering tissues of the brain) of the animal and causes progressive deterioration in brain functioning and, eventually, death. The virus is not known to cause human illness, but antibodies to the Borna disease virus have been measured in healthy humans. Although most animals infected with the Borna disease virus develop the rapidly fatal brain infection, some laboratory animals experimentally exposed to the virus have been observed to develop a persistent but low-grade infection that does not cause rapid death. Some of these animals develop behavior changes that bear some resemblance to bipolar disorder: periods of overactivity and of progressive apathy and withdrawn behavior.

There have been a number of studies testing mood-disorder patients and control groups for the presence of antibodies to the Borna disease virus. Several of these studies have found that a higher proportion of the mood-disorder patients have these antibodies compared with the control subjects.[10] This suggests that, in some patients at least, a virus similar to the Borna disease virus may contribute to the development of mood-disorder symptoms. Perhaps there is an interaction between viral infection and genetic vulnerability that can result in a mood disorder. Other illnesses are known to result from this interaction of genetic vulnerability and viral infection. For example, insulin-dependent diabetes, the severe form of diabetes that usually has its onset in childhood, is believed to occur when a combination of genetic factors and a viral infection brings about an abnormal immune reaction, causing the destruction of the insulin-producing cells of the pancreas. Perhaps a similar mechanism operates to cause some cases of mood disorders.

We now know that bipolar disorder is a "real" illness and that changes in the functioning of the nervous system cause the symptoms of the illness. By investigating mood syndromes that are caused by brain disease (like stroke) or hormonal problems, we are learning more about the biology of mood. By allowing us to picture the brain in finer detail and to visualize the brain at work, MRI and PET scanning techniques are teaching us more about how the brain might regulate mood and about the physical changes that occur in the brain because of episodes of bipolar disorder. Finally, work with viruses suggests that brain physiology may be only part of the picture and that understanding the role of viral infection will also be an important part of understanding the whole bipolar story.

CHAPTER 19

Bipolar Disorder and Creativity

ARISTOTLE SAID, "NO GREAT GENIUS HAS EVER EXISTED WITHOUT some touch of madness."[1] Most truisms contain a kernel of truth, and that of the "mad genius" seems to as well. Scholars who have studied the lives of highly creative people have discovered that there are unexpectedly high numbers of individuals with severe psychiatric illness among them. Clinicians involved in this work have concluded that bipolar disorder is by far the most common of these illnesses. It doesn't require extensive research to come up with a long list of writers, artists, and composers whose biographies indicate that they probably had a mood disorder. We'll begin this chapter with a glimpse into the lives of several of them.

George Gordon, Lord Byron (1788–1824) (see figure 19-1), had periods of fiery expansiveness and hollow despair throughout his life. The recorded observations of his friends and his physicians make a diagnosis of bipolar disorder all but certain in the great English poet. Lord Byron's family history is entirely consistent with the diagnosis of bipolar disorder—suicide, "madness," and murder can be traced back for several generations on both sides of his family tree.

Medical biographers of Vincent van Gogh (1853–90) have speculated for decades about the illness that drove him to self-mutilation and repeatedly confined him to the Asylum of Saint Paul at Saint-Rémy. The episodic nature of van Gogh's illness and the acceleration of its course toward the end of his life are highly suggestive of bipolar disorder. Van Gogh described his dreadful depressions in his letters and was diagnosed with mania by several

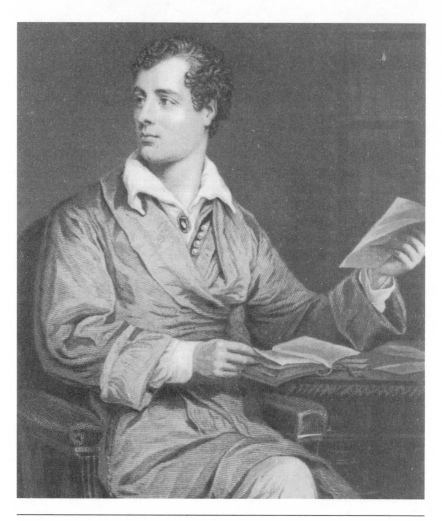

FIGURE 19-1 George Gordon, the English poet usually known as Lord Byron, suffered from severe mood symptoms throughout his life (as did several members of his family). "I must think less wildly," he wrote in his epic *Childe Harold's Pilgrimage.* "I have thought too long and darkly, till my brain became . . . a whirling gulf of phantasy and flame."
Source: Culver Pictures, Inc.

of his physicians. Van Gogh's family history, like Lord Byron's, seems to confirm the diagnosis of bipolar disorder: Vincent's brother Théo described his own struggles with depression in letters to Vincent, and a third brother, Cor, committed suicide. Doubters need only imagine the brilliant, swirling, sometimes frenzied colors and shapes of van Gogh's paintings as visual representations of his moods to clear up uncertainties as to what psychiatric illness best explains this artist's episodes of psychosis.

The Romantic composer Robert Schumann (1810–56) wrote of suicide at age eighteen, but only a year later reported, "I am so full of music, and so overflowing with melody that I find it simply impossible to write down anything." Schumann suffered his first major episode of psychiatric illness in 1844 at the age of thirty-four, but he had written a description of his depressions several years earlier in a letter to his future wife, Clara: "No one knows the suffering, the sickness, the despair, except those so crushed. In my terrible agitation I went to a doctor and told him everything—how my senses failed me so that I did not know which way to turn in my fright, how I could not be certain of not taking my own life when in this helpless condition." Schumann recovered from this episode to write some of his greatest musical works, including three of his four symphonies, but ten years later he suffered another collapse. In February 1854 Clara recorded that "in the night, not long after we had gone to bed, Robert got up and wrote down a melody which, he said, the angels had sung to him. Then he lay down again and talked deliriously the whole night. When morning came, the angels transformed themselves into devils and sang horrible music, telling him he was a sinner and that they were going to cast him into Hell."[2]

A few weeks later, probably in the grip of an episode of psychotic depression, Schumann ran out of their home and threw himself off a bridge into the icy waters of the Rhine. He was rescued by fishermen and placed in the asylum in Endenich, where he died a year later, possibly of self-starvation. As with van Gogh, biographers have quarreled at times about Schumann's diagnosis, but a glance at the opus numbers of his works grouped by year of composition (see figure 19-2) leaves little doubt that he suffered from bipolar disorder. What other illness could better explain these intense fluctuations of productivity, periods of intense creative energy that gave way to psychosis and despair?

The fact that a number of great artists have suffered from bipolar disorder does not in and of itself indicate a special link between bipolar disorder and creativity. There have certainly been many great artists, writers, and composers who as far as we can tell did *not* suffer from major psychiatric illnesses. Johannes Brahms, Schumann's musical protégé, who arguably went on to surpass his mentor's accomplishments as a composer, was as staid and steady a man as ever lived. Brahms took his dinner at the same restaurant in Vienna nearly every day for the last several *decades* of his life, often sitting at the same table and ordering the same items from the menu.

Nevertheless, several researchers who have performed psychobiographical surveys of groups of creative individuals have found that a striking and inordinate number of accomplished artists, writers, and musicians have suf-

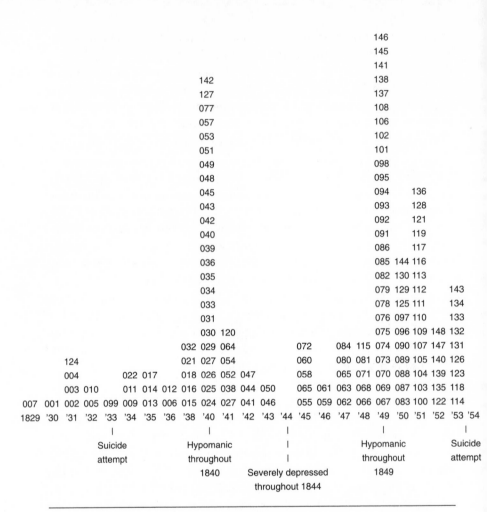

FIGURE 19-2 The severe fluctuations of the German Romantic composer Robert Schumann's musical productivity become strikingly apparent when his musical works (identified here by opus number) are arranged according to the year of their composition. Schumann died in an asylum a little more than a year after his suicide attempt in 1854.

Source: Adapted from Eliot Slater and Alfred Meyer, "Contributions to a Pathology of the Musician Robert Schumann," *Confinia Psychiatrica* 2 (1959): 65–94. Reproduced with the permission of S. Karger, AG, Basel.

fered from a bipolar disorder. Most studies have come up with prevalence rates of between 30 and 50 percent—nearly ten times the rate of mood disorders in the general population. Perhaps the most careful of these studies has been done by Kay Redfield Jamison, who examined autobiographical and biographical materials and, when available, the medical records of all major

British and Irish poets born between 1705 and 1805. Jamison concluded that over half of these writers suffered from a mood disorder, more than one-third from bipolar disorder. These numbers are so high that one can't help but wonder if there might be some bias in the research method: do the more tumultuous biographies of psychiatrically ill artists result in more biographical material being available, thus skewing the results? Studies of living writers, musicians, and artists picked by virtue of their having won literary and artistic prizes have been done to get around this possible problem—and have come up with virtually the same numbers. The prevalence of bipolar disorder is simply much higher in groups of accomplished artists than in the general population (see table 19-1).[3]

How can this striking finding be explained? Emil Kraepelin thought that manic-depressive illness could free a person from the inhibitions that might otherwise stifle creativity: "The volitional excitement which accompanies the disease may . . . set free powers which are otherwise constrained by all kinds of inhibition[s]."[4] Fear of failure, sensitivity to criticism, worry that one has nothing important to contribute—these kinds of inhibitions will, of course, vanish during periods of hypomania and mania.

One can argue that the extraordinary mental states experienced by persons with bipolar disorder provide them with rich raw materials for the pro-

TABLE 19-1 Artists, Writers, and Composers with Bipolar Disorders

Artists
  Paul Gauguin
  Vincent van Gogh*
  Mark Rothko*
Writers
  William Blake
  Lord Byron
  Ernest Hemingway*
  Robert Lowell*
  Sylvia Plath*
  Anne Sexton*
  Virginia Woolf*
Composers
  Hector Berlioz
  George Frederick Handel
  Robert Schumann*
  Hugo Wolf*

*Attempted or committed suicide.

duction of works of great creativity. As I tried to make clear in chapter 1 of this book, the clinical states of mania and major depression often bear little resemblance to normal mood states. They are not simply exaggerations of normal happiness and sadness but rather are normal moods transcended and transformed. Is it any wonder, then, that those who endure them have put such great effort into chronicling and communicating these remarkable experiences? Because of the relapsing and remitting course of the illness, a person who has recovered from mania or major depression can record what it was like. Individuals in the midst of an episode will usually be too disorganized or too lethargic to be very productive, but later, when their mood state returns to normal, they can express these almost inexpressible feelings and experiences in art, music, and poetry.

It has been suggested that the changes in thinking patterns that occur during the hypomanic and manic states are especially conducive to creative endeavor. When the thinking processes of highly creative individuals (with or without mood disorders) have been studied, it has been found that their thinking tends to be very fluid and divergent. Ideas spring from and give rise to other ideas only loosely connected by logic and convention. Unrelated ideas are merged and mingled in novel ways. Loss of logical progression in thinking and increased flow of loosely connected ideas are, of course, a fundamental aspect of the hypomanic state.

It has also been suggested that it is not any one mood state, normal or abnormal, that gives rise to the creative powers of these artists, but rather the flux and tensions between the different mood states. Constant changes in mood and temperament give the individual with cyclothymic mood changes a kaleidoscopic view of the world, always changing, always new. Perhaps bipolar disorder stimulates creativity in part because its sufferers experience the world through the emotional prisms of its many and shifting moods, some of them extreme, even violent. As the English poet John Keats observed, "What shocks the virtuous philosopher delights the chameleon poet."[5]

Individuals with bipolar disorder may be drawn to creative endeavors out of a need to understand and heal themselves through art and the act of creation. The French author and filmmaker Jean Cocteau said, "Art is science made clear."[6] When medicine and psychiatry fail to explain the inner experiences of the disease, when lithium and antidepressants and therapy all flounder and the terrible moods return again and again, people can find ways of understanding and transforming their suffering through poetry, music, and painting.

All these reasons help us to understand why this terrible and often destructive illness can also generate such intense creativity and artistic accomplishment. If creative work requires unique experiences, fluid imagination, confidence in one's abilities, and energetic excitement about the act of creation, bipolar disorder would seem to fit the bill.

But reading the biographies of these bipolar artists reveals the terrible price they often paid. Bipolar disorder was a mighty but malignant muse for Vincent van Gogh and Ernest Hemingway and Sylvia Plath, all of whom committed suicide. How many more symphonies would Robert Schumann have composed if, like his quiet, steady friend Brahms, he had lived into his sixties?

Perhaps the most intriguing question about the connection between bipolar disorder and creativity is whether or not the illness was somehow *essential* to the creative powers of these individuals. Van Gogh might have lived to paint many more paintings if he had not suffered from bipolar disorder, but would they have been great paintings? Would he have been a painter at all? Or would he have acquiesced to his father's wishes and contentedly applied himself to becoming a member of the clergy? This is, of course, an unanswerable question when historical figures are involved, but a related question poses a very real dilemma for many individuals with bipolar disorder and their physicians. Does the treatment of bipolar disorder with mood-stabilizing medication suppress creativity and dull the artistic spirit?

Several studies attempting to answer this question were done just after the introduction of lithium as a treatment for bipolar disorder in the 1970s (one of them by Morgans Schou, who, as you may remember from chapter 4, was a pioneer in lithium's use as a mood stabilizer). Artists and writers were asked whether they thought treatment with lithium had increased, decreased, or had no effect on their productivity. The results are fairly unequivocal and perhaps a little surprising. Over half (57 percent) reported that treatment of their mood disorder with lithium had *increased* their artistic productivity, and another 20 percent thought it had not affected their artistic output. Only one-quarter of these artists and writers felt that lithium had adversely affected their work.[7] Since one of the side effects of lithium in some persons is a dulling of thinking, it is also possible that these individuals were reporting the impact of a medication side effect rather than the impact of mood stabilization. Would artists treated with valproate or carbamazepine have reported the same results?

Over the years a very few of my patients have resisted taking mood stabilizers because they felt that their creative powers would be or actually were adversely affected by these medications. I have usually thought that these individuals were reluctant to take medications for other reasons: reluctance to accept a diagnosis of bipolar disorder, ambivalence about taking a medication that they felt would "control" them, and other understandable concerns that can usually be resolved with therapy and counseling (see chapter 20 for more discussion of these issues). People seize upon all kinds of reasons not to take medication; my impression is that this particular plausible-sounding reason is usually a substitute for facing and working through understandably conflicted feelings about taking medication.

The mysterious link between bipolar disorder and creativity, though unexplained by either psychiatrists or philosophers, is real. It poses challenges for patients and dilemmas for clinicians, and offers opportunities for researchers. Better understanding of this connection will not only expand our understandings of mood disorders but will perhaps lead us to new insights into the magic of artistry and the creative process.

PART IV

GETTING BETTER
AND STAYING WELL

There are millions of people living with bipolar disorder today. Many are living healthy, happy, and productive lives, but many others are not. This section of the book is intended to help you to maximize your chances of getting into and staying in the first category and staying out of the second.

If you're looking for a simple list of do's and don't's, I'm afraid you will be disappointed. Instead, in chapter 20, "Living with Bipolar Disorder," I've tried to lay out general principles that underlie the sorts of advice and recommendations that are usually given to patients in the doctor's office or clinic. I hope that after reading this chapter, you'll have a better understanding of why some of the do's and don't's that you hear from your doctor and therapist are so important.

In chapter 21 I have collected some principles for dealing with emergencies and have highlighted the types of emergency situations that in my experience patients and their families often fail to prepare for. It's so tempting to put off thinking about and planning for things we hope won't happen. In this chapter I talk about how important it is not to give in to this temptation, and how easy it is to be prepared for emergencies.

Bipolar disorder doesn't just affect the individual with the diagnosis of the illness. Inevitably, family and friends are affected in countless ways, both directly and indirectly. Chapter 22, "The Role of the Family," addresses this aspect of the illness. In this chapter I go over what family members can do—and just as important, what family members cannot and should not try to do—to help their loved one who has bipolar disorder.

We end with a short chapter that looks into the future and explores some of the exciting possibilities we hope will help us to better understand bipolar disorder, to better diagnose and treat it, and, yes, perhaps one day to *cure* this illness.

CHAPTER 20

Living with Bipolar Disorder

THERE IS NO ONE MEDICATION OR TREATMENT APPROACH FOR BIPOLAR disorder that works for everyone. The symptoms of the illness in a specific person are often as unique as the individual, and treatment must be carefully individualized to each patient and his or her particular symptom pattern. This said, I think there are some approaches and pieces of advice that are always going to be helpful. In fact, the principles I am going to lay out in this chapter are in my experience indispensable to staying well and having the best possible control of symptoms.

Confront and Accept the Illness

There is no cure for bipolar disorder, only treatment and management. It is a relentless illness whose symptoms inevitably and repeatedly return to torment its sufferers. The only way to keep it at bay is for the patient to be relentless as well—relentless about getting needed treatment and sticking to it. No other piece of advice I can give is as important as this one.

Human beings have an almost unlimited capacity to explain away the obvious. People who don't want to confront serious physical illnesses can ignore and explain away even the most alarming symptoms: the middle-aged man with a history of high blood pressure who doesn't pay attention to his repeated episodes of chest pain ("Oh, it's just heartburn; must have been something I ate"), the woman who feels a lump in her breast and tells herself, "It's probably just a cyst, I'm sure it will go away." Confronting a possibly life-threatening illness is perhaps the most frightening experience we can face. Small wonder we sometimes put ourselves through some impressive mental gymnastics to avoid the confrontation.

When there are no *physical* signs of illness, no pains or lumps or dizzy spells, it's perhaps all the easier to convince oneself that the symptoms of illness are something else. I don't know how many times I've had a patient ask if I thought he or she really needed to continue on a mood stabilizer after a manic episode had resolved: "After all, I was under a lot of stress, and I hadn't slept for weeks. Maybe I just need to take it easy." As we'll see, stress can indeed play a role in precipitating an episode of a mood disorder, *but it's not the cause.* Stress doesn't make people manic or send them into a major depression unless they have bipolar disorder. Neither does drinking too much or sleep deprivation or the loss of a job or the end of a love affair or the hundred other things that you can convince yourself explain your symptoms better than a diagnosis of bipolar disorder.

People with bipolar disorder can go through years of denial and anger about their illness. I have seen patients repeatedly stop taking medication and drop out of treatment and explain their repeated hospitalizations, shattered relationships, and ruined finances in all sorts of ways: "My wife has it in for me, she put me in the hospital again." "If my boss wouldn't put so much pressure on me, this wouldn't happen." "I think you need to check my thyroid again, I know that's the real problem." Or in its simplest form: "I don't need this medicine, because I'm not crazy."

If you have been diagnosed with bipolar disorder and you have read to this point in the book, you have almost certainly gotten past a great deal of this understandable denial and anger. This is a tremendous accomplishment and signals a turning point in your recovery. (If you're reading this book to better understand another person with bipolar disorder who hasn't yet made it past denial, chapter 22 is especially for you.) But there's a gap between complete denial and complete ability to confront and accept this illness. Unfortunately people sometimes try to hold on to the notion that nothing is seriously wrong by refusing to take the problem seriously. This is especially easy and especially problematic in bipolar disorder.

In bipolar disorder the patient ultimately determines how well *any* treatment is going to work—because it is the *patient* who puts treatment recommendations into action. It is the patient who will determine whether he or she takes *every* dose of medication, or just 90 percent of the doses, or 50 percent, or even less. The patient will determine whether his or her lithium or valproate blood level is drawn exactly twelve hours after the last dose, or whether he or she gets to the lab ten hours or fifteen hours after the last dose, throwing the results and the doctors' calculations off by 10 percent or 20 percent. The patient will determine how many appointments are kept with the doctor and therapist and how many are missed, and how many are shorter than scheduled because of tardiness. It's so easy to let your guard down, let treatment lapse in little ways, and convince yourself that missing a dose of medication here or there, having that second beer, ignoring a string of sleepless nights, isn't really important. To do so is to turn away from rather than to confront this disease, and often the turning away springs from ambivalence about the need for treatment: *less than complete acceptance of the diagnosis.* Not to accept, not to confront, this illness puts treatment success in jeopardy, because in bipolar disorder as perhaps in no other serious illness, it is the patient who administers the treatment most of the time.

Imagine that a surgeon is evaluating a patient with recurrent abdominal pain. He or she has done a physical examination and has ordered some lab tests and x-rays. All the evidence points to gall bladder problems, and the surgeon decides that the best treatment among several possibilities is gall bladder removal. Now imagine that the surgeon is in the middle of the operation and suddenly says to the OR nurse, "You know, this operating room's getting awfully hot, and besides, I'm hungry. I think we'll cancel the operation. I'll give our patient here the antibiotics for another week or so. Maybe we didn't stick with the medication approach long enough after all. Isn't there some new medication that's supposed to dissolve gallstones? Maybe I'll ask Dr. What's-his-name about that. But I just don't think I want to go on with this operation right now."

Sound far-fetched? (I certainly hope so!) Well, here's another scenario: A man with bipolar disorder has driven off with the family for their three-week vacation. The family has already traveled fifty miles when the wife says, "Honey, I packed Timmy's asthma medicine, but I didn't see your medication bottle in the cabinet; did you remember to bring your lithium?" The man realizes that he didn't. "Ah . . . sure I did," he tells his wife, and then says to himself, "Three weeks won't make any difference. Besides, I haven't felt depressed or anything in a long time. This is a vacation, after all. And if I get just a little high, it would be OK; I'm sure I could handle it."

Now, what do these scenarios have in common? In both cases, a treatment plan had been decided upon, presumably after much consideration and discussion as to the best course of action. In both cases, something comes up that makes continuing with the treatment a bit inconvenient. In both cases, rather than make a rational decision about the best course of action, the person in charge of the treatment uses flimsy logic—accompanied perhaps by a large measure of preexisting ambivalence about the treatment being the correct one in the first place—to justify doing what's easiest. Add in some misinformation—there *is* no medication that dissolves gallstones; three weeks without lithium *can* make a difference, and nobody can just "handle" evolving mania—and you have a recipe for disaster. No one would go back to a physician who treated him or her this way, and no one should treat himself or herself this way, either.

I am suggesting that making a commitment to treatment means (1) being active, not passive, in formulating a treatment plan with your providers, (2) taking charge of treatment implementation 100 percent of the time, and (3) making the decision that you will do everything possible to take control of this illness rather than be controlled by it.

But can a person be "on guard" all the time? In fact, who would *want* to be? What kind of life is it to be constantly worrying about one's mental health? A terrible one, of course. But worrying all the time is certainly not what I'm suggesting. Rather, accepting and confronting this illness means deciding to do whatever you need to do to be as healthy as you can possibly be. This means sticking with treatment and being frank and open with the treatment professionals. It also means more self-discipline and restraint than perhaps you're used to; it means making some lifestyle changes that I'll call *mood hygiene.*

Practice Mood Hygiene

Hygiene is a word that we perhaps don't use in medicine as much as we should, and we certainly don't use it as much as we used to. Hygeia was the Greek goddess of health, the daughter—or in some versions of the story, the wife—of Asclepias, the god of medicine (see figure 20-1).

Hygiene, or hygienics, is the science of *the establishment and maintenance of health*—as opposed to the treatment of disease—and concerns itself with conditions and practices that are conducive to health. The hygienic conditions and practices we think of today usually have to do with cleanliness, but the word really has a much broader meaning. Institutions like the Johns Hopkins University School of Hygiene and Public Health (founded in 1916) and the London University School of Hygiene and Tropical Diseases (1924) were founded to study methods for *preventing* disease and for promoting and improving the health of whole communities. Predating them both was the Mental Hygiene Association, founded in 1909 by former asylum inmate Clifford Beers (who probably had bipolar disorder). Now called the Mental Health Association, its purpose is to promote emotional health and well-being and to lobby for better and more readily available treatment for psychiatric illnesses.

So, what do I mean by *mood hygiene?* Simply put, practices and habits that promote good control of mood symptoms in persons with bipolar disorder. Several areas of research on bipolar disorder show just how important preventive measures can be for improving symptom control in bipolar disorder. Things like stress management and lifestyle regularity make a big difference.

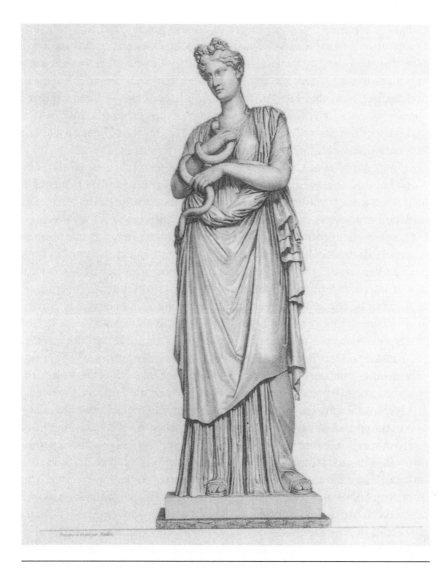

FIGURE 20-1 Hygeia, the Greek goddess of health
Courtesy of the National Library of Medicine

There is a lot of research that lends support to the *kindling* hypothesis in bipolar disorder. Emil Kraepelin noticed that early in the course of his manic-depressive patients' illnesses, their mood episodes often came on after a stressful event in their lives: "In especial, the attacks begin not infrequently after the illness or death of near relatives . . . Among other circumstances there are occasionally mentioned quarrels with neighbors or relatives, disputes with lovers . . . excitement about infidelity, financial difficulties . . . We must regard all alleged injuries as possible sparks for the discharge of individual attacks." Kraepelin was quick to point out that these events were triggers, not causes, and that "the real course of the malady must be sought in permanent internal changes which . . . are innate." Kraepelin noticed, however, that later in the course of the illness, attacks occurred "wholly without external influences," and he proposed that for patients at that stage of the illness "external influence[s] . . . must not be regarded as a necessary presupposition for the appearance of an attack."[1]

These observations have been borne out in later studies: initial and early mood episodes in patients with bipolar disorder are often related to psychological stressors, but after several episodes the illness can take on a life of its own, and episodes are more likely to arise spontaneously. This is now called the *kindling* phenomenon in bipolar disorder: a match held to a pile of wood will often start a small flame that quickly dies out, but if the process is repeated often enough, a fire is kindled, and no more matches are needed. An interesting parallel phenomenon is seen in animal experiments. An epileptic seizure can be triggered in an animal by applying a small electrical current to its brain. If this is repeated often enough, the animal will start having seizures even *without* the electrical stimulation. Seizures have been *kindled.*

Another interesting parallel in animals can be demonstrated by repeatedly giving animals small doses of stimulants such as cocaine. Over time, animals become *more* rather than less sensitive to the stimulant, and repeatedly giving the same small dose causes *increasing* amounts of behavioral stimulation in the animal. When these animals' brain cells are closely examined, it is found that a certain gene that had not been active previously had been turned on by the repeated stimulant exposure. This same gene can be made to turn on by stressing the animals—by depriving them of water, for example. This work with animals, showing that electrical and chemical stimulation as well as stress can bring about long-term changes in behavior—possibly through alterations in gene function—is thought by many experts to be highly relevant to the study of bipolar disorder.[2] One piece of evidence cited in support of this line of thinking is the observation that anticonvulsant medications, which have "antikindling" effects, are highly effective in treating bipolar disorder.

Several direct observations on patients indicate that kindling may occur in individuals with bipolar disorder: (1) Patients sometimes show more environmentally triggered mood episodes at first in the course of their illness and more spontaneously occurring episodes later. (2) They sometimes show an acceleration in their illness as they age, with episodes occurring more and more frequently as time goes on. (3) Mood episodes make patients more sensitive to stress and more likely to relapse than they might otherwise be. In a study of fifty-two patients with bipolar disorder followed for two years, those who relapsed during the time of the study were much more likely to have experienced some stressful event. In this group of patients, those with a greater number of prior episodes were *more* sensitive to these stresses: they were more likely to relapse under stress, and they relapsed more quickly.[3]

These observations mean several things for persons with bipolar disorder: (1) psychological stress can make a person with bipolar disorder more vulnerable to having a mood episode, and (2) as the person has more and more episodes, the symptoms can be triggered by smaller and smaller amounts of stress. However, (3) there may be a "point of no return" where the illness has become sufficiently "kindled" that stress management no longer has much of an impact, and episodes occur spontaneously and more and more frequently.

All of this means that one of the foundations of mood hygiene needs to be *relapse prevention.* And there should be no doubt in your mind at this point that the most effective relapse prevention tool is medication.

Persons with bipolar disorder should make peace with the idea of taking medication every day for the foreseeable future. This is an especially hard thing to do in this disease. The symptoms and the need for medication often start when people are in their twenties or at an even earlier age, when none of their peers have to bother with medication—when the only people they know who take medication are "old people" and "sick people." It's very difficult for a young, physically healthy person who's feeling well to take medication every day. The idea of taking medication to control one's moods and mental processes is also a daunting one. Remember, however, that in bipolar disorder the medication allows the patient to be in control of the moods rather than the other way around.

Each individual needs to work out for himself or herself a method for making sure that every single dose of every medication is taken. Pharmacies sell a variety of clever devices to help make this happen. There are pillboxes with built-in clocks and timers, with alarms that can be set to go off when it's time for the next dose. There are boxes that hold a whole week's worth of medication in little compartments, one for every dose, so that the answer to "Did I take my dose this morning?" is always clear and certain: if the little compartment is empty, the dose was taken. Or, ask your treating physician if your medication can be taken just once a day, or twice rather than three times a day. Ask about controlled-release forms of medications; a number are available, often making it possible to eliminate midday doses.

The body of evidence showing that medication prevents relapse cannot be argued with; it is simply overwhelming. But there is some evidence that persons who stop medication for bipolar disorder may run more than just the risk of a relapse. There have been a number of case reports of persons who stopped taking lithium for bipolar disorder having a relapse of the disorder *and then not responding to lithium when it was restarted.* Once the lithium had been stopped, it did not work very well for these patients when they started back on it, a phenomenon that has been called "lithium-discontinuation-induced refractoriness." In a series of fifty-four patients who stopped lithium, ten of them—nearly 20 percent—had a poor response when they restarted it. For these patients, lithium had lost some of its effectiveness.[4]

Next on the list of mood-hygiene practices is *stress and conflict management*. Most of us have very little control over when and how stress and conflict come into our lives. But we can learn how to manage stress and conflict better—and here I'll put in another plug for counseling and therapy. This is because I am talking about serious, *vigorous* attention to whatever ongoing sources of serious stress there may be: primary relationship and marital conflicts, job and career problems, and chronic financial or legal problems are good examples. The time of diagnosis with bipolar disorder may not be the time to deal with whatever ongoing and chronic problems of these sorts one might have. But several months later, after mood symptoms have been under good control for a time, would be a good point for some very serious stocktaking, and professional help is highly recommended.

By *stocktaking* I do not mean some process that can be described in a few paragraphs or distilled into the kinds of "helpful hints" and "do and don't" lists that you might find in a magazine article. Rather, I mean *serious examination and fundamental change.* This may involve changing jobs or even careers; selling a house you can't really afford, or declaring bankruptcy instead of struggling with an austerity budget; postponing or reconsidering marriage (or divorce); not going back to school. Just as a person who has had a heart attack would do some serious investigation and hard thinking before taking a job as, say, a high-level manager of a big company, the bipolar patient needs to go through the same process before making big decisions. The stress and strain involved in whatever is being considered should be seriously weighed in the decision-making process.

But serious attention to the "big stuff" doesn't mean that the details of everyday life will just take care of themselves. *Structuring your life* is a very important aspect of mood hygiene as well. In chapter 16 we reviewed the data and studies on the relationship between sleep and bipolar disorder. Remember that a properly synchronized sleep/wake cycle is important to the regulation of mood, and that periods of sleep deprivation precipitate hypomanic and manic symptoms. *Establishing and sticking to a personal schedule* is very important. This means establishing regular times for going to bed and getting up in the morning—seven days a week, if possible.

Research on sleep shows that many other lifestyle factors contribute to or detract from good sleep. Consider cutting caffeinated beverages out of your diet completely, or at least make a rule for yourself not to drink coffee, tea (including iced tea), or soft drinks containing caffeine after noon. Heavy meals late in the day should be avoided. Regular exercise has been shown to benefit sleep and has many other benefits as well on things like blood pressure. *Schedule* your daily walk, your Monday-Wednesday-Friday swim or visit to the gym. Don't exercise only when you "have the time" or "feel like it." Make it part of your regular week, not a luxury.

Don't allow yourself to procrastinate. Putting things off until the last moment invariably raises stress levels. Waiting until the eleventh hour to work on the income tax return and then staying up late tanked up on coffee, searching for receipts and W2 forms, is not something people with bipolar disorder should let happen to themselves. It's no fun for anybody, but for the bipolar individual, it's downright dangerous. File your taxes early, renew your driver's license early, get your car inspected early—you get the idea. Eliminate procrastination as a way of dealing with things, and you've gone a long way toward eliminating a lot of stress. This advice holds true for putting off dealing with interpersonal problems, too. Smoldering tensions in a relationship, chronic conflicts with a co-worker, neighbor, or landlord—these are chronic stresses that will inevitably take their toll on *anyone's* mental health and can exact a higher price on the individual with a mood disorder. Don't put off dealing with these problems, and if you don't know how to approach them, get the professional help you need, whether that means consulting a counselor or a therapist or an attorney.

Alcohol? As I've already said, *the less, the better.*

Some people find it helpful to keep a record of their moods, or a *mood chart.* This can be a journal or diary if you're so inclined, but simpler and less time-consuming techniques can work just as well. If you need to keep an appointment calendar anyway, it's a simple matter to make a notation of your mood every day using a numerical scale. Clinicians commonly ask patients to rate their mood on a 1 to 10 scale, with 1 being the most depressed they've ever felt, 10 the best mood they've ever had, and 5 a normal, neutral, everyday mood. If 1 to 10 seems too confining, use a scale of 1 to 100. It's important to rate your mood at the same time every day to control for diurnal mood variations. Simply record your mood ratings every day by jotting down a number in your appointment book, recording it in your computer time-management program, or marking it on a calendar you keep on your bedside table. Nothing could be simpler, and yet this record will provide you and your clinical team with invaluable information that can help show what medications are or are not working, determine whether there is a premenstrual or seasonal component to mood changes, and, of course, pick up evolving depressive or hypomanic episodes early.

All of this is much easier said than done for persons with bipolar disorder. Regularizing your life in this way may seem quite foreign and strange, not to mention boring. If throughout your life you've learned to wait for the good moods to get things done and just put off thinking about things during the inevitable return of the bad ones, this type of planning and regularity won't come easily. But a growing body of research supports the notion that external regulators like regular sleep and activity schedules help with mood stability.

Build Your Support System

Everyone should have a team of supporters and well-wishers to help him or her get through difficult times. Persons with bipolar disorder are no exception. All of the advice I've given you so far will be much easier to put into practice if you've got a team behind you.

Perhaps the most important members of the team are family and friends. A trusted family member or friend can be extremely helpful by acting as an objective observer of mood changes. One problem that persons with bipolar disorder all struggle with at one time or another is difficulty figuring out which mood changes are normal and which are not. I have seen patients go from one extreme to another in this regard, explaining away severe and obviously pathological mood changes as "normal ups and downs" while they are in denial about the illness, then overreacting and worrying that every period of normal low mood after a disappointment, every enthusiasm over a new project or relationship, means that their medication isn't working. The physician and the therapist can help with this, of course, but someone who is concerned and caring and closer to home can be an invaluable ally in this regard. An astute friend or family member who knows how to communicate observations in a caring, nonprovocative way upon noticing sustained changes in mood is one of the best supports you can have. You may need to give the person you choose permission to be blunt with you. The best person for this task might not be someone who lives in the same house with you; that person may be too close to the situation to be objective. Look around you and choose carefully.

This leads to the question, To whom should you disclose your diagnosis? Two good rules in this regard are that disclosure should be made only to those who *need to know* and to those who *can help and want to help.* The "need to know" category includes, of course, the family doctor, all treating physicians, and any health professional who might be in a position to prescribe medication—even dentists, for example. If you have an attorney or accountant who handles your affairs on an ongoing basis, that person probably needs to know, too.

With employers, things get a bit trickier. If you are asked to disclose conditions you are being treated for as part of receiving medical insurance or other benefits, then you need to disclose your diagnosis. Failure to do so can result in benefits being denied at a later date and claims for reimbursement of treatment costs not being paid. Disclosure up front can avoid a lot of problems down the line, whether this means sharing facts about diagnosis with a new employer or with the current employer at the time of diagnosis. Letting an employer know that shift changes, frequent long business trips, and late hours are things you will not be able to take on because of a medical condition seems to me to be fair to employer and employee alike. As in all relationships, basing the employer-employee relationship on openness and honesty is always good policy.

Although employers are legally prohibited from discriminating against individuals with medical problems in hiring and firing decisions, they can make life difficult for employees they want to get rid of. "Choose your battles" would seem to be good advice here. If you sense hostility at your place of work toward persons receiving psychiatric treatment, it might be doing yourself a favor to look for a different employer rather than for an employment-law attorney.

As for peers and co-workers on the job, the "helping" criterion would seem to be the applicable one, and careful consideration is necessary here. But if you find that you're telling co-workers about your diagnosis in order to get sympathy, to get special consideration, or to get out of unpleasant assignments, you're headed for trouble. There's no better way to breed resentment and conflict on the job. You don't want to develop a reputation as one of those people who use some factor beyond their control to get co-workers to cover for them in various ways. That's not building a support system; it's manipulation, and it will make things worse, not better.

I cannot speak too highly of *support groups* for persons with mood disorders. Under the auspices of several different national support organizations, hundreds of groups provide support to thousands of individuals with bipolar disorder. (See "Resources" at the end of this book for information on these organizations.) Support groups organized by and for individuals with mood disorders and their families not only provide peer support but also are great sources of accurate information about the resources available in a particular community for persons with mood disorders.

I sometimes hear a patient say that he or she doesn't want to attend a support group because "I don't want to sit and listen to other people's problems." Certainly, sitting through an hour of whining doesn't sound like something that could be helpful, but that's not what a support group is. Rather, a good support group brings together individuals who share a common problem and who want to learn from each other about coping with it better. It's one thing to ask your doctor about the side effects of a medication that you're contemplating starting, but talking to someone who is actually taking it for the same problem you have provides a very different and a very valuable perspective. Within a support group, you may have an opportunity to ask other persons with bipolar disorder how *they* told their boss or their children about their diagnosis, what *they* do to remember a complicated medication schedule, and a thousand other questions.

Don't Be a "Bipolar Victim"

Individuals with any incurable but treatable medical problem must learn how to walk the fine line between not taking their illness seriously enough and taking it *too* seriously. We psychiatrists see the consequences of not taking bipolar disorder seriously enough every day in our offices and clinics—and, more often than not, in hospitals and emergency rooms. Individuals who stop taking medication, who won't get the treatment they need for a substance-abuse problem, who ignore ongoing environmental stresses and interpersonal problems until they are overwhelmed by them—these individuals are truly victims of bipolar disorder who abdicate to the whims and erratic rhythms of their illness rather than do what they can to control their symptoms. But there's another kind of victim as well: the person who worries about his or her symptoms and illness all the time, who avoids challenges and withdraws from work and the community into a world of medications, blood tests, doctor's visits, and support-group meetings. I think most individuals with bipolar disorder spend some time on both sides of this fine line for a while as they sort out the impact of the illness on their view of themselves and figure out how to integrate what they need to do about the illness into their lifestyle. Neither extreme is healthy, and it takes time, good advice, and hard work to find the proper balance.

Perhaps the biggest obstacle to finding this balance is *stigma*. Sociologist Erving Goffman explained the grisly origins of the word in the introduction to his 1963 essay on the subject, *Stigma: Notes on the Management of Spoiled Identity:* "The Greeks, who were apparently strong on visual aids, originated the term *stigma* to refer to bodily signs designed to expose something unusual and bad about the moral status of the signifier. The signs were cut or burnt into the body and advertised that the bearer was . . . a blemished person, ritually polluted, to be avoided, especially in public places." Goffman had originally become interested in the issues of stigma, prejudice, and discrimination against physically handicapped individuals who had some immediately visible sign of their being different in some way: persons who were blind or disfigured or who had had a limb amputated. He soon came to realize, however, that the same issues were relevant, but became much more complicated, when there was no outward sign of the stigmatized condition, as in "the blemishes of individual character . . . mental disorder, imprisonment, addiction."[5]

Fortunately psychiatric conditions like bipolar disorder are not often considered "blemishes of individual character" anymore, but they are stigmatized just the same. Persons with psychiatric conditions are too often regarded as untreatable and thus unpredictable and dangerous, or at the very least unreliable and incompetent. Too many films and television programs still ridicule or demonize individuals with psychiatric illnesses, and words like *crazy* and *insane* are generalized terms of contempt that you can hear in any schoolyard during recess. Individuals with bipolar disorder have usually incorporated these prejudiced and negative views into their own way of thinking from a very young age. This means that when they themselves are diagnosed with bipolar disorder, they have to deal not only with the prejudices and unfair biases others may have toward them, but also with their *own* negative ideas and feelings about persons with a psychiatric illness. People can react to this in opposite ways, either not accepting the diagnosis and remaining in denial about the illness, or giving in to all of their negative thinking and feelings and becoming "a bipolar" rather than "a person who has bipolar illness," telling everyone and anyone about their illness and using it as an excuse to avoid responsibilities and challenges. In either case, the individual has become a victim of the illness.

How can you avoid becoming a victim? You've taken a big step by getting this book. Accurate information about what bipolar disorder is and is not provides an excellent defense against prejudiced thinking and bad decisions based on misinformation. A close second to getting accurate information is getting the support, feedback, and advice—and the opportunity to ask questions and just vent your fears and frustrations—that counseling, therapy, and support groups provide. No one needs to confront this problem and sort through all the conflicting emotions and feelings alone—and no one should.

CHAPTER 21

Planning for Emergencies

THE DECISIONS WE ARE FORCED TO MAKE IN A CRISIS ARE FREQUENTLY not the decisions we would have made under other circumstances. When an emergency arises for which we are unprepared, we are usually forced to improvise a response as we go along. In this chapter I want to identify several potential emergencies that may face the individual with bipolar disorder and his or her family and discuss how to prepare for and deal with them. One of the best ways to prepare for an emergency is to have a crisis plan ready to go.

Because we have such effective treatments available for bipolar disorder, we sometimes forget that this is a potentially lethal illness. And when you are dealing with a disease that has the potential to become life-threatening, the last thing you want is an improvised response to an emergency situation.

I could sense the frustration in Lisa's voice as I listened to her speaking into the emergency-room phone.

"I hear you, ma'am, but the magistrate won't approve a petition for involuntary treatment just because your husband isn't taking his medication. I need more information before we can—"

Suddenly she stopped and put the phone down. "I can't believe it; she hung up on me." Lisa looked down at her notepad, then turned to me. "Does the name Stanley Winters mean anything to you? That was his wife. She wanted someone to come out to their house and bring him into the emergency room. She said he's very depressed."

"The name doesn't ring any bells with me," I replied. "Let's try the computer to see if he's ever had any treatment here before. Maybe we've got some records. Then we can try calling her back." As Lisa stepped over to the emergency room's computer terminal, I glanced at my watch. It was almost noon, and I had a lunchtime lecture to give. "Lisa, I have to go give my lecture to the medical students. If we have a chart on Mr. Winters, can you order it from Medical Records? I'll be back a little after one, and we can see what we're dealing with and get back with Mrs. Winters."

It was just minutes past one when my beeper went off, with a message to call the emergency room.

"Frank, this is Lisa. Mr. and Mrs. Winters are here in the ER. Well, that's not exactly true. Mrs. Winters is here, but Mr. Winters won't get out of the car. Do you think you could come down?"

I hadn't done any parking-lot therapy for a while, and as I walked past the "Authorized Personnel Only Please" sign that guarded the door to the emergency room, I wondered who and what would be waiting for me. I walked into the nursing station and asked the secretary where the psychiatric nurse was. I had no sooner asked the question than Lisa walked in. "I went out and persuaded him to come in. They're in room 5. He's not doing too well; I think he'll need to be admitted. I'll call the unit and see if we have any beds."

"Has he been here before? Were you able to get a chart?" I asked.

"The last time he was here was about eight years ago, so the chart is on microfilm. We should have it soon, but the computer says he was admitted and the discharge diagnosis was bipolar disorder, manic episode."

"Well, that's some help. Let me go see them."

As soon as I opened the door to the interview room, I could see that (as usual) Lisa had sized up the situation pretty accurately. Mr. and Mrs. Winters looked to be in their early fifties. He was sitting in a corner, staring at the floor, and he looked as if he hadn't shaved in about a week. Mrs. Winters was sitting next to him but got up as I entered the room. "I practically had to carry him to get him into the car to come here," she said. "I've been desperate. He hasn't eaten anything in four days. We've only been married for a year, and I didn't realize—I mean, I didn't know how bad . . . I called his psychiatrist's office, but they said she wasn't practicing anymore."

It took a while to get Mrs. Winters calmed down, and even longer to get the whole story. Mr. Winters was obviously in the grip of serious depression and was barely able to talk, let alone give any kind of history of his problems.

When the microfilmed records arrived, they told us that Stan had been treated for mood problems since he was in his thirties. Our records of his treatment for a manic episode indicated that he had done well on lithium during the hospitalization. I recognized the name of the psychiatrist in the records as a colleague who had retired about six months before. I knew for a fact that she had sent letters announcing her retirement almost a year before she quit her practice group.

I was getting the more recent history from Stan's wife when I heard a knock on the door. Lisa peeked in. "Dr. Mondimore, can I see you for a moment?"

"Excuse me," I said and stepped outside. Lisa was holding the "preferred-provider" and HMO list that was posted on the ER bulletin board. "His insurance doesn't pay here. If he needs to be admitted, he'll have to go to Harris Memorial."

"Great," I grumbled. "He definitely needs to be in the hospital, but his wife had a terrible time getting him here. I don't think we should let her transport him. Can you have the secretary call the hospital transportation people?"

Lisa frowned. "Our transportation won't take patients to a hospital outside our system. We'll need to call an ambulance."

"That will cost these folks several hundred dollars. We can't use our people for a three-mile ride?" Lisa gave me her very best "I don't make the rules, I just follow them" look and said nothing. I took a deep breath and prepared to go tell the Winterses that it would probably be several more hours before Stan would be in the hospital.

People usually enjoy making plans—vacation plans, wedding plans, retirement plans. Planning for a psychiatric emergency is much less enjoyable but, unfortunately, much more important. Unlike vacation plans, these are plans that no one would be disappointed about not getting to use. But if you do need them, odds are you'll be very glad you made them.

Mr. Winters appeared to be operating under the assumption that his bipolar disorder had gone away for good (mistake #1). So when the letter came from the office of his psychiatrist announcing her retirement, he put off making arrangements to get hooked up with a new one. When the emergency came along, he had no treating physician familiar with his situation (mistake #2). He and his wife had obviously not had a very detailed discussion about bipolar disorder, about what she should do if symptoms flared up leaving Stan unable to make good decisions about treatment (mistake #3). Mrs. Winters was not familiar with the law and the procedures in their community regarding involuntary commitment of persons with psychiatric illness (mistake #4). And last but not least, the Winterses were unfamiliar with the requirements of their medical insurance plan and went to a hospital where their insurance would not approve hospitalization (mistake #5).

How long would it have taken to prevent all these mistakes? An hour or two? Maybe three? Obviously this would have been time well spent. Let's review some of the things it is important to know about in planning for this type of emergency.

Know Whom to Call for Help

I've always thought that the people who can handle almost anything are those who know when they need help and whom to call for it. Persons with bipolar disorder owe it to themselves to be under the care of a psychiatrist who is familiar with their symptoms and the course of their illness. This means establishing yourself with a new physician when you move to a new community or if any other factor, such as the retirement of your psychiatrist, leaves you "uncovered." Changes in insurance plans sometimes force a change in psychiatrists. Don't put off making an appointment to get established as a patient in a new community or with a new practice. Because it can sometimes take months for records to be transferred from one office to another, ask if you can be given a copy of your records or a letter of introduction that you can bring to your new doctor at the first appointment.

Don't hesitate to ask the psychiatrist how his or her practice is covered after hours. How easy is it to get a routine office appointment? Are appointments set aside that can be set up within a day or two for emergencies? Every psychiatrist or mental-health clinic should have some means of seeing patients within twenty-four hours in cases of true emergencies. One that does not is one to steer clear of.

Be sure you know how to contact the psychiatrist or his or her office at any time of the day or night and what arrangements are in place to handle emergencies. Does the psychiatrist see his or her own emergencies, or does everyone in the practice rotate emergency "on-call" duty? The on-call system, though not ideal, is often the standard in a practice, meaning that you may well see a doctor other than your regular one if you have an acute emergency. Are you prepared for such an arrangement in order to be under the care of a psychiatrist who comes highly recommended?

What hospitals does your psychiatrist or his or her practice have a relationship with? Does he or she admit to the hospital you prefer? To the hospital where your insurance covers in-patient psychiatric treatment?

If the answers to these questions are not satisfactory, consider your options. Ask your family doctor, family members, friends, or members of your support group for recommendations. Call the local chapter of the Mental

Health Association, the National Depressive and Manic-Depressive Association, or another advocacy group for a referral. (These groups are listed in "Resources" at the end of this book.) Sometimes your options are limited by medical insurance coverage—which brings us to another important aspect of being prepared.

Insurance Issues

Be familiar with the details of your medical insurance coverage for psychiatric illness. Unfortunately most plans treat psychiatric illnesses differently from nonpsychiatric illnesses. For example, they frequently have different and stricter limits on hospitalization coverage, the number of out-patient appointments they will pay for, and the percentage or amounts that patients must pay out of pocket for certain services ("co-payments"). Some insurance plans exclude coverage for treatment of psychiatric illness altogether or provide psychiatric coverage for an additional charge.

Do you have a lifetime "cap" on psychiatric services? This might be a limit on days of hospitalization or on number of out-patient appointments per year, or there might be a dollar-amount limit to coverage. Are you limited to or covered at a lower rate at certain hospitals or practice groups? If your insurance company denies coverage for a hospitalization or for several days of hospitalization, what are the procedures by which you can appeal the decision?

Hospital stays of all types are getting shorter, and psychiatric hospitalization is no exception. Hospitalization is reserved almost exclusively for life-threatening emergencies now, and patients are discharged as soon as possible. Patients are no longer hospitalized in a psychiatric unit or a psychiatric hospital for weeks or months. Does your psychiatrist have access to a *partial hospitalization* program (sometimes also referred to as a *day hospital*)? This alternative to traditional hospital treatment provides hospital-like monitoring and treatment during the day, or sometimes for only part of the day, but allows patients to return home in the evening and spend the night there. It is a very useful treatment option for bipolar disorder because it offers a way to provide daily monitoring of mood symptoms and treatment response without the disruption to personal and family life that staying in a hospital causes. Some insurers cover a partial hospitalization—even insist on it—but others do not. Know where your insurance company and your psychiatrist stand on partial hospitalization.

Everyone these days seems to be talking about "managed care." If you are a member of an HMO, you are part of the managed-care picture. (In a *health maintenance organization*, members pay a monthly fee to receive their medical care from the organization.) But even if you are not in an HMO, aspects of managed-care practice probably affect you in one way or another, no matter what kind of insurance you have.

Managed care means that the organization that is financially responsible for your medical care—your medical insurance company or HMO, for example—supervises or manages how much medical care you receive. This is accomplished in a variety of ways, some of which may be visible to you, some not. The main purpose of this management is to minimize your use of more expensive types of medical care, usually meaning hospitalization and treatment by specialists. In an HMO you may have to be referred by a primary physician to any specialists—including psychiatrists—in order to be covered. Lab tests may be covered only if your primary physician approves them (this can make it inconvenient to get the blood tests needed to monitor therapy with lithium and some other psychiatric drugs). If you are admitted to a hospital, your doctor may be called every few days by someone from the HMO or from the insurance company asking why you still need to be in the hospital, a function called *utilization review.* If this reviewer (usually a nurse) thinks you should be discharged, he or she will tell your doctor (and you) that coverage will be denied after a certain date and that you will be financially responsible for any additional in-patient treatment. (A variety of appeals procedures usually kick in at this point if your doctor disagrees.) Once usually limited to in-patient treatment, managed care is now becoming very interested in out-patient treatment as well, and psychiatrists are being asked to fill out forms specifying a treatment plan and requesting a certain number of office visits.

If the insurance plan includes coverage for pharmacy charges, you may not have a choice of brands of medication but will need to take whatever equivalent generic pharmaceutical the pharmacy stocks. Some HMOs have expanded on this theme and limit coverage to some members of a broadly defined class of medications, not permitting their doctors even to prescribe others. (For a while some insurance would not pay for SSRI antidepressants but would insist that tricyclic antidepressants be tried first.)

There was a time when medical treatment was controlled by doctors and patients. That time has passed. Managed-care methods save millions upon millions of health-care dollars. Some people argue that this means that more people have access to better medical care because the system is more efficient and effective. Others argue that "managed care" is an oxymoron. But whichever is the case, managed-care methods are used commonly in all types of insurance coverage now. Your type of medical insurance will almost certainly determine which hospital you can be admitted to, and it may determine which doctor you can see. Your insurance company will probably supervise the length of your hospitalizations and possibly control the number of office visits you can have, even which medications can be prescribed for you. All of this means that you should closely scrutinize all aspects of your insurance coverage for psychiatric illness, your existing policy and any new policies that you may have to choose from because of job changes. Don't put yourself in the position of getting an emergency-room surprise.

Safety Issues and Hospitalization

The most dangerous emergency situation for persons with bipolar disorder, and one that frequently leads to hospitalization, is the development of suicidal thoughts and behaviors. In studies from the 1940s, suicide rates of 30 and even 60 percent were reported in groups of bipolar patients. Thankfully, the availability of modern treatments for bipolar disorder has greatly changed these grim numbers. Nevertheless, the rate of suicide deaths in persons with bipolar disorder is many times that seen in the general population—in some studies, thirty to nearly eighty times higher.[1]

It may seem obvious to say that the most effective way of minimizing the risk of suicide in bipolar disorder is relapse prevention. But if I had said "*relapse* prevention is *suicide* prevention" in the last chapter, you might have thought I was just being dramatic. Do not *ever* lose sight of the fact that bipolar disorder is a potentially fatal disease: relapse prevention *is* suicide prevention.

Individuals with bipolar disorder should not have firearms in the home. There are any number of scientific studies showing that having a firearm in a home increases the chances of a violent death occurring in that home, either by suicide or by homicide.[2] Where an illness whose symptoms can include suicidal depression and heightened irritability with loss of inhibitions is concerned, there is never, *ever*, any justification whatsoever for having a gun of any type in the home. Period.

The emergence of self-destructive thoughts and impulses is frightening both to the patient and to those around him or her. The tremendous stigma and disgrace that have been associated with suicide for centuries still make people reluctant to discuss these thoughts when they occur. These ideas, and notions like "only crazy people kill themselves," complicate what is really a much simpler clinical issue: suicidal thinking is a serious symptom of this illness, which must be evaluated quickly by a professional and managed swiftly and effectively. Patients can be intensely ashamed of suicidal thoughts and feel that the development of self-destructive impulses is a kind of failure. Of course it is not a failing in any way; it is a symptom of an illness. It is important to see the development of suicidal feelings in a bipolar patient as a very dangerous symptom of serious illness, just like the onset of chest pains in a heart patient. When they occur, it's not time to wonder about what they mean, *it's time to call for help*. And just as with the development of chest pains in a heart patient, the development of suicidal feelings in a mood-disorder patient is often a reason for hospitalization.

Psychiatric hospitalization can be experienced as a terrible failure. Again, the clinical perspective tells us otherwise. Although we have gotten much better at treating bipolar disorder, our treatment methods are by no means perfect. Sometimes, despite everyone's very best efforts, relapses occur and serious symptoms like suicidal feelings emerge and require hospitalization. When this happens, it's not time for self-blame or questions like, What did I do wrong? Rather, it's time for healing.

Remember that the word we often used in the past for psychiatric hospitals was *asylum,* defined as "a place offering protection and safety."[3] Individuals whose will has been temporarily seized by this terrible illness and who are on the verge of terrible and desperate action deserve a place of protection and safety. No apologies are *ever* necessary, no reproach ever justified.

One more reminder: bipolar disorder can raise issues of personal safety. These issues need to be anticipated, discussed, planned for, and promptly addressed if and when they arise. Because family members are often a crucial part of dealing with these emergencies, I'll be discussing these issues further in the next chapter.

CHAPTER 22

The Role of the Family

THE CHALLENGES OF LIVING WITH BIPOLAR DISORDER ARE NOT LIM-
ited to those who have the disease. Family and friends face them as well. It's
intensely painful to see a loved one suffer from the desperate bleakness of
major depression, and just as painful and frightening to see him or her in the
frenzied grip of mania. As in any illness, the role of the family includes support, understanding, and encouragement of the person who is ill. The first
step in being able to provide this kind of support is understanding some very
important facts about the illness.

Recognizing Symptoms

Never forget that the person with bipolar disorder does not have control
of his or her mood state. Those of us who do not suffer from a mood disorder sometimes expect mood-disorder patients to be able to exert the same
control over their emotions and behavior that we ourselves are able to. When
we sense that we are letting our emotions get the better of us and we want to
exert some control over them, we tell ourselves things like "Snap out of it,"
"Get a hold of yourself," "Try and pull yourself out of it." We are taught that
self-control is a sign of maturity and self-discipline. We are indoctrinated to
think of people who don't control their emotions very well as being immature, lazy, self-indulgent, or foolish. But you can only exert self-control if the
control mechanisms are working properly, and in people with mood disorders, they are not.

People with mood disorders cannot "snap out of it," much as they would like to (and it's important to remember that they want *desperately* to be able to). Telling a depressed person things like "pull yourself out of it" is cruel and may in fact reinforce the feelings of worthlessness, guilt, and failure already present as symptoms of the illness. Telling a manic person to "slow down and get hold of yourself" is simply wishful thinking; that person is like a tractor trailer careening down a mountain highway with no brakes.

So the first challenge facing family and friends is to change the way they look at behaviors that might be symptoms of the illness—behaviors like not wanting to get out of bed, being irritable and short-tempered, being "hyper" and reckless or overly critical and pessimistic. Our first reaction to these sorts of behaviors and attitudes is to regard them as laziness, meanness, or immaturity and be critical of them. In a person with bipolar disorder, this almost always makes things worse: criticism reinforces the depressed patient's feelings of worthlessness and failure, and it alienates and angers the hypomanic or manic patient.

This is a hard lesson to learn. Don't always take behaviors and statements at face value. Learn to ask yourself, "Could this be a symptom?" before you react. Little children frequently say "I hate you" when they are angry at their parents, but good parents know that this is just the anger of the moment talking; these are not their child's true feelings. Manic patients will say "I hate you" too, but this is the illness talking, an illness that has hijacked the patient's emotions. The depressed patient will say, "It's hopeless, I don't want your help." Again, this is the illness and not your loved one rejecting your concern.

I'm now going to make things really difficult by warning against the other extreme: interpreting *every* strong emotion in a person with a mood disorder as a symptom. This other extreme is just as important to guard against. I have seen many couples in which one partner has a bipolar disorder and the healthy partner wields the diagnosis as a weapon to emotionally subdue the other. (Come to think of it, that doesn't sound very "healthy," does it?)

"Vicky's medication needs an adjustment. I'm sure of it."

Vicky stared down at the floor angrily as Peter went on. "She won't give up on this crazy idea about going back to college." I winced a little at Peter's use of the word *crazy*, a word that can make a person with a psychiatric illness feel like they've just been slapped in the face. I made a mental note to bring it to his attention later, but to do so now might make it look as if I was "taking sides."

"Peter," I said, "I'd like to hear from Vicky about this. She's been doing well for over two years now; I think it may be time to have a serious discussion about her idea."

Vicky looked up. "I was six months away from graduating from Bryn Mawr when I got sick the first time. I've called State, St. James College, and Everett, and I could get my degree with only a year of study at any of them."

Vicky was in her mid-thirties, an intense, vibrant woman who I suspected was probably brilliant as well. Peter had been transferred to town by his company a month after Vicky had gotten out of the hospital following a nearly lethal suicide attempt. It had taken three hospitalizations for her to be properly diagnosed as having bipolar disorder—after nearly ten years of roller-coaster moods. She had been treated for a depressive disorder, for a personality disorder, even for schizophrenia before she started on valproate and had a big turnaround. She had done so well, in fact, that I had seen her only half a dozen times over the past two years. About half the time her husband came along to her appointments. Every couple of months I noticed a book review she had written in the local newspaper, and on one visit she had mentioned working on a biography of Mary Todd Lincoln. Going back to college seemed well within her capabilities.

Peter sighed, then went on. "It makes me really nervous to see her up late at night looking at college entrance requirements over the Internet. And we've gotten dozens of college catalogs through the mail that she's called or written for. I'm afraid she's getting manic, and I just can't go through that again."

Vicky's eyes flashed, and she drew in her breath, then slowly released it. "Peter's not used to me being this confident and energized about anything. We've only been married for four years, and for nearly two of those I was more or less depressed. This is me, not mania." Her voice became just the slightest bit louder. "But he's treating me like a child, an incompetent." She looked over at her husband. "A lunatic, right? I'm finally getting back to *my* goals and career after ten years, and what did you call it? 'Crazy'?"

Now it was Peter's turn to look angry. "You see, Doctor? Do you see what I mean, how angry she gets? She's not usually like this. Before we came here today, she—"

"Oh, God, stop it." Vicky said quietly, through clenched teeth. Tears were flowing now.

"OK, you two, let's cool down for a moment," I said. I could sense that this was a continuation of a power struggle between Peter and Vicky that had probably been going on for weeks, maybe even months. But I also had the sense that Vicky was assessing herself accurately and that Peter was overreacting. Vicky was not being carried away by her feelings—not at the moment, at least; if anything she was showing a lot of restraint. Peter *was* treating her like a child.

"Vicky," I said, "perhaps Peter doesn't understand your reasons for wanting to go back to college."

"I admit it might seem like a waste of time," she said. "But that degree means a lot to me. I was devastated when I had to withdraw from college. I felt like a complete failure. Maybe I just need to prove to myself that I can do it. That I'm not . . ." She hesitated before spitting it out: "Not crazy."

Peter was calmer, too. "It's not that we can't afford it," he said. "I just worry that it will be too much for her, that she'll get sick again. And she gets so angry when we talk about it; she seems obsessed with this idea. That's not normal, is it?"

"I don't think trying to decide how much obsessiveness is normal or abnormal is going to help us here, Peter," I said. "It seems to me that the problem is that Vicky is investing a lot of time and emotional energy in a project that you don't think is worthwhile."

"That's right," Peter said decisively.

"But *I* think it's worthwhile," Vicky said. "Just because I have a psychiatric illness doesn't invalidate me as a person. It doesn't mean I need someone to make all my decisions for me."

"Honey, I'm just trying to help you, to protect you—"

Vicky snapped back, "I don't want to be protected, I want to have a real life."

"Wait a minute, wait a minute," I said. "I think we were getting somewhere. Let's go back to Vicky's reasons for wanting to go back to school."

This struggle between Peter and Vicky illustrates a very common problem that can come up in families in which an individual has been diagnosed with a bipolar illness. It's possible to jump to the conclusion that everything the person with the diagnosis does that might be foolish or risky is a symptom of illness, even to the point where the person is hauled into the psychiatrist's office for a "medication adjustment" every time he or she disagrees with spouse, partner, or parents. As with Peter and Vicky, a vicious cycle can get going wherein some bold idea or enthusiasm, or even plain old foolishness or stubbornness, is labeled as "getting manic," leading to feelings of anger and resentment in the person with the diagnosis. When these angry feelings get expressed, they seem to confirm the family's suspicion that the person is "getting sick again," leading to more criticism, more anger, and so on. "He's getting sick again" sometimes becomes a self-fulfilling prophecy: so much anger and emotional stress get generated that a relapse *does* occur because the person with the illness stops taking the medication that controls his or her symptoms, out of frustration and anger and shame: "Why bother staying well, if I'm *always* treated as if I were sick?"

So how does one walk this fine line between not taking every feeling and behavior at face value in a person with bipolar disorder and not invalidating "real" feelings by calling them symptoms? I think communication is the key: honest and open communication. Ask the person with the illness about his or her moods, make observations about behaviors, express concerns in a caring, supportive way. Go along with your family member to doctors' appointments, and share your observations and concerns during the visit in his or her presence. Above all, do not call the therapist or psychiatrist and say, "I don't want my _____ [husband, wife, son, daughter; fill in the blank] to know that I called you, but I think it's important to tell you that . . ." There's nothing more infuriating or demeaning than to have someone sneaking around reporting on you behind your back.

But it's also possible to err on the side of not being involved enough in treatment for fear of being a "tattletale," assuming that the clinicians will notice the same things you've noticed about changes in moods or behaviors. One of the most valuable ways a family member can help is to provide a clear, undistorted view of the situation to the clinical team treating the illness. In my experience, family members are frequently the first to pick up on subtle changes in behaviors and attitudes that signal the beginnings of a relapse. I don't know how many times I have seen patients in the clinic or even in the emergency room who reassured me that they were feeling fine, whose behavior and mood seemed normal, whom I sent on their way with a note in the chart that they were doing well, only to receive a panicked phone call from a spouse or other relative a few hours later: "Didn't she tell you that she's lost ten pounds?" ". . . that he hasn't slept in three nights?" ". . . that he got fired from his job?" Contrary to popular belief, psychiatrists cannot read minds! Become involved with treatment, and communicate your concerns openly, sincerely, and supportively—almost anything that might otherwise seem intrusive can be forgiven.

Remember that your goal is to have your family member trust you when he or she feels most vulnerable and fragile. He or she is already dealing with feelings of deep shame, failure, and loss of control related to having a psychiatric illness. Be supportive, and, yes, be constructively critical when criticism is warranted. But above all, be open, honest, and sincere.

Involuntary Treatment and Other Legal Issues

In every community there are laws and procedures to safeguard individuals who are unable to care for themselves. Laws allowing the removal of children from the care of parents who are abusing them are the most obvious example. Another set of laws are those allowing individuals to be treated for psychiatric illnesses against their will in certain circumstances. One of the most difficult things a person might be called on to do for a family member with bipolar disorder is to initiate involuntary treatment or commitment. But given the power of this illness (especially bipolar I) to cloud judgment and create dangerous situations, there is sometimes no choice but to force the treatment issue in this way. It is always a last resort, but it can literally be lifesaving.

Commitment laws are usually state laws and so vary from one state to another; in addition to these state-by-state variations, local procedures can vary from community to community. This means that I can't provide a step-by-step procedure here, only general principles. But in my experience it's not the procedures that confuse people, it's the general principles, so I think a brief discussion will be worthwhile.

Law and legal procedures governing the provision of psychiatric treatment—or any kind of medical treatment, for that matter—against a person's stated wishes are based on the knowledge that an individual whose judgment is clouded by the symptoms of an illness often does not make the same decisions about treatment that he or she would make otherwise. The delirious motor vehicle accident victim who has suffered massive blood loss may moan "I want to go home" as he or she loses consciousness on the stretcher, but the ER team will ignore such a statement and proceed to do what they have to do to save the person's life. It is presumed that if the person were alert and thinking clearly and understood the implications of "going home," he or she would not make such a request. Similar principles underlie psychiatric commitment law: treatment is given to persons against their will if clouded judgment prevents them from making good decisions about their treatment. Depressed individuals may be so hopeless that they feel treatment has no chance of helping. Thinking processes in mania can be so disorganized and scattered that seeking out and cooperating with treatment is not possible. In either case there are mechanisms to get needed treatment for persons whose psychiatric symptoms blind them to the need for it.

Fortunately these laws also have safeguards built in to prevent confinement in a psychiatric hospital for the wrong reasons. Decades ago it was very easy to invoke commitment law, and it often required only the signature of a relative or family physician to hospitalize a person for weeks or months, even years. People were hospitalized for all kinds of bogus reasons, and serious abuses of individual rights occurred. Laws became much stricter in the 1960s and 1970s to prevent these abuses. The main change was the addition of *dangerousness* as a commitment criterion. Unless an individual's behavior endangers himself or herself—usually meaning suicidal behavior—

or others, the person cannot be committed for involuntary psychiatric treatment.

Requests or petitions for involuntary commitment do not necessarily mean that the person who is alleged to be psychiatrically ill will be hospitalized. Friends and relatives cannot sign a patient in to a hospital; only a doctor can do so. The family's request for involuntary commitment usually will allow the patient to be transported to an emergency room, where a physician will make a decision about hospitalization. The patient may be released if he or she does not meet legal criteria for commitment.

Involuntary commitment is a legal procedure in which an individual is confined against his or her will and temporarily loses some rights of self-determination. For this reason the law and the courts take involuntary psychiatric treatment very seriously, and many safeguards against abuses are built in to the procedures. The person requesting the involuntary commitment must usually appear in person at the local courthouse or police station to give information and, in some jurisdictions, make a sworn statement before a judge or magistrate. Family or friends will be asked for very specific and detailed information about behaviors. This is often frustrating for those trying to get help for their loved one. They may feel that it's uncaring for them to be asked such a lot of questions or that their judgment or motives are being questioned. It's important to remember that in the days when individuals could be confined to psychiatric hospitals simply because a relative or doctor "thought it was best" for them, there were significant abuses of civil rights. When there is serious attention on the part of the issuing magistrate or judge to documenting the facts and close questioning of the need for involuntary treatment, it means that the system is working.

There is a judicial review (a "commitment hearing") at some point (usually a few days after hospitalization) wherein a judge or hearing officer determines that the commitment procedure was done properly and legally. Although this is a legal proceeding, it is not a big courtroom scene. Usually a conference room in the hospital is used, only a few people are present, and the proceedings are kept confidential (they are not a matter of public record). The patient is allowed legal representation; in fact an attorney will be appointed to represent the patient if he or she cannot afford to hire one.

Involuntary commitment for psychiatric treatment does not usually affect a person's other legal rights. Wills or other legal instruments he or she has executed are not invalidated, and patients do not become legally "incompetent" in other areas. Hospitalization and treatment are the only issues that are addressed in commitment hearings.

Occasionally I have seen individuals with severe, poorly controlled bipolar disorder whose families make legal arrangements to safeguard the individuals' financial assets in case another severe episode of the illness comes upon them. This can involve actually having a legally appointed guardian who might control access to bank accounts, prevent the sale of property or other assets, and so forth. Although rarely necessary, this is a valuable option that can go a long way toward preventing financial ruin caused by manic spending sprees. A document called a *power of attorney* can convey certain specific responsibilities and powers—and not others—and does not constitute guardianship. Careful consideration and consultation with an attorney are, of course, necessary so that legally binding documents with safeguards appropriate to the situation can be drafted.

I am aware that the topic of this section of the chapter is a very frightening one, especially to persons with bipolar disorder to whom it might seem that liberty and the right of self-determination can be taken away all too easily. At the risk of sounding glib, however, I want to reassure you that involuntary commitment of an individual is *not* a quick and easy procedure. On the contrary, in my experience most people are surprised at how difficult it is to invoke these laws, how many safeguards are built in to the procedures, and how seriously the strict interpretation of the laws is taken by everyone involved. These laws have been carefully written in the interest of helping, not simply confining, people with severe psychiatric illnesses. In my experience they are effective at doing just that.

More on Safety

Never forget that bipolar disorder can occasionally precipitate truly dangerous behavior. Kay Jamison writes of the "dark, fierce and damaging energy" of mania,[1] and the even darker specter of suicidal violence haunts those with serious depression. Violence is often a difficult subject to deal with because the idea is deeply imbedded in us from an early age that violence is primitive and uncivilized and represents a kind of failure or breakdown in character. Of course we recognize that the person in the grip of psychiatric illness is not violent because of some personal failing, and perhaps because of this there is sometimes a hesitation to admit the need for a proper response to a situation that is getting out of control: when there is some threat of violence, toward either self or others.

I've already talked a bit about suicidal thinking, and it bears repeating that people with bipolar disorder are at much higher risk for suicidal behavior than the general population. Although family members cannot and should not be expected to take the place of psychiatric professionals in evaluating suicide risk, it is important to have some familiarity with the issue. As I've already mentioned, patients who are starting to have suicidal thoughts are often intensely ashamed of them. They will often hint about "feeling desperate," about "not being able to go on," but may not verbalize actual self-destructive thoughts. It's important not to ignore these statements but rather to clarify them. Don't be afraid to ask, "Are you having thoughts of hurting yourself?" People are usually relieved to be able to talk about these feelings and get them out into the open where they can be dealt with. But they may need permission and support in order to do so.

Remember that the period of recovery from a depressive episode can be one of especially high risk for suicidal behavior. People who have been immobilized by depression sometimes develop a higher risk for hurting themselves as they begin to get better and their energy level and ability to act improve. Patients having mixed symptoms—depressed mood and agitated, restless, hyperactive behavior—may also be at higher risk for self-harm. In fact there is some evidence that mixed or dysphoric mania is the most dangerous mood state in this regard.[2]

Another factor that increases risk of suicide is substance abuse, especially alcohol abuse. Alcohol not only worsens mood, it lowers inhibitions. People will do things when drunk that they wouldn't do otherwise. Increased use of alcohol increases the risk of suicidal behaviors and is definitely a worrisome development that needs to be confronted and acted upon.

The development of serious suicidal risk calls for action. Have an emergency plan, and be prepared to use it. Don't hesitate to invoke involuntary commitment procedures if you are really worried and the patient is disputing the need for evaluation.

A less frequent but nevertheless very real risk of violence is the violence toward others that can occur in mania. Friends and family members should not hesitate to call for police help if they feel threatened. "What will the neighbors think?" should not be an issue where safety is concerned. If the situation is becoming dangerous, don't call the psychiatrist's office or the local emergency room; dial 911. Police officers are accustomed to dealing with psychiatrically ill individuals. They know safe physical-restraint techniques, and they will be familiar with psychiatric emergency services in the community. In my experience police officers will have the same goals you will in the situation: transporting the patient quickly and safely to the appropriate health-care facility so that he or she can receive proper treatment.

Getting Support

It's important that family members recognize their own need for support, encouragement, and understanding in dealing with this illness. Mental-health professionals go home every day and leave their work of dealing with psychiatric illnesses behind, an option that family members often do not have. It can be exhausting to live with a hypomanic person and frustrating to deal with a seriously depressed person day after day. The changes and unpredictability of the moods of someone with bipolar disorder intrude into home life and can be the source of severe stress in relationships, straining them to the breaking point.

Perhaps the most difficult challenge is that posed by a family member with bipolar disorder who is resistant to getting treatment. The most astonishing learning experience that medical students and interns have is with their first patient who repeatedly refuses to continue with a treatment that will keep him or her well and out of the hospital. I remember as a resident reading the chart of a bipolar patient who had been admitted to the hospital dozens of times after stopping lithium. Why on earth, I wondered, would a person make such a foolish decision again and again? I remember thinking that taking three capsules of lithium a day seemed a very small inconvenience compared with spending what added up to several years of this patient's life in a psychiatric hospital. I've since learned that making peace with the illness and with the idea of staying in treatment is much more difficult than healthy people realize (see chapter 20). But the harder lesson is learning that there is no way anyone can *force* a person to take responsibility for his or her treatment. Unless the patient makes the commitment to do so, no amount of love and support, sympathy and understanding, cajoling or even threatening, can make someone take this step. Even family members who understand this at some level may feel guilty, inadequate, and angry at times dealing with this situation. These are very normal feelings. Family members should not be ashamed of these feelings of frustration and anger but rather get help with them.

Even when the patient does take responsibility and is trying to stay well, relapses can occur. Family members might then wonder what *they* did wrong. Did I put too much pressure on? Could I have been more supportive? Why didn't I notice the symptoms coming on sooner and get him or her to the doctor? A hundred questions, a thousand "if only's," another round of guilt, frustration, and anger.

On the other side of this issue is another set of questions: How much understanding and support for the bipolar person might be too much? What is protective, and what is overprotective? Should you call your loved one's boss with excuses as to why he or she isn't at work? Should you pay off credit card debts from hypomanic spending sprees caused by dropping out of treatment? What actions constitute helping a sick person, and what actions are helping a person to be sick? These are thorny, complex questions that have no easy answers.

For all these reasons it's vital that family members go along with the patient to support groups—and go to support groups themselves even if the patient will not go—and consider getting counseling or therapy for themselves to deal with the stresses caused by this illness. Comprehensive programs for the treatment of persons with bipolar disorder are increasingly emphasizing family involvement.

Like many chronic illnesses, bipolar disorder afflicts one but affects many in the family. It's important that *all* those affected get the help, support, and encouragement they need.

CHAPTER 23

Looking Ahead

WE ARE MAKING ENORMOUS PROGRESS IN THE FIELD OF PSYCHIATRY.
The diagnosis of bipolar disorder and other psychiatric illnesses is becoming
more accurate all the time. The available treatments for these illnesses are
more effective, and there are more of them. But these advances have come
about through trial and error, not through a better scientific understanding
of the causes of these diseases. In the not too distant future, however, this situation is likely to change. Thousands of scientists are working on two great
enterprises that will eventually lead to a fuller understanding of these illnesses and to new and more effective treatment approaches.

The first of these is the field of *neuroscience:* the study of the biology and
chemistry of the brain and nervous system. At the beginning of the twentieth century, the physical and psychiatric examination of patients with brain
disorders and the microscopic study of brain tissue obtained from them after death were the only available methods to investigate the diseases of the
brain. Animal experiments complemented these studies, but this work resulted in only the vaguest outline of the organization of brain function. The
location of brain areas important for speech, movement, vision, and so forth
were discovered, but psychiatric illnesses remained so mysterious that ideas
that had nothing to do with biology, theories such as psychoanalysis, were
the only ones that seemed to offer any hope of understanding these problems.

By the end of the century, however, breakthrough followed upon breakthrough, mostly in the field of the chemistry of brain functioning, as neuro-

transmitters were discovered, more powerful electron microscopes allowed the visualization of synapses and other cellular structures, and sophisticated chemical probes allowed scientists to work out the mechanisms by which neurons grow and communicate with each other. The understanding of the fine details of how neurons develop and link to and communicate with each other through complex networks, and how brain cells and their networks adapt and change in the living organism in response to experience, continues to grow.

Now, new technologies for brain imaging such as PET (positron emission tomography) and SPECT (single photon emission computed tomography) are allowing scientists to see the brain at work in living persons for the first time. These imaging techniques can show changes in blood flow within the brain, locate areas that are hyperactive or abnormally low in activity, or detect abnormally high or abnormally low levels of brain chemicals like serotonin and dopamine. This information is revealing how the interplay of activity between different brain areas is important in the regulation of mood and is making possible the identification of the responsible circuitry. These techniques are allowing us to see how the brain of the person with a mood disorder functions differently from that of a person who does not have the disorder and, perhaps even more beneficially, what changes occur when a person receives treatment and is beginning to feel well again.

The second of these great scientific enterprises is the field of *genetics.* Here again, it is the development of new biochemical methods and molecular probes that has made this research possible. With the announcement that the Human Genome Project had mapped almost all of the genetic material in the human chromosomes, a new era in the understanding of genetics began. The discovery of new genes is announced every day, and it is only a matter of time before the genetic mechanisms of mood disorders are unraveled. But the identification of the genes responsible for mood disorders is only one of the goals of work in this field. Just as important will be understanding the mechanisms by which genes turn on and off and other mechanisms that regulate the expression and work of the instructions encoded in the DNA molecule.

As the genetic basis of the mood disorders is discovered, it may turn out that our classification system for these disorders is all wrong and a whole new diagnostic system will be needed for psychiatric illnesses, perhaps one based on the genes that are involved in individual patients. Instead of "bipolar disorder II" we may be diagnosing patients with something like "21q22 mood disorder," a diagnostic label derived from the location of a gene.

A new field within the larger one of genetics is that of *pharmacogenetics.* Rather than looking for genes that are linked to specific illnesses, this field concerns itself with genes that are associated with therapeutic responses to particular medications, an approach that promises to take the guesswork out of psychiatric therapies. The promise of pharmacogenetics is the development of simple blood tests that will indicate which medication will work best for a particular patient, ending the lengthy and frustrating trial-and-error approach we now must use to find the right medication for patients.

The two fields of neuroscience and psychiatric genetics are closing in on the causes and mechanisms of mood disorders from different directions. As these two enterprises advance, they will begin to inform each other—that is, advances in one field will lead to advances in the other. The discovery that a gene for a particular protein is linked to a mood disorder will tell neuroscientists that the protein is important in the regulation of mood. The discovery of an enzyme in neurons that is important in neuroplasticity will tell geneticists to focus on the gene for that enzyme in their association studies. Little by little the whole picture will become increasingly clear.

As our understanding of the biology of mood disorders improves, we get closer to better diagnostic methods and safer and more effective treatments. The number of new medications continues to grow, and many more new pharmaceuticals are "in the pipeline," some of them based on clues about the biological causes of these illnesses. The era of finding new medications essentially by accident may be coming to a close, and soon we will be able to design treatments more effectively and more rationally. More sophisticated use of nonpharmaceutical treatments like transcranial magnetic stimulation may make it possible to use lower doses of medications or may help medications work more quickly.

As we take the step from isolating genes to determining the function of those genes, there is the possibility of *gene therapy:* repairing the code in the DNA that causes mood disorders. The obstacles to be overcome before we can look for this type of cure can only be called monumental, even daunting. But scientists are closing in on these illnesses little by little, and with enough time and enough hard work, a cure might be possible.

As the mechanisms of illness development become known and the genetic vulnerabilities are identified, another exciting possibility emerges: *prevention.* Genetic data and a better understanding of what triggers the illness may allow the development of programs aimed at preventing the development of illness in individuals known to be at higher risk for a particular disorder.

So, there is much reason to expect great strides in our ability to diagnose and effectively treat bipolar disorder. But we have *already* made great strides—individuals with bipolar disorder must not let denial or fear stand in the way of taking advantage of the very good treatments that are now available. Ignorance is no excuse, either. Support organizations provide up-to-date information about bipolar disorder through newsletters, brochures, websites, and, most importantly, in the support groups they sponsor (see the list of resources that follows this chapter). With the ever-growing on-line resources now available, anyone with access to a computer can, with the click of a mouse, get the very latest information on new pharmaceuticals and other treatments.

Like many serious illnesses, bipolar disorder can be life threatening. Unlike some others, however, it has a unique capacity to rob individuals of their spirit, to take over their humanity. And yet, some of its sufferers have taken inspiration from their struggle with this illness to produce music and art and literature that have inspired and exhilarated the world.

People with bipolar disorder frequently ask me, Will I have to take medication for the rest of my life? I always tell them that no one knows the answer to that question because no one knows exactly what the treatment of mood disorders might be in the future. Physicians practicing in the 1930s probably could not have imagined that vaccines would one day practically eliminate diphtheria, polio, measles, and other childhood diseases, the common, frequently crippling, and sometimes fatal illnesses they diagnosed so frequently in their patients but were so helpless to treat. The astonishing developments in neuroscience and genetics hold just this much promise for people afflicted with mood disorders. There is every reason to expect that the time is not too far off when treatments for bipolar disorder will be more effective than *we* can now imagine.

Resources

SUGGESTED READING

Barondes, Samuel H. *Mood Genes: Hunting for the Origins of Mania and Depression.* New York: Oxford University Press, 1999.
   A clearly written and engrossing account of the tough science involved in the search for the genetic basis of mood disorders. An excellent introduction to the science of genetics.

Hedaya, Robert. *The Antidepressant Survival Guide: The Clinically Proven Program to Enhance the Benefits and Beat the Side Effects of Your Medication.* New York: Three Rivers Press, 2001.
   An ambitious program for avoiding medication side effects that includes prescriptions for diet, exercise, and other lifestyle changes.

Jamison, Kay Redfield. *Touched with Fire: Manic-Depressive Illness and the Artistic Temperament.* New York: Free Press, 1993.
   A thorough survey of creative individuals who suffered from bipolar disorder, and an excellent discussion of the connections between creativity and mood disorders.

Jamison, Kay Redfield. *An Unquiet Mind: A Memoir of Moods and Madness.* New York: Vintage Books, 1996.
   A powerful and moving narrative written with grace and wit by an international expert on the illness who suffers from it herself. This treasure of a book contains some of the most engrossing and vivid descriptions of the experience of bipolar disorder ever written. A "must read" for anyone touched by bipolar disorder.

Kraepelin, Emil. *Manic-Depressive Insanity and Paranoia*. Trans. R. M. Barclay, ed. G. M. Robertson. 1921; reprint, New York: Arno Press, 1976.

Many college and university libraries have a copy of this book. Arguably the very first textbook on the illness ever written, it is definitely worth reading.

Miklowitz, David. *The Bipolar Disorder Survival Guide: What You and Your Family Need to Know*. New York: Guilford Press, 2002.

This book emphasizes the patient's role in managing bipolar disorder symptoms, in simple and easy-to-understand terms. A good introduction.

Mondimore, Francis Mark. *Adolescent Depression: A Guide for Parents*. Baltimore: Johns Hopkins University Press, 2002.

OK, I'm biased in favor of this one. But if you're looking for a book that focuses on the diagnosis and treatment of, and coping with, mood disorders (including bipolar disorder) in young people, I think this is the one to buy!

Rosenthal, Norman E. *Winter Blues: Seasonal Affective Disorder, What It Is and How to Overcome It*. New York: Guilford Press, 1993.

A comprehensive and highly readable discussion of seasonal affective disorder.

Styron, William. *Darkness Visible: A Memoir of Madness*. New York: Random House, 1990.

I recommend this book to medical students as one of the best accounts of the symptoms of depression available. A good book for family members to read to better understand the experience of serious depression.

SUPPORT AND ADVOCACY ORGANIZATIONS

All of the following organizations provide information and resources, and many offer referrals to support groups as well as to clinicians in your community who are skilled in treating mood disorders. Contact them all and become a member! In addition to the direct services they provide to consumers, they are active in combating the stigmatization of psychiatric illnesses, in lobbying for better medical insurance coverage for psychiatric disorders, and in supporting research.

Depression and Bipolar Support Alliance (DBSA)
730 North Franklin Street
Chicago, IL 60610
800-82-NDMDA
www.dbsalliance.org

The Depression and Related Affective Disorders Association (DRADA)
2330 West Joppa Road, Suite 100
Lutherville, MD 21093
410-583-2919
www.drada.org

National Alliance for the Mentally Ill (NAMI)
Colonial Place 3
2107 Wilson Blvd., Suite 300
Arlington, VA 22201
800-950-6264
www.nami.org

The National Foundation for Depressive Illness, Inc.
P.O. Box 2257
New York, NY 10116
800-239-1265
www.depression.org

National Mental Health Association (NMHA)
2001 N. Beauregard Street
12th Floor
Alexandria, VA 22311
800-969-NMHA
www.nmha.org

INTERNET RESOURCES

All of the support and advocacy groups listed in the previous section have sites on the World Wide Web, and the astonishing range of resources on the Internet continues to grow. Remember, however, that there are also inaccurate information, bias, and just plain nonsense on the Internet, and that it's important to consider information sources very carefully.

Here are some excellent resources:

The American Psychiatric Press, Inc.
www.appi.org
> Access to several of the most important and influential professional publications for psychiatrists: the *American Journal of Psychiatry,* the *Journal of Neuropsychiatry and Clinical Neurosciences,* and others (scientific publications written for physicians and scientists).

Internet Mental Health
www.mentalhealth.com
> An excellent site with information on many different disorders and their treatments, information on many psychiatric medications, and hundreds of reference articles from popular and professional publications.

Medscape
www.medscape.com
> This is primarily a news site for medical professionals, but it also has a "patient information" section with many useful articles and links to other resources.

Moodswing.org

www.moodswing.org

> Many resources on bipolar disorder, including reading materials, an "FAQ" (frequently asked questions) section on bipolar disorder, and links to many other sources.

Pendulum Resources

www.pendulum.org

> Another storehouse of information on bipolar disorder with an on-line bookstore and links to other useful sites.

PubMed

www.ncbi.nlm.nih.gov/entrez/query.fcgi

> Free access to the most comprehensive medical database in the world, maintained by the U.S. National Library of Medicine. Anyone can use PubMed to search through fifteen million scientific journal citations on any and every medical topic. The vast majority of the citations include an abstract of the article (a short summary), and your local public library can often help you obtain a copy of the complete text.

Support Group.com

www.supportpath.com

> Dozens of pages on different disorders, including several on bipolar disorder. Bulletin boards and "chats" for patients, for significant others, and "Bipolar Teens." Well-organized and, judging from the number of people leaving messages, a popular and useful resource for a lot of people.

WebMD

www.webmd.com

> One of the best sources of information on just about any medical problem. Organized into "Condition Centers," including ones for bipolar disorder and depression, that pull together many resources for common illnesses.

Notes

1. For a discussion of the diagnosis of bipolar disorder in these historical personalities, see Kay Redfield Jamison, *Touched with Fire: Manic-Depressive Illness and the Artistic Temperament* (New York: Free Press, 1993).

2. Gabor Keitner, Ivan Miller, M. Tracie Shea, and Martin Keller, "Course of Illness and Maintenance Treatments for Patients with Bipolar Disorder," *Journal of Clinical Psychiatry* 56, no. 1 (1995): 5–13.

3. "National Survey of NDMDA Members Finds Long Delay in Diagnosis of Manic-Depressive Illness," in "News and Notes," *Hospital and Community Psychiatry* 44, no. 8 (1993): 800–801.

4. Frederick K. Goodwin and Kay Redfield Jamison, *Manic-Depressive Illness* (New York: Oxford University Press, 1990), 228.

CHAPTER 1. NORMAL AND ABNORMAL MOOD

1. *Webster's Ninth New Collegiate Dictionary,* ed. Frederick C. Mish (Springfield, Mass.: Merriam-Webster, 1984).

2. Although I have made these clinical vignettes as realistic as possible by using symptom details culled from many patients, they are fictitious and do not portray any person living or dead.

3. The word *mania* has very ancient origins, deriving from the Greek word *mainesthai,* which means simply "to be insane." Very early English physicians sometimes used the word *madness* to describe the syndrome of disorganized hyperactivity that we now call mania. But during the eighteenth and nineteenth centuries, European physicians writing about mental disorders increasingly used the term *mania*

(in French *la manie* and in German *die Manie*). When Emil Kraepelin used the term *manic-depressive insanity* in his ground-breaking work on bipolar disorder, the use of the term *mania* for the excited phase of the disorder became firmly established.

4. Henry J. Berkley, *A Treatise on Mental Diseases* (1900; reprint, New York: Arno Press, 1980), 143.

5. Kay Redfield Jamison, *An Unquiet Mind: A Memoir of Moods and Madness* (New York: Vintage Books, 1996), 36.

6. Frederick K. Goodwin and Kay Redfield Jamison, *Manic-Depressive Illness* (New York: Oxford University Press, 1990), 23.

7. Quoted in ibid., 26–27.

8. Emil Kraepelin, *Manic-Depressive Insanity and Paranoia,* trans. R. M. Barclay, ed. G. M. Robertson (1921; reprint, New York: Arno Press, 1976), 31. This is a translation of volumes 3 and 4 of the eighth edition (1913) of Kraepelin's textbook *Psychiatrie,* which originally appeared in 1896.

9. Goodwin and Jamison, *Manic-Depressive Illness,* 29.

10. Kraepelin, *Manic-Depressive Insanity,* 31.

11. For a discussion of the concept of motivated behaviors in psychiatry, see Paul McHugh and Philip Slavney, *The Perspectives of Psychiatry* (Baltimore: Johns Hopkins University Press, 1986), 105–7.

12. Kraepelin, *Manic-Depressive Insanity,* 62.

13. Ibid., 56, 64.

14. J. D. Campbell, *Manic-Depressive Disease: Clinical and Psychiatric Significance* (Philadelphia: J. D. Lippincott, 1953), 159–60, quoted in Goodwin and Jamison, *Manic-Depressive Illness,* 24.

15. Jamison, *Unquiet Mind,* 83.

16. Kraepelin, *Manic-Depressive Insanity,* 70.

17. Berkley, *Treatise on Mental Diseases,* 160.

18. Gabrielle Carlson and Frederick Goodwin, "The Stages of Mania," *Archives of General Psychiatry* 28 (1973): 221–28.

19. Quoted in Edward Hare, "The Two Manias: Study of the Evolution of the Modern Concept of Mania," *British Journal of Psychiatry* 138 (1981): 89–99.

20. Norman Endler, *Holiday of Darkness: A Psychologist's Personal Journey out of His Depression* (New York: John Wiley and Sons, 1982), 4.

21. Ibid., 86.

22. William Styron, *Darkness Visible: A Memoir of Madness* (New York: Random House, 1990), 19.

23. Endler, *Holiday of Darkness,* 48–49.

24. Johann Wolfgang von Goethe, *The Sorrows of Young Werther,* trans. Elizabeth Mayer and Louise Bogan (New York: Random House, 1971), 114.

25. Quoted in Kay Redfield Jamison, *Touched with Fire: Manic-Depressive Illness and the Artistic Temperament* (New York: Free Press, 1993), 21.

26. Styron, *Darkness Visible,* 17.

27. Endler, *Holiday of Darkness,* 29.

28. Kraepelin, *Manic-Depressive Insanity,* 75.

29. F. Scott Fitzgerald, *The Crackup* (New York: New Directions, 1956), 75.

30. Styron, *Darkness Visible*, 17.

31. Endler, *Holiday of Darkness*, 54.

32. Styron, *Darkness Visible*, 44.

33. Endler, *Holiday of Darkness*, 46.

34. Kraepelin, *Manic-Depressive Insanity*, 84.

35. Ibid., 89.

36. Styron, *Darkness Visible*, 58.

37. Kraepelin, *Manic-Depressive Insanity*, 97.

38. Jamison, *Unquiet Mind*, 45.

39. Kraepelin, *Manic-Depressive Insanity*, 104.

40. Because some patients in an otherwise typical manic episode develop desperate, anxious, distraught symptoms as they become sicker, some researchers have made the case that mixed states can be thought of as a very severe stage of mania ("stage III mania" as described above in the section "The Manic Syndrome").

41. Kraepelin, *Manic-Depressive Insanity*, 99.

CHAPTER 2. THE DIAGNOSIS OF BIPOLAR DISORDER

Epigraph: Emil Kraepelin, *Manic-Depressive Insanity and Paranoia*, trans. R. M. Barclay, ed. G. M. Robertson (1921; reprint, New York: Arno Press, 1976), 193.

1. Frederick K. Goodwin and Kay Redfield Jamison, *Manic-Depressive Illness* (New York: Oxford University Press, 1990), 132.

2. Modern diagnostic classifications are usually different from those that were used when these older studies were done. In most cases, however, patients with "manic-depressive illness" in these studies had full-blown manic episodes and severe depressions and thus would today probably be diagnosed with bipolar I. Nevertheless, cases that would today be diagnosed differently (as bipolar II, for example) may have been mixed in. Thus, the findings and statistics must be interpreted with some caution.

3. Thomas A. C. Rennie, "Prognosis in Manic-Depressive Psychosis," *American Journal of Psychiatry* 98 (1942): 801–14, quoted in Goodwin and Jamison, *Manic-Depressive Illness*, 133.

4. Kraepelin, *Manic-Depressive Insanity*, 136.

5. Ibid., 3, 137.

6. G. Winokur, P. Clayton, and T. Reich, *Manic-Depressive Illness* (St. Louis: C. V. Mosby, 1969), quoted in Goodwin and Jamison, *Manic-Depressive Illness*, 141.

7. Athansio Koukopoulas, Daniela Reginaldi, Giampolo Minnai, Gino Serre, Luca Pani, and Neil Johnson, "The Long Term Prophylaxis of Affective Disorders," in *Depression and Mania: From Neurobiology to Treatment*, ed. G. Gessa, W. Fratta, L. Pina, and G. Serre (New York: Raven Press, 1995), 127–47.

8. William Coryell, Nancy Andreasen, Jean Endicott, and Martin Keller, "The Significance of Past Mania or Hypomania in the Course and Outcome of Major Depression," *American Journal of Psychiatry* 144 (1987): 309–15.

9. G. Cassano, H. Akiskal, M. Savina, L. Musetti, and G. Perugi, "Proposed Subtypes of Bipolar II and Related Disorders: With Hypomanic Episodes (or Cyclothymia) and with Hyperthymic Temperament," *Journal of Affective Disorders* 26 (1992): 127–40.

10. See Sylvia Simpson, Susan Folstein, Deborah Meyers, Francis McMahon, Diane Brusco, and J. Raymond DePaulo, "Bipolar II: The Most Common Bipolar Phenotype?" *American Journal of Psychiatry* 150 (1993): 901–3.

11. Hagop Akiskal, Jack Maser, Pamela Zeller, Jean Endicott, William Coryell, Martin Keller, Meredith Warshaw, Paula Clayton, and Frederick Goodwin, "Switching from 'Unipolar' to Bipolar II: An Eleven-Year Prospective Study of Clinical and Temperamental Predictors in 559 Patients," *Archives of General Psychiatry* 52 (1995): 114–23.

12. Goodwin and Jamison, *Manic-Depressive Illness*, 69.

13. Simpson, Folstein, Meyers, McMahon, Brusco, and DePaulo, "Bipolar II: The Most Common Bipolar Phenotype?"

14. Kraepelin, *Manic-Depressive Insanity*, 131.

15. Hagop S. Akiskal, "The Prevalent Clinical Spectrum of Bipolar Disorders: Beyond DSM-IV," *Journal of Clinical Psychopharmacology* 16, suppl. (1996): 4S–14S.

16. Kraepelin, *Manic-Depressive Insanity*, 132.

17. H. Akiskal, M. K. Khani, and A. Scott-Strauss, "Cyclothymic Temperamental Disorders," *Psychiatric Clinics of North America* 2 (1979): 527–54.

18. Robert Howland and Michael Thase, "A Comprehensive Review of Cyclothymic Disorder," *Journal of Nervous and Mental Disease* 181 (1993): 485–93.

19. Akiskal, "Prevalent Clinical Spectrum of Bipolar Disorders."

20. Howland and Thase, "Comprehensive Review of Cyclothymic Disorder."

21. Kraepelin, *Manic-Depressive Insanity*, 2.

22. Hagop Akiskal and Gopinath Mallya, "Criteria for 'Soft' Bipolar Spectrum: Treatment Implications," *Psychopharmacology Bulletin* 23, no. 1 (1987): 68–73.

23. Akiskal, "Prevalent Clinical Spectrum of Bipolar Disorders."

24. American Psychiatric Association, *Diagnostic and Statistical Manual of Mental Disorders*, 4th ed. (Washington, D.C.: American Psychiatric Association, 1994), 390–91.

25. See Goodwin and Jamison, *Manic-Depressive Illness*, 136–38.

26. R. W. Cowdry, T. A. Wehr, A. Zis, and F. K. Goodwin, "Thyroid Abnormalities Associated with Rapid Cycling Bipolar Illness," *Archives of General Psychiatry* 40 (1983): 414–20, and T. A. Wehr and F. K. Goodwin, "Rapid Cycling in Manic-Depressives Induced by Tricyclic Antidepressants," *Archives of General Psychiatry* 36 (1979): 555–59.

27. A. Koukopoulos, B. Caliari, A. Tundo, G. Floris, D. Reginaldi, and L. Tondo, "Rapid Cyclers, Temperament, and Antidepressants," *Comprehensive Psychiatry* 24, no. 3 (1983): 249–58.

28. William Coryell, Jean Endicott, and Martin Keller, "Rapid Cycling Bipolar Disorder: Demographics, Diagnosis, Family History, and Course," *Archives of General Psychiatry* 49 (1992): 126–31.

CHAPTER 3. A SUMMARY OF THE DIAGNOSTIC CATEGORIES
OF BIPOLAR DISORDER IN *DSM IV*

1. American Psychiatric Association, *Diagnostic and Statistical Manual of Mental Disorders*, 4th ed. (Washington, D.C.: American Psychiatric Association, 1994), xvii. Note that "epilepsy" was at the time considered to be a mental illness.

2. Alfred Kinsey, Wardell Pomeroy, and Clyde Martin, *Sexual Behavior in the Human Male* (Philadelphia: W. B. Saunders, 1948), 678, 639.

CHAPTER 4. THE MOOD DISEASE

1. Quoted in Stanley W. Jackson, *Melancholia and Depression, from Hippocratic Times to Modern Times* (New Haven: Yale University Press, 1986), 251 ("peevish," "complain[ed]," "At the height"), and in Frederick K. Goodwin and Kay Redfield Jamison, *Manic-Depressive Illness* (New York: Oxford University Press, 1990), 58 ("in my opinion").

2. Quoted in Jackson, *Melancholia and Depression,* 253–54.

3. Quoted in ibid., 257.

4. See ibid., 262–63.

5. Emil Kraepelin, *Manic-Depressive Insanity and Paranoia,* trans. R. M. Barclay, ed. G. M. Robertson (1921; reprint, New York: Arno Press, 1976), 1.

6. Jackson, *Melancholia and Depression,* 272.

7. Henry J. Berkley, *A Treatise on Mental Disorders* (1900; reprint, New York: Arno Press, 1980), 179.

8. John F. J. Cade, "Lithium Salts in the Treatment of Psychotic Excitement," *Medical Journal of Australia* 36 (1949): 349–52.

9. Ibid., 350–51.

10. For a superb account of this shameful story, see Götz Aly, Peter Chroust, and Christian Pross, *Cleansing the Fatherland: Nazi Medicine and Racial Hygiene* (Baltimore: Johns Hopkins University Press, 1994).

11. Ronald R. Fieve, *Moodswing: The Third Revolution in Psychiatry* (New York: Bantam Books, 1975), 3.

12. M. Schou, N. Juel-Nielsen, E. Strömgren, and H. Voldby, "The Treatment of Manic Psychoses by the Administration of Lithium Salts," *Journal of Neurology, Neurosurgery, and Psychiatry* 17 (1954): 250–60.

13. Roland Kuhn, "The Treatment of Depressive States with G 22355 (Imipramine Hydrochloride)," *American Journal of Psychiatry* 115 (1958): 459–64, at 461.

14. Schou, Juel-Nielsen, Strömgren, and Voldby, "Treatment of Manic Psychoses by the Administration of Lithium Salts," 256. Emphasis added.

CHAPTER 5. THE BRAIN: NEURONS, NEUROTRANSMITTERS, AND MORE

1. Nancy C. Andreasen, *The Broken Brain: The Biological Revolution in Psychiatry* (New York: Harper and Row, 1985).

2. I. C. Reid and C. A. Stewart, "How Antidepressants Work: New Perspectives on the Pathophysiology of Depressive Disorder," *British Journal of Psychiatry* 178 (2001): 299–303.

CHAPTER 6. MOOD-STABILIZING MEDICATIONS

1. Anastase Georgotas and Samuel Gershon, "Historical Perspectives and Current Highlights on Lithium Treatment in Manic-Depressive Illness," *Journal of Clinical Psychopharmacology* 1, no. 1 (1981): 27–31.

2. Paul Baalstrup and Morgans Schou, "Lithium as a Prophylactic Agent: Its Effect against Recurrent Depressions and Manic-Depressive Psychosis," *Archives of General Psychiatry* 16, no. 2 (1967): 162–72.

3. B. Blackwell and M. Shephard, "Prophylactic Lithium: Another Therapeutic Myth?" *Lancet* 1 (1968): 968–71.

4. P. Baalstrup, J. Poulsen, M. Schou, K. Thomsen, and A. Amdisen, "Prophylactic Lithium: Double-Blind Discontinuation in Manic and Recurrent-Depressive Disorders," *Lancet* 2 (1970): 326–30.

5. American Psychiatric Association, "Practice Guidelines for the Treatment of Bipolar Disorder," *American Journal of Psychiatry* 151, suppl. (1994): 6.

6. To be more precise, the therapeutic index is the ratio of the largest dose producing no toxic symptoms to the smallest dose routinely producing the desired therapeutic effects.

7. Alan Gelenberg, John Kane, Martin Keller, Phillip Lavori, Jerrold Rosenbaum, Karyl Cole, and Janet Lavelle, "Comparison of Standard and Low Levels of Lithium for Maintenance Treatment of Bipolar Disorder," *New England Journal of Medicine* 321, no. 22 (1989): 1489–93.

8. Morgans Schou, "Forty Years of Lithium Treatment," *Archives of General Psychiatry* 54 (1997): 9–13.

9. Ibid., 11.

10. For an excellent review, see M. Gitlin, "Lithium and the Kidney: An Updated Review," *Drug Safety* 20, no. 3 (1999): 231–43.

11. American Psychiatric Association, "Practice Guidelines for the Treatment of Bipolar Disorder," 7.

12. Frederick K. Goodwin and Kay Redfield Jamison, *Manic-Depressive Illness* (New York: Oxford University Press, 1990), 707.

13. See Charles Bowden and Susan McElroy, "History of the Development of Valproate for the Treatment of Bipolar Disorder," *Journal of Clinical Psychiatry* 56, suppl. 3 (1995): 3–5.

14. American Psychiatric Association, "Practice Guidelines for the Treatment of Bipolar Disorder," 9.

15. Paul Keck, Azmi Nabulsi, Jennifer Taylor, Curtis Henke, Joseph Chmiel, Sean Stanton, and Jerry Bennett, "A Pharmaco-economic Model of Divalproex versus Lithium in the Acute and Prophylactic Treatment of Bipolar I Disorder," *Journal of Clinical Psychiatry* 57, no. 5 (1996): 213–22.

16. Susan McElroy, Paul Keck, Karen Tugrul, and Jerry Bennett, "Valproate as a Loading Treatment in Acute Mania," *Neuropsychobiology* 27 (1993): 146–49.

17. Charles L. Bowden, "Predictors of Response to Divalproex and Lithium," *Journal of Clinical Psychiatry* 56, suppl. 3 (1995): 25–29.

18. Susan McElroy, Paul Keck, Harrison Pope, and James Hudson, "Valproate in Psychiatric Disorders: Literature Review and Clinical Guidelines," *Journal of Clinical Psychiatry* 50, suppl. 3 (1989): 23–29.

19. American Psychiatric Association, "Practice Guidelines for the Treatment of Bipolar Disorder," 21. See also Alan Swann, Charles Bowden, David Morris, Joseph Calabrese, Frederick Petty, Joyce Small, Steven Dilsaver, and John Davis, "Depression

during Mania: Treatment Response to Lithium or Divalproex," *Archives of General Psychiatry* 54 (1997): 37–42.

20. American Psychiatric Association, "Practice Guidelines for the Treatment of Bipolar Disorder," 10.

21. See Frederick Jacobsen, "Low-Dose Valproate: A New Treatment for Cyclothymia, Mild Rapid-Cycling Disorders, and Premenstrual Syndrome," *Journal of Clinical Psychiatry* 54, no. 6 (1993): 229–34. Also J. A. Delito, "The Effect of Valproate on Bipolar Spectrum Temperamental Disorders," *Journal of Clinical Psychiatry* 54, no. 8 (1993): 300–304.

22. Gary Sachs, "Bipolar Mood Disorder: Practical Strategies for Acute and Maintenance Phase Treatment," *Journal of Clinical Psychopharmacology* 16, no. 2, suppl. 1 (1996): 32S– 47S.

23. J. C. Ballenger and R. M. Post, "Carbamazepine in Manic-Depressive Illness: A New Treatment," *American Journal of Psychiatry* 137, no. 7 (1980): 782–90.

24. B. Lerer, M. Moore, E. Meyendorff, S. R. Cho, and S. Gershon, "Carbamazepine versus Lithium in Mania: A Double-Blind Study," *Journal of Clinical Psychiatry* 48, no. 3 (1987): 89–93.

25. Robert Post, Thomas Uhde, James Ballenger, and Kathleen Squillace, "Prophylactic Efficacy of Carbamazepine in Manic-Depressive Illness," *American Journal of Psychiatry* 140, no. 12 (1983): 1602–4.

26. R. H. Weisler, A. H. Kalali, and T. A. Ketter, "A Multicenter, Randomized, Double-Blind, Placebo-Controlled Trial of Extended-Release Carbamazepine Capsules as Monotherapy for Bipolar Disorder Patients with Manic or Mixed Episodes," *Journal of Clinical Psychiatry* 65, no. 4 (2004): 478–84.

27. F. Centorrino, M. J. Albert, J. M. Berry, J. P. Kelleher, V. Fellman, G. Line, A. E. Koukopoulos, J. E. Kidwell, K. V. Fogarty, and R. J. Baldessarini, "Oxcarbazepine: Clinical Experience with Hospitalized Psychiatric Patients," *Bipolar Disorders* 5, no. 5 (2003): 370–74.

28. Jonathan Sporn and Gary Sachs, "The Anticonvulsant Lamotrigine in Treatment-Resistant Manic-Depressive Illness," *Journal of Clinical Psychopharmacology* 17, no. 3 (1997): 185–89.

29. Joseph R. Calabrese, S. Hossein Fatemi, and Mark J. Woyshville, "Antidepressant Effects of Lamotrigine in Rapid Cycling Bipolar Disorder," *American Journal of Psychiatry* 153, no. 9 (1996): 1236.

30. C. L. Bowden, J. R. Calabrese, G. Sachs, L. N. Yatham, S. A. Asghar, M. Hompland, P. Montgomery, N. Earl, T. M. Smoot, and J. DeVeaugh-Geiss (Lamictal 606 Study Group), "A Placebo-Controlled 18-Month Trial of Lamotrigine and Lithium Maintenance Treatment in Recently Manic or Hypomanic Patients with Bipolar I Disorder," *Archives of General Psychiatry* 60, no. 4 (2003): 392.

31. J. R. Calabrese, C. L. Bowden, G. Sachs, L. N. Yatham, K. Behnke, O. P. Mehtonen, P. Montgomery, J. Ascher, W. Paska, N. Earl, and J. DeVeaugh-Geiss (Lamictal 605 Study Group), "A Placebo-Controlled 18-Month Trial of Lamotrigine and Lithium Maintenance Treatment in Recently Depressed Patients with Bipolar I Disorder," *Journal of Clinical Psychiatry* 64, no. 9 (2003): 1013–24.

32. G. M. Goodwin, C. L. Bowden, J. R. Calabrese, H. Grunze, S. Kasper, R. White,

P. Greene, and R. Leadbetter, "A Pooled Analysis of 2 Placebo-Controlled 18-Month Trials of Lamotrigine and Lithium Maintenance in Bipolar I Disorder," *Journal of Clinical Psychiatry* 65, no. 3 (2004): 432–41.

33. M. A. Frye, M. J. Gitlin, and L. L. Altshuler, "Unmet Needs in Bipolar Depression," *Depression and Anxiety* 19, no. 4 (2004): 199–208.

34. J. R. Calabrese, J. R. Sullivan, C. L. Bowden, T. Suppes, J. F. Goldberg, G. S. Sachs, M. D. Shelton, F. K. Goodwin, M. A. Frye, and V. Kusumakar, "Rash in Multicenter Trials of Lamotrigine in Mood Disorders: Clinical Relevance and Management," *Journal of Clinical Psychiatry* 63, no. 11 (2002): 1012–19.

35. Sean P. Stanton, Paul E. Keck, Jr., and Susan L. McElroy, "Treatment of Acute Mania with Gabapentin," *American Journal of Psychiatry* 154, no. 2 (1997): 287.

36. M. A. Frye, T. A. Ketter, T. A. Kimbrell, R. T. Dunn, A. M. Speer, E. A. Osuch, D. A. Luckenbaugh, G. Cora-Ocatelli, G. S. Leverich, and R. M. Post, "A Placebo-Controlled Study of Lamotrigine and Gabapentin Monotherapy in Refractory Mood Disorders," *Journal of Clinical Psychopharmacology* 20, no. 6 (2000): 607–14.

37. A. C. Pande, J. G. Crockatt, C. A. Janney, J. L. Werth, and G. Tsaroucha, "Gabapentin in Bipolar Disorder: A Placebo-Controlled Trial of Adjunctive Therapy. Gabapentin Bipolar Disorder Study Group," *Bipolar Disorders* 2, no. 3, pt. 2 (2000): 249–55.

38. D. Marcotte, "Use of Topiramate, a New Anti-Epileptic, as a Mood Stabilizer," *Journal of Affective Disorder* 50, no. 2–3 (1998): 245–51.

39. One of these reports discusses three patients with bipolar disorder also taking other medications who became profoundly depressed shortly after starting on topiramate. Within days of discontinuing the drug, these symptoms resolved. (See A. Klufas and D. Thompson, "Topiramate-Induced Depression," *American Journal of Psychiatry* 158, no. 10 [2001]: 1736.) Another report is of a thirty-one-year-old woman who started taking topiramate for epilepsy. This patient had previously experienced "mild seasonal depressions" that had required antidepressant therapy, but she had never had manic or hypomanic symptoms. Within two weeks of starting on topiramate, she required hospitalization for manic symptoms including severe agitation, decreased need for sleep, pressured speech, and "intense suicidal ideation." Within two days of discontinuing topiramate the symptoms resolved. (See F. Schlatter, C. Soutullo, and S. Cervera-Enguix, "First Break of Mania Associated with Topiramate Treatment," *Journal of Clinical Psychopharmacology* 2, no. 4 [2001]: 464–65.)

40. T. Suppes, "Review of the Use of Topiramate for Treatment of Bipolar Disorders," *Journal of Clinical Psychopharmacology* 22, no. 6 (2002): 599–609.

41. C. A. Zarate, Jr., J. A. Quiroz, J. B. Singh, K. D. Denicoff, G. De Jesus, D. A. Luckenbaugh, D. S. Charney, and H. K. Manji, "An Open-Label Trial of the Glutamate-Modulating Agent Riluzole in Combination with Lithium for the Treatment of Bipolar Depression," *Biological Psychiatry* 57, no. 4 (2005): 430–32.

CHAPTER 7. ANTIDEPRESSANT MEDICATIONS

1. H. S. Lee, D. H. Song, C. H. Kim, and H. K. Choi, "An Open Clinical Trial of Fluoxetine in the Treatment of Premature Ejaculation," *Journal of Clinical Psychopharmacology* 16, no. 5 (1996): 379–82.

CHAPTER 8. ANTIPSYCHOTIC MEDICATIONS

1. Jeffrey Lieberman, Allan Safferman, Simcha Pollack, Sally Szmanski, Celeste Johns, Alfreda Howard, Michael Kronig, Peter Bookstein, and John Kane, "Clinical Effects of Clozapine in Chronic Schizophrenia: Response to Treatment and Predictors of Outcome," *American Journal of Psychiatry* 151, no. 12 (1994): 1744–52.

2. In a study of 11,555 patients treated with clozapine, 73 developed agranulocytosis (of whom 2 died of the infectious complications of the condition). See Jose Alvir, Jeffrey Lieberman, Allan Safferman, Jeffrey Schwimmer, and John Schaaf, "Clozapine-Induced Agranulocytosis: Incidence and Risk Factors in the United States," *New England Journal of Medicine* 329 (1993): 162–67.

3. Joseph R. Calabrese, Herbert Y. Meltzer, and Paul J. Markovitz, "Clozapine Prophylaxis in Rapid Cycling Bipolar Disorder," *Journal of Clinical Psychopharmacology* 11, no. 6 (1991): 396–97.

4. Joseph Calabrese, Susan Kimmel, Mark Woyshville, Daniel Rapport, Carl Faust, Paul Thompson, and Herbert Meltzer, "Clozapine for Treatment-Refractory Mania," *American Journal of Psychiatry* 153, no. 6 (1996): 759–64.

5. Carlos Zarate, Jr., Mauricio Tohen, Michael Banov, Michelle Weiss, and Jonathan Cole, "Is Clozapine a Mood Stabilizer?" *Journal of Clinical Psychiatry* 56, no. 3 (1995): 108–12.

6. T. Baptista, N. M. Kin, S. Beaulieu, and E. A. de Baptista, "Obesity and Related Metabolic Abnormalities during Antipsychotic Drug Administration: Mechanisms, Management, and Research Perspectives," *Pharmacopsychiatry* 35, no. 6 (2002): 205–19.

CHAPTER 9. MORE MEDICATIONS, HORMONES, AND DIETARY SUPPLEMENTS

1. S. Dubovsky, R. Franks, and M. Lifschitz, "Effectiveness of Verapamil in the Treatment of a Manic Patient," *American Journal of Psychiatry* 139 (1982): 502–3.

2. For an overview of these studies, see Steven Dubovsky and Randall Buzan, "Novel Alternatives and Supplements to Lithium and Anticonvulsants for Bipolar Affective Disorder," *Journal of Clinical Psychiatry* 58 (1997): 224–42.

3. See, for example, Kishore Gadde and K. Ranga Rama Krishman, "Recent Advances in the Pharmacologic Treatment of Bipolar Illness," *Psychiatric Annals* 27 (1997): 496–506.

4. American Psychiatric Association, "Practice Guidelines for the Treatment of Patients with Bipolar Disorder," *American Journal of Psychiatry* 151, suppl. (1994): 14.

5. See the section on the use of "stimulants and euphoriants" in the treatment of acute bipolar depression in Frederick K. Goodwin and Kay Redfield Jamison, *Manic-Depressive Illness* (New York: Oxford University Press, 1990), 652, for a discussion and list of references on trials of psychostimulants in various depressive disorders. See also P. S. Masand, P. Pickett, and G. B. Murry, "Psychostimulants for Secondary Depression in Medical Illness," *Psychosomatics* 32 (1991): 203–8.

6. American Psychiatric Association, "Practice Guidelines for the Treatment of Patients with Bipolar Disorder," 14.

7. See M. Peet and S. Peters, "Drug Induced Mania," *Drug Safety* 12 (1995):

146–53, and P. S. Masand, P. Pickett, and G. B. Murry, "Hypomania Precipitated by Psycho-stimulant Use in Depressed Medically Ill Patients," *Psychosomatics* 36 (1995): 145–47.

8. Barbara Bartlik, Peter Kaplan, James Kocsis, Carol Roeloffs, Richard Friedman, and Alan Cohen, "Stimulants for SSRIs-Induced Sexual Dysfunction," poster presented at the 149th Annual Meeting of the American Psychiatric Association, May 4–6, 1996 (NR644).

9. M. S. Bauer, P. C. Whybrow, and A. Winokur, "Rapid Cycling Bipolar Affective Disorder I: Association with Grade I Hypothyroidism," *Archives of General Psychiatry* 47, no. 5 (1990): 427–32.

10. H. A. Oomen, A. J. Schipperijn, and H. A. Drexhage, "The Prevalence of Affective Disorder and in Particular of a Rapid Cycling of Bipolar Disorder in Patients with Abnormal Thyroid Function Tests," *Clinical Endocrinology* 45, no. 2 (1996): 215–23.

11. D. P. Cole, M. E. Thase, A. G. Mallinger, J. C. Soares, J. F. Luther, D. J. Kupfer, and E. Frank, "Slower Treatment Response in Bipolar Depression Predicted by Lower Pretreatment Thyroid Function," *American Journal of Psychiatry* 159, no. 1 (2002): 116–21.

12. Joseph R. Calabrese and Mark J. Woyshville, "A Medication Algorithm for Treatment of Bipolar Rapid Cycling?" *Journal of Clinical Psychiatry* 56, suppl. 3 (1995): 11–18.

13. K. Linde, G. Ramirez, C. D. Mulrow, A. Pauls, and W. Weidenhammer, "St. John's Wort for Depression—An Overview and Meta-Analysis of Randomised Clinical Trials," *British Medical Journal* 313, no. 7052 (1996): 253–58.

14. R. C. Shelton, M. B. Keller, A. Gelenberg, D. L. Dunner, R. Hirschfeld, M. E. Thase, J. Russell, R. B. Lydiard, P. Crits-Christoph, R. Gallop, L. Todd, D. Hellerstein, P. Goodnick, G. Keitner, S. M. Stahl, and U. Halbreich, "Effectiveness of St. John's Wort in Major Depression: A Randomized Controlled Trial," *Journal of the American Medical Association* 285, no. 15 (2001): 1978–86.

15. A. J. Gelenberg, R. C. Shelton, P. Crits-Christoph, M. B. Keller, D. L. Dunner, R. M. Hirschfeld, M. E. Thase, J. M. Russell, R. B. Lydiard, R. J. Gallop, L. Todd, D. J. Hellerstein, P. J. Goodnick, G. I. Keitner, S. M. Stahl, U. Halbreich, and H. S. Hopkins, "The Effectiveness of St. John's Wort in Major Depressive Disorder: A Naturalistic Phase 2 Follow-Up in Which Nonresponders Were Provided Alternate Medication," *Journal of Clinical Psychiatry* 65, no. 8 (2004): 1114–19.

16. A. L. Stoll, W. E. Severus, M. P. Freeman, S. Rueter, H. A. Zboyan, E. Diamond, K. K. Cress, and L. B. Marangell, "Omega 3 Fatty Acids in Bipolar Disorder: A Preliminary Double-Blind, Placebo-Controlled Trial," *Archives of General Psychiatry* 56, no. 5 (1999): 407–12.

17. Joseph R. Calabrese, Daniel J. Rapport, and Melvin D. Shelton, "Fish Oils and Bipolar Disorder: A Promising but Untested Treatment," *Archives of General Psychiatry* 56, no. 5 (1999): 413–14.

CHAPTER 10. ELECTROCONVULSIVE THERAPY
AND RELATED TREATMENTS

1. Emil Kraepelin, *Manic-Depressive Insanity and Paranoia*, trans. R. M. Barclay, ed. G. M. Robertson (1921; reprint, New York: Arno Press, 1976), 97.

2. C. Freeman and R. E. Kendell, "ECT I: Patients' Experiences and Attitudes," *British Journal of Psychiatry* 137 (1980): 8–16.

3. Larry Squire, Pamela Slater, and Patricia Miller, "Retrograde Amnesia and Bilateral Electroconvulsive Therapy, Long Term Follow-up," *Archives of General Psychiatry* 38 (1981): 89–95.

4. C. L. Freeman, D. Weeks, and R. E. Kendell, "ECT II: Patients Who Complain," *British Journal of Psychiatry* 137 (1980): 17–25.

5. Larry R. Squire and Pamela C. Slater, "Electroconvulsive Therapy and Complaints of Memory Dysfunction: A Prospective Three-Year Follow-up Study," *British Journal of Psychiatry* 142 (1983): 1–8.

6. American Psychiatric Association, "Practice Guidelines for the Treatment of Patients with Bipolar Disorder," *American Journal of Psychiatry* 151, suppl. (1994): 15.

7. Frederick K. Goodwin and Kay Redfield Jamison, *Manic-Depressive Illness* (New York: Oxford University Press, 1990), 661.

8. Sukdeb Mukherjee, Harold Sackeim, and David Schnur, "Electroconvulsive Therapy of Acute Manic Episodes: A Review of Fifty Years' Experience," *American Journal of Psychiatry* 151 (1994): 169–76.

9. S. Mukherjee, H. Sackeim, and C. Lee, "Unilateral ECT in the Treatment of Manic Episodes," *Convulsive Therapy* 4 (1988): 74–80.

10. Much of the work comparing the effectiveness of ECT with that of medication compares it with treatment with lithium. As studies comparing it with treatment with newer agents (such as the anticonvulsants) are done, statements about ECT's superiority to medical treatments for mania may need to be revised. However, given that the new mood stabilizers are perhaps *less* effective than lithium for depression, ECT's claims as a more predictably effective treatment for bipolar depression remain unchallenged.

11. See Mark S. George, Eric Wasserman, and Robert Post, "Transcranial Magnetic Stimulation: A Neuropsychiatric Tool for the Twenty-first Century," *Journal of Neuropsychiatry and Clinical Neurosciences* 8 (1996): 373–82.

12. Mark George, Eric Wasserman, Tim Kimbrell, John Little, Wendol Williams, Aimee Danielson, Benjamin Greenberg, Mark Hallett, and Robert Post, "Mood Improvement Following Daily Left Prefrontal Repetitive Transcranial Magnetic Stimulation in Patients with Depression: A Placebo Controlled Crossover Trial," *American Journal of Psychiatry* 154 (1997): 1752–56.

13. A. Pascual-Leone, B. Rubio, F. Pallardo, and M. D. Catala, "Beneficial Effect of Rapid-Rate Transcranial Magnetic Stimulation of the Left Dorsolateral Prefrontal Cortex in Drug-Resistant Depression," *Lancet* 348 (1996): 233–37, and Charles Epstein, Gary Figiel, William McDonald, Jody Amazon-Leece, and Linda Figiel, "Rapid Rate Transcranial Magnetic Stimulation in Young and Middle-Aged Refractory Depressed Patients," *Psychiatric Annals* 28 (1998): 36–39.

14. A. J. Rush, M. S. George, H. A. Sackeim, L. B. Marangell, M. M. Husain, C. Giller, Z. Nahas, S. Haines, R. K. Simpson, Jr., and R. Goodman, "Vagus Nerve Stimulation (VNS) for Treatment-Resistant Depressions: A Multicenter Study," *Biological Psychiatry* 47, no. 4 (2000): 276–86.

15. L. B. Marangell, A. J. Rush, M. S. George, H. A. Sackeim, C. R. Johnson, M. M.

Husain, Z. Nahas, and S. H. Lisanby, "Vagus Nerve Stimulation (VNS) for Major Depressive Episodes: One Year Outcomes," *Biological Psychiatry* 51, no. 4 (2002): 280–87.

CHAPTER 11. COUNSELING AND PSYCHOTHERAPY

1. Jan Scott, "Psychotherapy for Bipolar Disorder," *British Journal of Psychiatry* 167 (1995): 581–88.

2. Nick Kanas, "Group Psychotherapy with Bipolar Patients: A Review and Synthesis," *International Journal of Group Psychotherapy* 43 (1993): 321–33.

3. L. E. Pollack, "Content Analysis of Groups for Inpatients with Bipolar Disorder," *Applied Nursing Research* 6 (1993): 19–27.

4. Many articles on this type of therapy now use the term *cognitive-behavioral therapy* to describe it. Psychologist Donald Meichenbaum has written extensively on Beck's cognitive therapy as well as on other types of therapy that use the techniques of behavioral psychology to help change thinking patterns (cognition). He is perhaps most responsible for creating the broader category of "cognitive-behavioral therapy." (See Donald Meichenbaum and Roy Cameron, "Cognitive-Behavior Therapy," in *Contemporary Behavior Therapy: Conceptional and Empirical Foundations,* ed. G. Terence Wilson and Cyril M. Franks [New York: Guilford Press, 1982], 310– 37.) Although some researchers and theoreticians will describe subtle differences between the terms *cognitive therapy* and *cognitive-behavioral therapy,* they now seem to be used interchangeably by most clinical psychologists—at least they are by five out of the five psychologist colleagues of mine whom I asked about it—and by researchers as well.

5. The area of comparison studies of psychotherapy and medication in the treatment of depression can be accurately described as a hornet's nest of controversy. It's not difficult to find a study to support any possible view: superiority of medication over psychotherapy, superiority of psychotherapy over medication, and equal efficacy for both. A nicely designed and well-executed study that found cognitive therapy to be as helpful as imipramine for 107 patients with major depressive disorder is Steven Hollon, Robert DeRubeis, Mark Evans, Marlin Wiemer, Michael Garvey, William Grove, and Vincente Tuason, "Cognitive Therapy and Pharmacotherapy for Depression, Singly and in Combination," *Archives of General Psychiatry* 49 (1992): 774–81. Readers who would like to jump into the hornet's nest feet first are referred to Jacqueline Persons, Michael Thase, and Paul Crits-Chistoph, "The Role of Psychotherapy in the Treatment of Depression: Review of Two Practice Guidelines," *Archives of General Psychiatry* 53 (1996): 283–90, and to the four (yes, four) accompanying rebuttal/commentary articles in the same issue of *Archives.*

6. A. T. Beck, A. J. Rush, B. F. Shaw, and G. Emory, *Cognitive Therapy of Depression* (New York: Guilford Press, 1979), 11.

7. The linguistic purist in me wants the plural of *schema* to be *schemata* or perhaps *schemae*. But *schemas* is the plural used in cognitive-therapy literature.

8. See Jan Scott, "Cognitive Therapy of Affective Disorders: A Review," *Journal of Affective Disorders* 37 (1996): 1–11.

9. David J. Miklowitz, "Psychotherapy in Combination with Drug Treatment for Bipolar Disorder," *Journal of Clinical Psychopharmacology* 16, suppl. (1996): 56S–66S.

10. E. Frank, S. Hlastala, A. Ritenour, P. Houck, X. M. Tu, T. H. Monk, A. G.

Mallinger, and D. J. Kupfer, "Inducing Lifestyle Regularity in Recovering Bipolar Disorder Patients: Results from the Maintenance Therapies in Bipolar Disorder Protocol," *Biological Psychiatry* 15 (1997): 1165–73.

11. Kay Redfield Jamison, *An Unquiet Mind: A Memoir of Moods and Madness* (New York: Vintage Books, 1996), 88–89.

CHAPTER 12. TREATMENT APPROACHES IN BIPOLAR DISORDER

1. The word *empirical* is derived from the Greek word *empeirikos,* which means "a doctor relying on experience alone." It also has the archaic meaning—at least I hope it's archaic—of "charlatan."

CHAPTER 13. BIPOLAR DISORDER IN CHILDREN AND ADOLESCENTS

1. Barbara Geller, Kai Sun, Betsy Zimerman, Joan Luby, Jeanne Frazier, and Marlene Williams, "Complex and Rapid-Cycling in Bipolar Children and Adolescents: A Preliminary Study," *Journal of Affective Disorders* 34 (1995): 259–68.

2. Roselind Neuman, Barbara Geller, John Rice, and Richard Todd, "Increased Prevalence and Earlier Onset of Mood Disorders among Relatives of Prepubertal versus Adult Probands," *Journal of the American Academy of Child and Adolescent Psychiatry* 36 (1997): 466–73.

3. American Academy of Child and Adolescent Psychiatry, "Practice Parameters for the Assessment and Treatment of Children and Adolescents with Bipolar Disorder," *Journal of the American Academy of Child and Adolescent Psychiatry* 36 (1997): 138–57. Studies cited on 140.

4. See Barbara Geller and Joan Luby, "Child and Adolescent Bipolar Disorder: Review of the Past Ten Years," *Journal of the American Academy of Child and Adolescent Psychiatry* 36 (1997): 1168–76.

5. Geller, Sun, Zimerman, Luby, Frazier, and Williams, "Complex and Rapid-Cycling in Bipolar Children and Adolescents: A Preliminary Study."

6. M. Strober and G. Carlson, "Bipolar Illness in Adolescents with Major Depression: Clinical, Genetic, and Psychopharmacologic Predictors in a Three- to Four-Year Prospective Follow-Up Investigation," *Archives of General Psychiatry* 39, no. 5 (1982): 549–55.

7. T. Spencer, J. Biederman, and T. Wilens, "Attention-Deficit/Hyperactivity Disorder and Comorbidity," *Pediatric Clinics of North America* 46, no. 5 (1999): 915–27.

8. J. Biederman, S. Faraone, E. Mick, J. Wozniac, L. Chen, C. Ouellette, A. Marrs, J. Garcia, D. Mennin, and E. Lelon, "Attention-Deficit Hyperactivity Disorder and Juvenile Mania: An Overlooked Comorbidity?" *Journal of the American Academy of Child and Adolescent Psychiatry* 35, no. 8 (1996): 997–1008.

9. S. V. Faraone, J. Biederman, D. Mennin, J. Wozniak, and T. Spencer, "Attention-Deficit Hyperactivity Disorder with Bipolar Disorder: A Familial Subtype?" *Journal of the American Academy of Child and Adolescent Psychiatry* 36, no. 10 (1997): 1378–87.

10. See American Academy of Child and Adolescent Psychiatry, "Practice Parameters for the Assessment and Treatment of Children and Adolescents with Bipolar Disorder."

11. M. Strober, M. DeAntonio, S. Schmidt-Lackner, R. Freeman, C. Lampert, and

J. Diamond, "Early Childhood Attention Deficit Hyperactivity Disorder Predicts Poorer Response to Acute Lithium Therapy in Adolescent Mania," *Journal of Affective Disorders* 51, no. 2 (1998): 145–51.

12. T. A. Henderson, "Mania Induction Associated with Atomoxetine," *Journal of Clinical Psychopharmacology* 24, no. 5 (2004): 567–68.

13. T. Spencer and J. Biederman, "Non-Stimulant Treatment for Attention-Deficit/ Hyperactivity Disorder," *Journal of Attention Disorders* 6, suppl. 1 (2002): S109–19.

14. M. Strober, S. Schmidt-Lackner, R. Freeman, S. Bower, C. Lampert, and M. DeAntonio, "Recovery and Relapse in Adolescents with Bipolar Affective Illness: A Five-Year Naturalistic, Prospective Follow-up," *Journal of the American Academy of Child and Adolescent Psychiatry* 34 (1995): 724–31.

CHAPTER 14. WOMEN WITH BIPOLAR DISORDER:
SPECIAL CONSIDERATIONS

1. All three studies are described and referenced in Ellen Leibenluft, "Women with Bipolar Illness: Clinical and Research Issues," *American Journal of Psychiatry* 153 (1996): 163–73.

2. Douglas Maskall, Raymond Lam, Shala Misri, Lakshmi Yatham, and Athanasios Zis, "Seasonality of Symptoms in Women with Late Luteal Phase Dysphoric Disorder," *American Journal of Psychiatry* 154 (1997): 1436–41.

3. Leibenluft, "Women with Bipolar Illness: Clinical and Research Issues."

4. Ibid., 164.

5. Ibid., 166.

6. Victoria Hendrick, Vivien Burt, and Lori Altshuler, "Psychotropic Guidelines for Breast-Feeding Mothers," *American Journal of Psychiatry* 153 (1996): 1236–37.

CHAPTER 15. ALCOHOLISM AND DRUG ABUSE

1. D. A. Reger, M. E. Farm, and D. S. Rae, "Comorbidity of Mental Disorders with Alcohol and Other Drug Abuse: Results from the Epidemiologic Catchment Area Study," *Journal of the American Medical Association* 264 (1990): 2511–18.

2. Results quoted in Kathleen Brady and Susan Sonne, "The Relationship between Substance Abuse and Bipolar Disorder," *Journal of Clinical Psychiatry* 56, suppl. 3 (1995): 19–24.

3. Susan Sonne, Kathleen Brady, and W. Alexander Morton, "Substance Abuse and Bipolar Affective Disorder," *Journal of Nervous and Mental Disease* 182 (1994): 349–52.

4. Markus Henriksson, Hillevi Aro, Mauri Marttunnen, Martti Heikkinen, Erkki Isometsä, Kimmo Kuoppasalmi, and Jouko Lönnqvist, "Mental Disorders and Comorbidity in Suicide," *American Journal of Psychiatry* 150 (1993): 935–40.

CHAPTER 16. SEASONAL AFFECTIVE DISORDER
AND CHRONOBIOLOGY

1. A. J. Lewy, H. A. Kern, N. E. Rosenthal, and T. A. Wehr, "Bright Artificial Light Treatment of a Manic-Depressive Patient with a Seasonal Mood Cycle," *American Journal of Psychiatry* 139 (1982): 1496–98.

2. Emil Kraepelin, *Manic-Depressive Insanity and Paranoia,* trans. R. M. Barclay, ed. G. M. Robertson (1921; reprint, New York: Arno Press, 1976), 139.

3. Norman E. Rosenthal, *Winter Blues: Seasonal Affective Disorder, What It Is and How to Overcome It* (New York: Guilford Press, 1993), 6.

4. Ibid., 9.

5. Curt Paul Richter, *Biological Clocks in Medicine and Psychiatry* (Springfield, Ill.: Charles C Thomas, 1965), 3.

6. Ibid., 14–15. Emphasis added.

7. Diane Boivin, Charles Czeisler, Derk-Jan Dijk, Jeanne Duffy, Simon Folkard, David Minors, Peter Totterdell, and James Waterhouse, "Complex Interaction of the Sleep-Wake Cycle and Circadian Phase Modulates Mood in Healthy Subjects," *Archives of General Psychiatry* 54 (1997): 145–52.

8. Michael Terman, Leora Amira, Jiuan Terman, and Donald Ross, "Predictors of Response and Non-response to Light Treatment for Winter Depression," *American Journal of Psychiatry* 153 (1996): 1423–29.

9. Alexander Neumeister, Nicole Praschak-Rieder, Barbara Heßelmann, Marie-Luise Rao, Judith Glück, and Siegfried Kasper, "Effects of Tryptophan Depletion on Drug-Free Patients with Seasonal Affective Disorder during a Stable Response to Bright Light Therapy," *Archives of General Psychiatry* 54 (1997): 133–38.

10. Alan O. Kogan and Patricia Guilford, "Side Effects of Short-Term 10,000-Lux Light Therapy," *American Journal of Psychiatry* 155 (1998): 293–94.

11. Scott Campbell and Patricia Murphy, "Extraocular Circadian Phototransduction in Humans," *Science* 279 (1998): 396–99.

12. Dan A. Oren and Michael Terman, "Tweaking the Human Circadian Clock with Light," *Science* 279 (1998): 333–34.

13. A comprehensive and very readable discussion of SAD is Rosenthal, *Winter Blues.*

14. Frederick K. Goodwin and Kay Redfield Jamison, *Manic-Depressive Illness* (New York: Oxford University Press, 1990), 556–57. Chapter 19 of that volume, "Sleep and Biological Rhythms," has a comprehensive discussion of the issues presented in this chapter.

15. F. Benedetti, B. Barbini, A. Lucca, E. Campori, C. Colombo, and E. Smeraldi, "Sleep Deprivation Hastens the Antidepressant Action of Fluoxetine," *European Archives of Psychiatry and Clinical Neuroscience* 247 (1997): 100–103.

16. T. Wehr, D. Sack, and N. Rosenthal, "Sleep Reduction as a Final Common Pathway in the Genesis of Mania," *American Journal of Psychiatry* 144 (1987): 201–4.

CHAPTER 17. THE GENETICS OF BIPOLAR DISORDER

1. Emil Kraepelin, *Manic-Depressive Insanity and Paranoia,* trans. R. M. Barclay, ed. G. M. Robertson (1921; reprint, New York: Arno Press, 1976), 165.

2. For a more detailed account that includes references to the original articles, see Eliot Marshall, "Manic Depression: Highs and Lows on the Research Roller Coaster," *Science* 264 (1994) 1693–95.

3. A. Ram, F. Guedj, A. Cravchik, L. Weinstein, Q. Coa, J. Badner, L. Goldin, N. Grisaru, H. Manji, R. Belmaker, E. Gershon, and P. Gejman, "No Abnormality in the

Gene for the G Protein Stimulatory Alpha Subunit in Patients with Bipolar Disorder," *Archives of General Psychiatry* 54, no. 1 (1997): 44–48.

4. Elliot Gershon, "Genetics," in *Manic-Depressive Illness*, ed. Frederick K. Goodwin and Kay Redfield Jamison (New York: Oxford University Press, 1990), 373–401.

CHAPTER 18. BIPOLAR BIOLOGY

1. Marshall Folstein, Susan Folstein, and Paul McHugh, "Mood Disorder as a Specific Complication of Stroke," *Journal of Neurosurgery and Psychiatry* 40 (1977): 1018–20.

2. R. Robinson and T. Price, "Post-stroke Depressive Disorders: A Follow-up Study of 103 Patients," *Stroke* 13 (1982): 635–41.

3. For an in-depth discussion of the relationship between mood disorders and stroke, see Robert G. Robinson and Javier I. Travella, "Neuropsychiatry of Mood Disorders," in *Neuropsychiatry*, ed. Barry S. Fogel, Randolph B. Schiffer, and Stephen M. Rao (Baltimore: Williams and Wilkins, 1996), 287–305.

4. M. Shetty and D. Lynn, "Valproate as Prophylaxis for Steroid-Induced Mood Disturbance: A Case Report," poster #51 presented at the Second International Conference on Bipolar Disorder, sponsored by the University of Pittsburgh School of Medicine, Center for Continuing Education in the Health Sciences, Pittsburgh, June 19, 1997.

5. Lori Altshuler, John Curran, Peter Hauser, Jim Mintz, Kirk Denikoff, and Robert Post, "T_2 Hyperintensities in Bipolar Disorder: Magnetic Resonance Imaging Comparison and Literature Meta-analysis," *American Journal of Psychiatry* 152 (1995): 1139–44.

6. Monte Buchsbaum, Toshiyuki Someya, Joseph Wu, Cheuk Tang, and William Bunney, "Neuroimaging Bipolar Illness with Positron Emission Tomography and Magnetic Resonance Imaging," *Psychiatric Annals* 27 (1997): 480–95.

7. Hady Shimon, Galila Agam, R. H. Belmaker, Thomas Hyde, and Joel Kleinman, "Reduced Frontal Cortex Inositol Levels in Postmortem Brain of Suicide Victims and Patients with Bipolar Disorder," *American Journal of Psychiatry* 154 (1997): 1148–50.

8. E. Fuller Torrey, Robert Rawlings, Jacqueline Ennis, Deborah Merrill, and Donn Flores, "Birth Seasonality in Bipolar Disorder, Schizophrenia, Schizoaffective Disorder, and Stillbirths," *Schizophrenia Research* 21 (1996): 141–49.

9. Robert H. Yolken, "Molecular Analysis of Brains from Individuals with Bipolar Disorder: Evidence of Viral Infections," paper presented at the Second International Conference on Bipolar Disorder, sponsored by the University of Pittsburgh School of Medicine, Center for Continuing Education in the Health Sciences, Pittsburgh, June 21, 1997.

10. Zhen Fang Fu, Jay D. Amsterdam, Moujahed Kao, Vidya Shankar, Hilary Koprowski, and Bernhard Dietzschold, "Detection of Borna Disease Virus-Reactive Antibodies from Patients with Affective Disorders by Western Immunoblot Technique," *Journal of Affective Disorders* 27 (1993): 61–68.

CHAPTER 19. BIPOLAR DISORDER AND CREATIVITY

1. Aristotle, attributed by Seneca in *Moral Essays*, "De tranquillitate animi" (On Tranquility of Mind), sec. 17, subsec. 10, quoted in *The Columbia Dictionary of Quotations* (New York: Columbia University Press, 1993; CD ROM ed., 1994).

2. Quoted in Kay Redfield Jamison, *Touched with Fire: Manic-Depressive Illness and the Artistic Temperament* (New York: Free Press, 1994), 203–5.

3. These studies are described and cited in ibid.

4. Emil Kraepelin, *Manic-Depressive Insanity and Paranoia*, trans. R. M. Barclay, ed. G. M. Robertson (1921; reprint, New York: Arno Press, 1976), 17.

5. Quoted in Jamison, *Touched with Fire*, 126.

6. Jean Cocteau, "Le coq et l'arlequin," in *Le rappel à l'ordre* (1926), quoted in *Columbia Dictionary of Quotations*, CD ROM ed.

7. These studies are cited and described in Frederick K. Goodwin and Kay Redfield Jamison, *Manic-Depressive Illness* (New York: Oxford University Press, 1990), 365–66.

CHAPTER 20. LIVING WITH BIPOLAR DISORDER

1. Emil Kraepelin, *Manic-Depressive Insanity and Paranoia*, trans. R. M. Barclay, ed. G. M. Robertson (1921; reprint, New York: Arno Press, 1976), 179–81.

2. For a complete discussion of these animal models of the kindling phenomenon, see Robert Post, "Transduction of Psychosocial Stress into the Neurobiology of Recurrent Affective Disorder," *American Journal of Psychiatry* 149 (1992): 999–1010.

3. Constance Hammen and Michael Gitlin, "Stress Reactivity in Bipolar Patients and Its Relation to Prior History of Disorder," *American Journal of Psychiatry* 154 (1997): 856–57.

4. Mario Maj, Raffaele Pirozzi, and Lorenza Magliano, "Non-response to Reinstituted Lithium Prophylaxis in Previously Responsive Bipolar Patients: Prevalence and Predictors," *American Journal of Psychiatry* 152 (1995): 1810–11. A similar study concluded that "the efficacy of lithium did not differ significantly" when it was started a second time in patients who had stopped it. But almost 13 percent of these patients needed *another* medication added to the lithium to achieve remission the second time around. (This seems to me to indicate that the lithium was *not* as effective the second time around.) See Leonardo Tondo, Ross Baldessarini, Gianfranco Floris, and Nereida Rudas, "Effectiveness of Restarting Lithium Treatment after Its Discontinuation in Bipolar I and Bipolar II Patients," *American Journal of Psychiatry* 154 (1997): 548–50.

5. Erving Goffman, *Stigma: Notes on the Management of Spoiled Identity* (Englewood Cliffs, N.J.: Prentice-Hall, 1963), 1, 2.

CHAPTER 21. PLANNING FOR EMERGENCIES

1. Frederick K. Goodwin and Kay Redfield Jamison, *Manic-Depressive Illness* (New York: Oxford University Press, 1990), 228–30.

2. See, for example, J. E. Bailey, A. L. Kellerman, G. W. Somes, J. G. Banton, F. Rivara, and N. Rushforth, "Risk Factors for Violent Death of Women in the Home," *Archives of Internal Medicine* 157 (1997): 777–82.

3. *American Heritage Dictionary of the English Language*, 3d ed. (New York: Houghton Mifflin, 1992).

CHAPTER 22. THE ROLE OF THE FAMILY

1. Kay Redfield Jamison, *An Unquiet Mind: A Memoir of Moods and Madness* (New York: Vintage Books, 1996), 120.

2. Stephen Strakowski, Susan McElroy, Paul Keck, and Scott West, "Suicidality among Patients with Mixed and Manic Bipolar Disorder," *American Journal of Psychiatry* 153 (1996): 674–76.

Index

Eldepryl, 109
electroconvulsive therapy (ECT), 25, 129–38, 161; development of, 129–31; side effects of, 131–33
Emsam, 109
Endler, Norman, 16–17, 19–20, 21, 23
EPA, 127
episode number, 34, 36
Epitol. *See* carbamazepine
Epival. *See* valproate
EPS. *See* extrapyramidal symptoms
Equetra. *See* carbamazepine
escitalpram, 106
extrapyramidal symptoms (EPS), 114–15

Falret, Jean-Pierre, 63–64
Fieve, Ronald, 71
fish oil, 126–28
Fitzgerald, F. Scott, 22
flight of ideas, 10
fluoxetine, 80, 106
fluphenazine, 114
fluvoxamine, 106
folie circulaire, 63–64
Freud, Sigmund, 64, 67–68, 140
functional psychiatric illnesses, 68, 140

gabapentin, 101
Gabatril, 102
GAF. *See* Global Assessment of Functioning scale
gamma amino butyric acid (GABA), 93
"general paresis of the insane," 66
genetics, 40–41, 198–204
Geodon, 116
George Gordon, Lord Byron, 217–18
Global Assessment of Functioning (GAF) scale, 59
glutamate, 82
Goethe, Johann Wolfgang von, 20
Goffman, Erving, 238
G proteins, 81–82
Greek descriptions of mood disorders, 62–63
group therapy, 142–43
guanfacine, 170

Haldol, 114
half-life of pharmaceuticals, 87–88

hallucinations: in depression, 24; in mania, 13; in schizoaffective disorder, 52–54
haloperidol, 114
hemoglobin, 200–201
herbal therapies, 125–26
heredity. *See* genetics
hippocampus, 83
"humoral theory" of bipolar disorder, 62–63
Hygeia, 230–31
hypericum, 125–26
hypersexuality, 11
hypersomnia, 21
hyperthymic temperament, 49
hyperthyroidism, 211–12
hypochondria, 23
hypomania, 16–18
hypothyroidism, 211–12

imipramine, 72–73, 105
individual psychotherapy, 149
insight-oriented psychotherapy, 149
interpersonal and social rhythm therapy (IP/SRT), 147–48
involuntary commitment, 252–55

James, Robert, 63
Jamison, Kay Redfield, 14, 25, 148, 220–21
Johns Hopkins University, 1, 40, 186, 230

kindling hypothesis, 232–33
Klonopin, 120
Kraepelin, Emil, 1, 12–14, 25–27, 28, 35, 43–44, 64–65, 185, 221, 231–32
Kuhn, Roland, 72, 80, 105

Lamictal, 98–101
lamotrigine, 98–101
legal issues, 252–55
Lexapro, 106
Librium, 120
light therapy, 186, 192–94
lithium: blood levels, 88–89; discovery of, 69–73; therapy, 84–92
Lorazepam, 120
Luvox, 106

magnetic resonance imaging (MRI), 213
major depression: *DSM* categories, 59–61; symptoms of, 18–25

Two Becoming One *provides a blueprint for marriage. It has revolutionized our marriage. I believe your marriage will be blessed if you read and apply the faith concepts found in this book.*

    Joe Gibbs
    President, Joe Gibbs Racing
    Former head coach, three-time Super Bowl
    champion Washington Redskins

Is it realistic? Is it scriptural? Is it balanced? Is it believable? Two Becoming One *combines all four ingredients. This is an honest book with practical content.*

    Charles Swindoll
    President of Dallas Theological Seminary
    Speaker, Insight for Living radio program

If I had it within my power, Two Becoming One *would be required reading for every couple.*

    Dennis Rainey
    President of FamilyLife Ministry,
    Host of Family Life Today radio programs

Don and Sally Meredith are two of God's choicest servants and longtime friends. This book is must reading for all who desire to experience a rich and God-blessed marriage.

    Bill Bright
    Founder and President,
    Campus Crusade for Christ

Don and Sally Meredith apply sound, biblical wisdom to the tough issues of marriage—communication, how to grow in oneness, finances, facing trials, romance, and sorting out the biblical roles of husbands and wives. This material is so good that we will include it in our new Resourceful Living Series curriculum.

    Larry Burkett
    Founder and CEO
    Christian Financial Concepts

This is a wonderful tool for bringing godly principles into a marriage. I don't think there is a more important issue than oneness in marriage, whether in finances, communication, or romance. Numerous Crown leaders have gone through this study, and I highly recommend Two Becoming One *to couples.*

Howard Dayton
CEO
Crown Ministries

These materials are rock solid, Bible centered, Christ honoring, practical, and comprehensive. We use these materials and find an excellent response to them.

Pastor Jim Henry
First Baptist Church of Orlando

This book has helped numerous couples, including us, to understand the foundational principle of moving from a performance-based relationship to one of faith. We recommend it highly.

Bob and Connice Dyar,
President, Carolina Sports Outreach
and NASCAR team chaplain

We strongly recommend the Two Becoming One *book and the study to all couples. When we took the class, God gave us a biblical foundation, strengthened our relationship, and brought us closer to Him.*

Jimmy and Patti Makar
Crew Chief of Bobby LaBonte NASCAR team

BECOMING 2ONE

God Designed
MARRIAGE
He Can Make it Work.

DON & SALLY MEREDITH

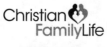

Christian
FamilyLife

Nashville, Tennessee

ISBN 0-9657965-2-3

1 3 5 7 9 10 8 6 4 2

Printed in the United States of America

*To our children
who have blessed our lives incredibly
and now have become our best friends:*

*Todd and Sara Meredith
Scott and Carmen Gertz
Brandon and Kathryn Ruby
Brad and Tiffany Haines*

Contents

Foreword

◈ PAT AND I HAVE BEEN MARRIED FOR OVER THIRTY years now. We're both professing Christians, and we actively seek God's direction in our lives. But I'll be the first to admit that I'm not always the world's best husband. Pat can readily attest to this. And she'd tell you that she's not always the perfect wife. We try, but though we deeply love each other, we sometimes fail.

I'll level with you: Sometimes I used to put my career as an NFL football coach above everything, occasionally even God! And the pressures of running our NASCAR team have made me difficult to be around at times. As for Pat, every now and then her frustration in defining her role, now that our kids have grown up, surfaces. Yet, there was the time when she faced a serious, life-threatening illness and her faith never wavered. I love her for the way she responded to God.

Through it all, we believe that God made our marriage, and that He has a plan for it. That's why we strongly recommend, and practice, the marriage principles that Don and Sally lay out in *Two Becoming One.*

This book provides a biblical blueprint for marriage. Don and Sally show God's commitment to marriage and our responsibility to Him and each other. They call this commitment a "faith relationship," and it has revolutionized our marriage. God does have a plan and practical solutions for your marriage, whether you are happily married, have hit some painful trials, or wonder if you're married to someone you believe is not God's best for you. Whatever your situation, *Two Becoming One* will set you straight. It will give you biblical hope and direction.

Don and Sally are dear friends, and our families are very close. We've spent enough time together to know that they use these principles in their own marriage. So do our married children. Pat and I, our son J. D. and his wife, Melissa, took the twelve-week Becoming One course. We highly recommend the *Two Becoming One Workbook,* based on that course, after you finish this book.

This material has blessed thousands of marriages. The material presented in this book is the foundation for two fine ministries: Christian Family Life, which focuses on marital counseling and small groups, and the Family Life Ministry of Campus Crusade, which holds the tremendous weekend marriage conferences.

I believe your marriage will be blessed if you read and apply the faith concepts described in *Two Becoming One.* It has blessed our lives and those of our children. We will forever be grateful to the Merediths for sharing the faith-relationship concept with us.

JOE GIBBS
President, Joe Gibbs Racing
Former head coach, three-time Super Bowl
champion Washington Redskins

Acknowledgements

SALLY AND I ARE VERY AWARE OF THE INDIVIDUALS and groups who have influenced our lives and this book over the years. We know that the Holy Spirit has used each one of these friends to contribute insights to this message. We are very thankful for each person.

Howard Hendricks, professor emeritus of Dallas Theological Seminary, has greatly impacted the development of this book. During my (Don's) years of study under him, I learned valuable lessons and received great encouragement.

Two groups have been equally important to us. First, we owe significant gratitude to the original founders of Christian Family Life. Many of the insights in this book are directly attributable to them. We are especially grateful to Dr. Barry Leventhal, our faithful friend, who has always taken time to help us biblically. We are also thankful to Dennis Rainey and the Family Life Ministry staff of Campus Crusade for Christ and particularly grateful that they teach these faith concepts at their seminars.

Over the years, numerous good friends have contributed individual help in typing and editing. Others have contributed over the last thirty-five years through their financial and prayer support for our ministry. We owe a debt of gratitude to each of you.

part one

WHY MARRIAGES FAIL

CHAPTER ONE

"But Sally it's third and eight!"

◈ DO YOU KNOW A COUPLE WITH A GREAT MARRIAGE, one so solid that you would trade your marriage for theirs? Probably not. Most counselors that we have known agree that the majority of marriages today are either hurting badly or are on the verge of breaking up. Marriages are failing in tremendous numbers.

All things considered, marriage today is a risky proposition. In recent times, applications for divorce number about the same as applications for marriage licenses in most major U.S. cities. "In 1990, there were forty-eight divorces for each one-hundred marriages," reported researcher George Barna.[1] In the nineties there has been one divorce for every 1.8 marriages. Divorce cases affect more than one million children each year, and "13 million children under eighteen have one or both parents missing." [2] As alarming as those figures are, additional research reveals that many marriages not visited by divorce are hurting; the parents are attempting to "hang in there" for the sake of the children.

Is the situation hopeless? No. Not only is marriage as an institution not hopeless, it can succeed beyond one's expectations. The successful marriage, though, begins with an attitude and a dedication: *Happy marriages are made, not found.* Begin now to earnestly seek the answers on how to succeed in marriage. Both married couples and those planning to marry must recognize that romantic feelings or good intentions are not enough. Couples must work to strengthen marriages. The good news is: God designed marriage, so He can make it work!

Before we look at God's plan for making marriage work, let us introduce ourselves and look at how marriages begin to deteriorate (the focus of part 1). Sally and I have been married more than thirty years, and we continue to be amazed by the love and satisfaction we feel for each other. Even though we are just human beings with strengths and weaknesses, God has shown us the key to loving by faith. As our faith has grown, God has given us the ability to love with a love that honors and gives hope to the other.

Happy marriages are made, not found.

Each of us has weaknesses, as do all husbands and wives. Sally's shortcomings used to really bother me, and mine upset her too. But we now see our weaknesses in a realistic way, and we experience an exhilarating love for each other. That's a miracle. It hasn't always been that way. In 1967, when we married, such love was foreign to us. At that time our love was based on performance. And unfortunately, we each began to fall short of the other's expectations beginning on our wedding day.

MY FOOTBALL BRIDE
(DON'S STORY)

After a three-month engagement, our wedding day arrived. Because we were both twenty-seven and had been Christians longer than most newlyweds, we thought marriage would be a little bit easier for us. Frankly, we were naïve and overconfident. We struggled from the very first day.

Our different backgrounds surfaced on the day of the wedding. The ceremony was scheduled at 4:00 on a Saturday afternoon in the early fall. Since I (Don) was ahead of schedule, I flipped on the television to catch the first University of Texas football game of the season. I hadn't seen a game in six months. Before I knew it, it was 3:45 and I wasn't completely ready. Frustrated that I had to leave the game before halftime, I rushed off to the wedding. Go ahead and chastise me, women. I realize that I deserve it.

After the ceremony in Boulder, Colorado, we left for Vail, where we had reservations in a lovely hotel. As soon as we pulled out of the church parking lot, I quickly switched on the radio, trying to catch the end of the Texas game. The experts said 1967 would be the "year of the Horns" (Texas Longhorns). I just had to know the score!

No luck. The mountains limited the radio reception, throwing me into a "sports panic." I decided to stop short of Vail and find another motel just so I wouldn't miss the 10:00 news and the Texas score. To me, one hotel was as good as another. When I suggested that we stop early, Sally thought I was anxious for the honeymoon night. Well, I was. But the Texas score, now *that* was a really important issue! Mind you, I didn't intend to hurt Sally with my fixation on Texas football. Why, I was behaving like any red-blooded, twenty-seven-year-old Texan would! Unfortunately, I was giving first place to football over my new bride. This wasn't the first or the last time I did this.

We stopped forty miles east of Vail, checked into a motel, had dinner, and got back to the room about 10:15—just in time for the sports report. My adrenaline was pumping—to discover the Texas football score. As my bride disappeared into the bathroom to prepare for our wedding night, I quickly clicked on the television and learned the big news of the day: *Texas had been defeated.* I was literally sick! I can still remember trying to regain my composure as Sally entered the room. She had no idea how important football was in my life, and how upset I was by the opening-day Texas tragedy. Of course, I had never communicated any of this to her.

The very next day brought more conflicts. That morning, on our first full day of married life, we drove on to Vail. Sally had envisioned us spending time together by hiking in the mountains—a romantic outdoors-type honeymoon in the breathtaking mountains of Colorado. But after two hours of walking around gazing at trees, my mind began drifting to thoughts of the NFL, completed passes, and touchdowns. *After all,* I told myself, *when you've seen one tree, you've seen them all.* Wouldn't you know, the Dallas Cowboys and the Green Bay Packers were scheduled to play that afternoon!

Feeling perfectly justified and believing that Sally wanted to watch football also, I began speeding toward Denver in order to find a hotel—and a television with the big game. I knew if we stopped for lunch, we'd miss the start of the game. So we bought some cheese and crackers at a country store and headed for Denver. Of course, I got a speeding ticket along the way. By this time Sally was a very disappointed bride. She sat in silence in the car. No problem; I just figured she didn't have anything to say.

When we arrived in Denver, I suggested that we buy some Kentucky Fried Chicken and take it to the room. She bought a magazine to read while I watched the game. To my dismay, she wasn't very excited about all the big plays. It dawned on me that Sally knew nothing about football when she commented, "Hey, that guy has the same name as you," speaking of the all-pro Dallas Cowboy quarterback, Don Meredith. I remember looking at her and saying, "You've got to be kidding. Do you know anything about football?" to which she replied, "I could care less." Wouldn't you know, the Cowboys lost that day, and I was sick again!

From Sally's viewpoint, the honeymoon (perhaps even the marriage) was a total disaster. The discussion we had that night was mild compared to the ones we had throughout the rest of the football season. Every Saturday and Sunday I could be found sitting in front of the tube watching football games.

17

Sally actually had nothing against football; she had just never thought much about it. Her idea of a pleasant autumn day was walking or riding through the woods, enjoying the changing colors of trees and smelling the brisk autumn air. Again, I thought, *Trees are trees. What's the big deal about trees?*

Already seeds of conflict were beginning to germinate in our marriage. Now, neither of us was right or wrong; well, maybe I was a bit entranced—obsessed?—with football, but my desire to be with Sally was no less. We both meant well; we didn't want to hurt each other. But we did! Clearly our differing backgrounds were beginning to collide and damage our relationship.

Another discouraging force was *our tendency to focus on performance.* We began to notice every failure and weakness in each other. It became absurd. For example, Sally was a good housekeeper, but if she didn't do one particular thing like my mother had, I became critical and drilled her about that one point. I was mature enough to know better, but I couldn't seem to help my critical attitude. She, on the other hand, would criticize the fact that I read the sports page the first thing each morning instead of the Bible. She wanted a "spiritual leader," but all I could think about was football!

The purpose of this book is to help couples avoid ever reaching this unfortunate and unnecessary point in marriage.

Several things stood out. I was amazed at how my feelings of love for her could change so quickly when I was hurt. A jolted marriage relationship can be intensely painful. Rejection, insults, insecurities, and lost devotion can ravage one's emotions. I found that after being wounded emotionally, my strongest feelings of love could quickly change to bitterness.

In spite of our good intentions, we began to find it hard to live together. I can remember thinking to myself that I just couldn't let things continue in the direction they were going. But they did. In just two years, our very best intentions for a model Christian marriage had become, at best, a memory of the past. Things were just mediocre.

The purpose of this book is to help couples avoid ever reaching this unfortunate and unnecessary point in marriage. Tragically, most couples naïvely feel this sort of situation will never happen to them. "We are different. We love each other so much!" they say.

By God's grace, our marriage did not remain mired in mediocrity. During our third year of marriage, while we were involved in a college campus ministry, I noticed that a number of students were getting involved in foolish dating relationships. I saw a need for someone to teach the students some biblical guidelines for dating. So I began to page through the Bible to discover those key insights. It was during this study of dating and marriage that Sally and I discovered our own need.

God changed our marriage. Perhaps those students don't remember much of what we said, but for the Merediths, marriage has never been the same.

TRANSFORMING TRUTHS

The rest of this book is our attempt to describe the biblical truths that transformed our marriage. We've seen the same principles work for countless other couples as well. Believe me, our improvement has not been based on personal strengths. These discoveries stand on the certainty of the Scriptures and God's statement that He intends for marriage to be a blessing. That call for people to bless each other was stated by Peter to the New Testament church, and it certainly applies to the relationship between Christian husbands and wives: "To sum up, all of you be harmonious, sympathetic, brotherly, kind-hearted, and humble in spirit; not returning evil for evil or insult for insult, but giving a blessing instead; for you were called for the very purpose that you might inherit a blessing" (1 Peter 3:8–9).

The first step in solving a problem is to recognize what causes it. For this reason, part 1 of this book attempts to answer the question, "Why are so many marriages failing?" We will discuss six major reasons marriages disintegrate and trace what happens if the causes are not confronted and corrected. Allow me one old football saying: "The best defense is a good offense." If you understand how to recognize and respond to these six factors, you will be much better prepared to thrive in your marriage.

Part 2 describes the spiritual insight necessary to make lasting commitments and changes in marriage. God's purpose for creating marriage will be evident as partners understand His creation plan. This plan can help empower you to experience permanent and fulfilling love. Questions like these will be answered:

- What is God's blueprint for marriage?
- What is love and how can I experience it?
- Did He design my mate for me? If so, why are we struggling so much?
- What part does the Holy Spirit play in marriage?
- What qualities in my life are necessary for me to be a loving spouse?
- How do the roles of the husband and wife work in harmony?

Part 3 gives directions on how to apply these biblical patterns to everyday married life. This section integrates the spiritual and practical sides of marriage. Questions like these will be covered:

- In what ways do men and women differ? How do these differences create conflict?
- How can your sexual expression grow?
- What should be your perspective on trials?
- How can you overcome in-law problems?
- How can you transform financial issues from dividing your marriage to becoming a source of unity?

Couples who understand why marriages fail as well as how God intends marriage to work have a significant advantage. They are well on the road to a growing and thriving marriage. *God not only designed marriage, He can make it work!*

NOTES
1. George Barna, *The Future of the American Family* (Chicago: Moody, 1993), 67–68.
2. Armand Nicholi Jr., in George A. Rekers, ed., *Family Building* (Ventura, Calif.: Gospel Light, 1985), as cited in Bill Bright, *The Coming Revival* (Orlando: New Life, 1994), 54.

CHAPTER TWO

Six Reasons Marriages Fail

◈ WHAT STANDS BETWEEN YOU AND DIVORCE? MOST couples confidently reply:

- "Our love is more mature than most other couples."
- "We are wiser."
- "We are better educated."
- "We have been Christians longer."
- "We know each other so well."

Even though all of those factors will help marriages, they cannot ensure success in marriage. Good intentions will not divorce-proof your marriage. After all, no one gets married expecting the marriage to self-destruct. Yet 50 percent of all divorces occur within three years of saying "I do."[1] Remarkable, isn't it? From "I do" to "Get out!" in less than three years! Among couples who remain married, countless thousands suffer in icy silence, needs unmet, and complete discouragement —a far cry from the joy that God intends for marriage.

So why do marriages fail? This chapter will alert you to the six most common reasons that marriages break up. During more than two decades of counseling literally thousands of couples, Sally and I have seen these six tearing away at marriages and often destroying them. All six reasons represent powerful forces; left unchecked, they will silently undermine your most valued human relationship.

We challenge you to learn what these powerful forces are, how to safe-guard your marriage, and spread your new insights to extended family and friends. Interestingly, the more confident that couples are concerning their love and commitment, the more closed-minded they are to help or suggestion. The apostle Paul wrote, "Therefore let him who thinks he stands take heed that he does not fall" (1 Corinthians 10:12). Jesus exhorted His followers to count the cost prior to undertaking a significant life commitment. "For which one of you, when he wants to build a tower, does not first sit down and calculate the cost to see if he has enough to complete it? Otherwise, when he has laid a foundation and is not able to finish, all who observe it begin to ridicule him, saying, 'This man began to build and was not able to finish'" (Luke 14:28–30).

Most people complete twelve to sixteen years of schooling to learn a career. But few ever take a course on marriage. No wonder marriages fail—people are not prepared for the most important relationship on this earth.

Have you counted the cost for a successful marriage? Are you prepared to overcome the six most common reasons marriages fail?

REASON ONE:
DIFFERING BACKGROUNDS, HOMES, AND ENVIRONMENTS

Our melting-pot society results in many couples getting married with very different backgrounds. These cultural and family differences often result in immediate disagreements, which lead to conflict and hurt. At first, couples find that it's fun making up. As the differences become more personal and numerous, however, couples begin to focus on the performance of their mate. Over time, this progression begins to undermine their commitment to each other. These differences may touch every activity or belief of the couple.

Early in our marriage, Sally and I had to face adjustments due to family differences. We married after a short engagement, only to discover we really did not know each other very well. Remember, women, as you read this, please do not give up on me! I really didn't intend to hurt Sally.

I grew up in Texas where my parents were outgoing people of modest means. Because Dad was in sales, we were often involved in community-wide social events. We did not have a great deal of money, but I was fairly free financially. Sally, on the other hand, grew up in the mountains of Colorado. Her family had close friends and relatives, but weren't active in social circles. In addition, she was very different in the way she approached finances. I felt considerably freer about spending money, while she was more conservative in her money management.

When my family took vacations, we usually got up early in the morning and drove all day. We stopped at new motels that were certain to be clean and comfortable. We were the "no-surprises" people. Thirty years ago, Holiday Inn fit the bill perfectly. We seldom stopped to eat at expensive restaurants, preferring burgers and fries instead. When we traveled, we were very goal oriented. The vacation started after we arrived at our destination.

By contrast, Sally's family considered the drive as part of the vacation. Since they enjoyed eating out, they splurged on good meals. To afford that, they economized in other areas, primarily in their choice of motels. They shopped motels to find the best deal. I've learned since that many people do that, but at the time it was a real jolt to my country-club pride. Sally always seemed to head for those old, beige-colored stucco motels—you know, the kind with the creaky furniture, the 1926 chenille bedspreads, and the everyday low prices.

The first two days of our honeymoon we stayed in what I considered nice motels. On the third day, we headed for Tulsa. To Sally's great disappointment, I had decided to cut the honeymoon short. After all, there were no more football games, and who wants to look at the trees? Being a Holiday Inn man, I kept driving trying to find one. I wasn't about to lower my standards. It didn't occur to me that in that sparsely populated area of the country, there might not be a Holiday Inn. And since we were still ignorant of each other's choices, Sally couldn't understand why I wouldn't stop. She fell asleep in the car. After driving through town after town with no Holiday Inn, we found ourselves nearly out of gas at two o'clock in the morning. Fortunately, we were close to a small New Mexico town, one hundred miles from nowhere.

It's likely you have married . . . someone very different from yourself. These differ- ences . . . can lead your spouse and you down the road to hurt and rejection.

There were only three motels in town. To me, they were all the old, unpredictable kind that didn't appeal to my senses at all. To Sally there was nothing unacceptable about them. In fact, she encouraged me to check each motel at 2:00 a.m. for rates! Much to my discomfort, we had to stay, since no gas stations were open at that time of the morning. I lay awake thinking bugs were going to eat me while Sally slept like a baby.

Throughout our travels later that fall, there were many opportunities to stay in motels. Sally, motivated to be a good steward of God's money, just didn't feel right about paying Holiday Inn prices. I didn't want to settle for anything less. Note that it wasn't so much an issue of right or wrong, but of two people with different perspectives. That first year, we experienced some real hurt and conflict over such differences. Because of my strong logical reasoning, I was able to maneuver her toward my thinking, but in the process I unknowingly destroyed some of her respect for me.

Another example of a difference that caused almost immediate struggle involved our intellectual pursuits. As someone interested in sports activities more than reading, I almost never read a book. I was a *Cliffs Notes* man. I don't think I had read ten books in my entire life up to that point. My bride, on the other hand, was the intellectual in our family. Indeed, she still is an excellent student who loves to read. She came from a family who read constantly.

Later we discovered another difference: Sally is more group-oriented while I am a one-on-one person.

We have since learned to value our differences and learn from one another. I now enjoy reading and even writing, while she has learned to enjoy various sports activities with me. But in those early days, our divergent intellectual and social pursuits were a real problem. We simply placed different values on different things.

When people get married, they're usually at the peak of emotional love. Their intentions are so good, they would do anything for the other. Yet, immediately after the wedding day, they begin to recognize many differences. The examples mentioned above, differences in lodging preferences and in intellectual and social pursuits, may seem small by themselves. But if multiplied by ten other issues, the couple can quickly become overwhelmed with obstacles.

In our diversified American society, it's likely you have married (or will marry) someone very different from yourself. These differences, if not properly anticipated, can lead your spouse and you down the road to hurt and rejection. And for many couples, there's the added emotional baggage from a previous marriage. If stepchildren are also involved, the blending process often can take years to work through.

REASON TWO:
THE DECEPTIVE "FIFTY-FIFTY" RELATIONSHIP

Marriage, many believe, is a "fifty-fifty" relationship. That belief sounds good and seems to make sense. There's just one problem—it doesn't work.

That proposition is the second major reason marriages fail. Here's why: Thinking our spouse must do his or her 50 percent leads us to focus on the other person's performance. Over time, each mate wants to ensure that the *other* does *his or her part*. Human nature demands it. Unfortunately, there is no way to know who met whom halfway. It is impossible to know if the other mate cared as much, worked as hard, or felt as strongly. Ultimately, couples are drawn into deeper levels of examination and criticism. Furthermore, the fifty-fifty concept actually promotes independence: "You do your part; I'll do mine."

Once couples start measuring each other's performance, disappointment follows close behind, leading to feelings of rejection and hurt. Some mates react with anger; others respond with a deafening silence. Either way, a cycle

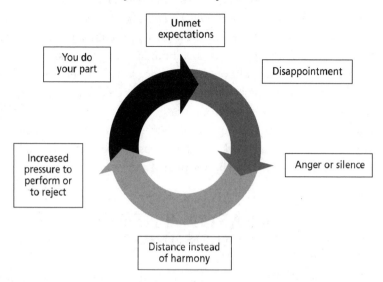

Figure 1
The Cycle of Unmet Expectations

Unmet expectations

You do your part

Disappointment

Increased pressure to perform or to reject

Anger or silence

Distance instead of harmony

begins (above) resulting in distance.

The resulting frustration reveals the fallacy of the fifty-fifty notion. It is impossible to believe *that the other person has actually met you halfway.* The minute one mate believes the other is not meeting him halfway, condemnation and conflict usually follow.

As newlyweds, Dave and Ruth experienced the cycle above. They became so tense and uptight that they regularly overstated things and made hurtful accusations, such as "Well, maybe we shouldn't have gotten married," or "Maybe I'm not the person you thought I was!" As the arguments escalated, Ruth resorted to cutting remarks, only to have David retaliate. Eventually, Ruth would start crying, march to the bedroom, and slam the door shut. At that, David would get in the car and drive around town, his stomach in a knot. After an hour or so, he'd return home in hopes of making up to Ruth.

Early in the marriage, they actually enjoyed the making-up scenes, believing them to be evidences of a growing maturity and ability to handle differences. But with the passing of time, the fun of making up faded and their resentment began to slowly build. *If David knew how badly I was hurting, he'd stop yelling at me,* she thought to herself. *He doesn't understand how hurt I am.* Strangely, David had similar thoughts. He could never believe that Ruth cared as much as he did. And he felt he was always the first to give in. Resentment and hostility continued to smolder in each partner, making it more difficult to say, "I'm sorry" and really mean it.

With the cycle in full gear, resentment soon led to anger. David began keeping a mental tally on how Ruth responded. She kept her own score. He studied her every move, looking for an opportunity to criticize. If she didn't respond "properly," that is, *according to David's standard of performance,* he pounced on her mistake. Ruth withdrew into a protective shell of silence.

Maybe you're thinking, "Christians shouldn't have those kind of problems." No, they shouldn't, but, believe us, they do. We find very little difference between Christian and non-Christian couples in our counseling. Entering marriage naïvely, planning to only meet your mate halfway, will guarantee the same results as David and Ruth experienced: bitter frustration and aloneness. The fifty-fifty relationship may work in other areas of life, but it miserably fails in marriage. God has an infinitely better plan!

REASON THREE:
SELFISHNESS

The third reason most marriages fail is outright selfishness. The natural human way is to look out for number one first. The Bible tells us that every person has an inborn sense of selfishness that is capable of incredible devastation. "The heart is more deceitful than all else and is desperately sick; who can understand it?" (Jeremiah 17:9). We don't really believe that about our own hearts, do we? Yet strong, self-centered agendas appear in most marriages, and the mate almost always resists and retaliates against the agenda.

You may think you're right; indeed, perhaps you are. But the Lord Jesus calls us to serve one another, [to put] the well-being of our mate first.

If you aren't yet married or are newly married, you're probably thinking, *That doesn't describe my mate,* or *That's too strong.* Most couples naïvely enter marriage believing their mates are incapable of such actions. But the failure to deal openly with this human tendency frequently leads to disappointment and dissatisfaction in marriage.

The Bible says we all have this innate tendency to look out for ourselves first, and calls it *the flesh, old man, and old nature.* It also calls it sin. For that reason, only Jesus Christ is able to break this bondage to self and give us a supernatural, divine nature. But even after becoming Christians, we need to mature in the Spirit to rise above selfishness.

There will be times in marriage when you really want your way. You may think you're right; *indeed, perhaps you are.* But the Lord Jesus calls us to serve one another, and that specifically means putting the well-being of our mate first.

Couples who marry without a firm commitment to sacrifice selfish rights in order to serve the other will invariably inflict emotional pain on one another. Two people with sinful natures who marry don't make for greater peace; rather, great strife and destruction follow.

During counseling, we typically hear statements like, "He doesn't understand me anymore" or "I thought she was a Christian. How can she act that way?" With eyes welling up in tears, some women say, "I can't repeat the words he called me." Some altercations become physically violent with punches thrown and threats to kill. But not everyone is outwardly aggressive. Some seethe in silence, resolving to get even. Christians marry with the best of intentions, only to discover that their lifelong mates are capable of inflicting great hurt, often with little remorse. Feelings of love are replaced with fear. Romance sours. Hostile environments mushroom like ominous summer thunderstorms, reinforcing the tendency to serve oneself first.

Everyone has a choice to make: We can be either a mirror that reflects approval, appreciation, and encouragement to our mates, or we can reflect failure and disappointment. What does your mate get from you? If your reflection is negative, the result will be fear and retaliation. Over time, feelings will become frozen and attitudes critical. And our harsh words and attitudes can be destructive: "'The poison of asps is under their lips; whose mouth is full of cursing and bitterness; their feet are swift to shed blood, destruction and misery are in their paths, and the path of peace they have not known'" (Romans 3:13–17).

Strong words, right? But turn on the nightly news and listen to the description of family life in America. How can one spouse come to the point of killing the one he once loved? *Every family tragedy mentioned above started with good intentions.* The root cause is nothing less than sinful, selfish behavior, and only Christ can deliver. The apostle Paul described the struggle—and the solution—in Romans 7:22–8:2:

> *For I joyfully concur with the law of God in the inner man, but I see a different law in the members of my body, waging war against the law of my mind and making me a prisoner of the law of sin which is in my members. Wretched man that I am! Who will set me free from the body of this death? Thanks be to God through Jesus Christ our Lord! So then, on the one hand I myself with my mind am serving the law of God, but on the other, with my flesh the law of sin. Therefor there is now no condemnation for those who are in Christ Jesus. For the law of the Spirit of life in Christ Jesus has set you free from the law of sin and of death.*

So take heart. The balance of this book reveals God's plan for a successful, lasting, and joyful marriage. We will see that a successful marriage depends on the Holy Spirit freeing us from our selfish, sinful attitudes.

REASON FOUR:
INABILITY TO COPE WITH LIFE'S TRIALS

I used to believe that successful Christians dodged trials like soldiers running through a field of land mines. The people who missed the most mines were successful. Trials were for the unfortunate or unfaithful. As a result, when I married Sally, I had given no thought to facing trials. Although I knew there would be tough times, I expected them to be few and momentary. Most couples marry with a similar perspective, particularly younger newlyweds. We're no longer surprised to hear, "If I had known then what I know now, I would have never gotten married."

This inability to anticipate or cope with the normal trials of life represents the fourth major cause of marriage failure. When couples enter marriage with a naïve perception of trials, it's not long before each partner begins to say, "Well, I must have married the wrong person. I never thought marriage would be like *this*." Doubt, division, and distance replace the unity and strength God desires for trials to produce in the marriage.

When this became an issue early in our marriage, we began a study of what God's Word had to say about trials, primarily because of our own desperate need. Our first reality shock came from reviewing 1 Peter 2:21: "For you have been called for this purpose, since Christ also suffered for you, leaving you an example for you to follow in His steps." The passage clearly teaches that God will allow Christians to suffer trials. God also gave us Christ as our model to overcome trials.

As Christians, we gladly accept the blessing of salvation through Christ's suffering. Yet we quickly reject any thought of joining in His suffering. Like the culture around us, we come to see our mission in life as avoiding pain or anything uncomfortable. But if our Lord suffered through trials, shouldn't we expect to experience them? The Bible teaches that God uses trials to cultivate the character of Christ in us. James explained that trials produce endurance, which leads to maturity. Therefore we are to "consider it all joy . . . when [we] encounter various trials" (James 1:2). The joy in this passage means a deep abiding peace that transcends difficult circumstances.

Sally and I repeatedly see couples in counseling who think their marriage is in trouble because of the trials they face. When they can't eliminate the trials, they attribute the resulting frustration and stress to their mate or marriage. *Blaming replaces unity.*

The truth is, life will almost always present us with trials. Most couples will experience them. Because they are so predictable, mental preparation is a must for wise couples. And though we can never be fully prepared for the unexpected, knowing that God is in control and that He has a plan for us can radically change the outcome. Recognizing suffering will come and giving thanks in the midst of it is a prerequisite to success in marriage.

When we got married, Sally had been a Christian for a number of years and was a very effective counselor on several college campuses. After a few years, our first child graced our home, followed by our second a year later. Through her contacts with students, Sally enjoyed a handy network of baby-sitters. The college girls needed the money, and Sally was able to continue her counseling ministries. It was a dream setup.

Shortly after our second child arrived, however, we moved to another city. With both children in diapers and each demanding more time and care, Sally's life totally changed. Her network of child-care help evaporated since it was difficult to become acquainted with people in the new neighborhood. My work required me to travel frequently, supervising staff in a large five-city area. The brunt of the move fell on Sally, who lost her counseling ministry, all her child-care support, and began a new era as a full-time mother.

My attitude was destroying what little self-respect she had left. . . . Sally did pull through this difficult life change, but with precious little help from me!

Her stress level skyrocketed. Often when I came home, her frustration was so high that we quickly had blowups, and I didn't understand why. Unresolved tension rapidly drained our "feelings" during this period. Like so many couples, we blamed the pain of life on each other, and we generalized: All of the frustration is because of our marriage, we thought.

I began to feel like Sally didn't love me. She sure wasn't much fun to be around anymore. I resented her negative changes when everything was going so well for me professionally—finding great success in my work, growing in the Christian life, and gaining respect among my peers. And since I didn't understand normal trials in life, it was as though I was blind to her sufferings. To make matters worse, I actually developed spiritual pride and said things like, "Sally, you've been acting like this for months! When are you going to snap out of it? What's the matter with you? You used to be such a stable Christian."

Actually, Sally was then—and is now—a godly woman, but my attitude was destroying what little self-respect she had left. The confidence she had in her relationship with Christ began to fade away. After much prayer and perseverance, Sally did pull through this difficult life change, but with precious little help from me! Having God's perspective on trials would have made things so much easier. We weren't out of God's will because we moved to another city, because we had two children so close together, or by our daily routines being changed so much. Instead, I failed to lift Sally up in the midst of this trial because we were unprepared for it.

Major lifestyle changes, such as having a child, moving, changing jobs, or even the death of a family member will trigger various degrees of trials. Daily living presents its own set of trials and sufferings. Isn't that what we confessed in our marriage vows when we said "for better or for worse, in sickness and in health?" So the issue is not how to avoid trials, but rather how to face them together.

Are you prepared to stand together? Having studied marriages for years, we have observed that trials stimulate growth in successful marriages. In less successful marriages, trials become a source of struggle, bitterness, and division. (In the final chapter, we will consider in depth how to confront some of the major trials in marriage.)

REASON FIVE:
FANTASY VIEW OF LOVE

With a troubled tone, Harry stammered, "After sixteen years of marriage, how could she fall in love with another man? How could she spend time alone with Jim? She should have known better. Now she wants him instead of me. I've been faithful; why can't she be?"

"It's his fault," Sue replied. "For two years he said he didn't care. I thought I would go crazy. Finally, in desperation, I turned to Jim and he was so understanding. We didn't plan on it, but we fell in love."

The fifth major cause of marriage failure today is what I call "fantasy love." It is based on feelings more than anything else. It is the kind of love we read about or see in movies and on television, represented by an emotional "high" that causes us to daydream and fantasize, or sends chills up our spines.

It is true that God created us with emotions, and they are an important element of human love. But *emotions are a terrible basis for a relationship*. The tragedy of fantasy love is that it is primarily based on feelings. If a person doesn't feel it anymore, he or she concludes that love has disappeared. Poof—it's gone! Like the couple I just mentioned, most couples today define love in terms of how they feel. There can be no weaker foundation for a relationship.

One of the primary contributors to fantasy love is unrestrained sexual expression. Our culture has encouraged the abuse of one of God's greatest gifts by encouraging people to prematurely become sexually active. Few issues can obscure an important decision more than sex. Encouraged by physical intimacy, emotions will flare instantly beyond normal proportions. Couples easily mistake lust for love. A relationship based solely on sex is bound for disaster. Today in a majority of troubled marriages, couples list sexual problems as one contributing factor. One study found that "virgin brides . . . are less likely to divorce than women who lost their virginity prior to marriage."[2] For many, these problems started long before their marriage began. Living together before marriage does not insure the adjustment or the relationship. Statistics prove just the opposite. "Couples who live together before marriage are about 48% more likely to divorce than those who don't," according to a *USA Today* article that reported the findings of a Rutgers University study. The research also found that unmarried couples have lower levels of happiness and a higher risk of domestic violence for the women.[3]

Most couples define love in terms of how they feel There can be no weaker foundation for a relationship.

Some time ago a single woman came to ask my advice about a man with whom she was "terribly in love." I talked with her for about thirty minutes, and it was apparent she believed the relationship was really serious. At one point I made several suggestions on how to improve communications with her friend. Much to my surprise, she answered, "Oh, I haven't actually talked to him yet." Can you believe it? She had created a complete love relationship with a man she had never talked to! She was deeply in love with a myth! Today, easy access to the Internet allows long-distance computer love affairs with those we do not really know—the ultimate example of fantasy love!

Instead of risking the disappointment of rejection by a real person, some people create fantasies to bring them emotional pleasure. Not long ago I read in the newspaper that television soap operas have become such an important part of American women's lives that when news stories preempt the soap operas, the TV networks are deluged with complaints. The article went on to say that women are so caught up in these stories that when a marriage or death occurs on the screen, TV stations across the nation actually receive flowers or condolence cards. The end result of such fantasies is often personal mysticism and deep depression.

David's relationship with Bathsheba in the Old Testament is another example of fantasy love. As you recall, David had decided to stay home rather than fulfill his military duty. One day, while strolling on the palace roof, he noticed a woman bathing. He began to lust and have a fantasy relationship; then he had to have her. After learning who Bathsheba was, David had her husband, Uriah (a part of David's inner guard; 2 Samuel 23:8, 39), dispatched to war with sinister plans for him to purposely be killed. The ensuing affair would transform David into a liar, adulterer, and even a murderer. It is not an overstatement to say that affairs are based on lies and deception and may even lead to murder. They plunge honorable people into disgrace.

All fantasy love relationships, whether real or imagined, are simply counterfeit ways of trying to meet our needs. On the other hand, God's definition of love provides the real basis for permanent feelings. The Bible teaches that permanent feelings are only possible when couples learn to love by faith. Part 2 of this book describes that kind of love.

REASON SIX:
LACK OF A VITAL RELATIONSHIP WITH JESUS CHRIST

According to Colossians 1:16, "All things have been created through Him and for Him." That includes marriage. Your marriage exists primarily to bring honor and glory to God. Even before you list your hopes, dreams, and needs for marriage, God is the first reason for your union. That's what it means to call Jesus Christ *preeminent:* He gets first place in all things, including your relationship.

The fundamental reason why marriages fail is because many couples lack a vital relationship with Jesus Christ. Only Jesus Christ can unlock the deepest dimensions of human intimacy that occur at the spiritual level. If Jesus Christ does not dwell in your life, you're living at a reduced level of intimacy in your marriage. This is necessarily so since you're spiritually dead until Christ gives you life (see Ephesians 2:1). As shown in figure 2 (page 38), "Finding True Spiritual Intimacy," only Jesus Christ can take individuals and couples to their deepest level of intimacy—the intimacy of spirit.

Spiritual death in our lives limits intimacy in our marriages. Early in Genesis we see this principle at work. The death that God warned Adam about in Genesis 2:17 was realized later when the first couple together rebelled against God. Their fall in Genesis 3 did not bring immediate physical death. However, their fellowship was severed and they experienced spiritual death. Note that both Adam and Eve hid "themselves"; literally, their core selves were masked from God and one another. No longer did they enjoy the transparency and vulnerability described in Genesis 2:25. Instead, shame and blame replaced the perfect fellowship they once experienced.

You may experience various degrees of intimacy with one another physically,

Figure 2
Finding True Spiritual Intimacy

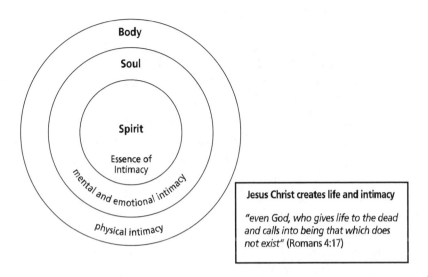

mentally, and emotionally in marriage. But only Jesus Christ can bring life to your core inner being—*your spirit*. Life at the spiritual level is most essential since God opens to the believing Christian a vast reservoir of supernatural capabilities for love, forgiveness, mercy, and all the fruits of the Holy Spirit. If you think you love your spouse now, just try loving him or her with the agape love of God!

The prerequisite to loving your spouse with God's agape love is maintaining a vibrant, intimate relationship with Jesus Christ. Many people know *about* God, have joined the church, been baptized, but really overlook knowing God *personally*. Others have become Christians and have a personal relationship with God through Christ, yet lack a vibrant, daily relationship with Him. Like getting to know a new friend, knowing God involves communicating with Him frequently, as well as having a growing appreciation for His attributes—holiness, mercy, love, kindness, and so on. When we know God in this intimate way, He is able to transform our lives by His love, thus equipping us to love our spouses even better.

It is possible to have Jesus Christ in your heart, but neglect a personal relationship with Him. To illustrate, suppose two people married, but immediately parted company after the wedding ceremony. One moved to New York and the other to Los Angeles, and the two lived with this arrangement for years. Are they legally married? Yes! But do they know one another very well? Hardly. Intimacy requires the investment of time and effort. It involves sharing yourself and becoming intimately acquainted with your spouse. Making Christ preeminent in your marriage requires that you first cultivate your intimate relationship with Him in your prayer life and Bible study time.

FROM GOOD INTENTIONS
TO CRITICISM AND FAILURE

As we noted earlier, good intentions cannot assure a successful marriage. Good intentions quickly give way to self-centered natures. As feelings subside, the couple slips into a fifty-fifty plan of responsibilities. Unsure that your mate is doing his part, you begin to watch your spouse's performance. A short list of observed failures begins to grow. You may soon conclude that you're stuck with a loser, an attitude certain to offend the mate. Critical attitudes deepen, and the cycle spins deeper and deeper. When you factor in trials common to most marriages, frustrations explode. Instead of standing together in adversity, the trials drive you farther apart as a couple.

So you see how easy it is for couples to plummet from marital bliss to shocking criticism and failure. Fantasy love has long evaporated, and they begin to think, "There's someone else out there who can better meet my needs."

The good news is that if you find yourself in this cycle, God has made a way for you to break free. If you're newly married, you don't have to get caught up in this destructive cycle. Regardless of how tempting each of the six reasons for marital failure noted above is, you can overcome all of them in Christ. Parts 2 and 3 will demonstrate that God not only created marriage; *He can make marriage work!*

NOTES

1. Larry Whitham, "Study of Successes Leads to Scoring of Couples' Chances," *The Washington Times,* 2 April 1996, A3.

2. "The Trouble with Premarital Sex," *U.S. News & World Report,* 19 May 1997, 60.

3. Karen S. Peterson, "Live-in Couples May Miss Out," *USA Today,* 1 February 1999, D1.

CHAPTER THREE

How the Flame Fades

WE OFTEN FACE COUPLES WHOSE DREAMS ARE being destroyed by one or more of the six factors discussed in chapter 2. Yet a person may understand all of the pitfalls and work to address them and still become ensnared in a problem marriage.

The flame that warmed romantic love and spurred a deeper love doesn't fade overnight; the fires and the dreams die gradually and subtly. In almost thirty years of working closely with couples and individuals, we have observed a progression toward bitterness and isolation in marriage that typically includes the following four stages:

- Stage One: The Days of Romance
- Stage Two: The Days of Reality
- Stage Three: The Days of Resentment
- Stage Four: The Days of Rebellion

While the stages are not absolute, they exist in most problem marriages. We could subtitle this chapter, "Predictable Stages of Marital Decline," as the stages are common and often cause the flame of marital love to flicker and fade. We will look at each.

STAGE ONE:
THE DAYS OF ROMANCE

Our media is presently bombarding Americans with an unprecedented blitz that delivers one prevailing message: Experience the finest, most tantalizing things in life without taking personal responsibility. That is the ultimate fantasy, and its message comes constantly, delivered by the ever-present TV, and for the typical American, "six hundred advertising messages each day."[1] Years of this programming have resulted in a society that is looking for an experience or romance. The purpose of each message is to make you dissatisfied with what you have so you'll buy what the advertisers are selling.

Nowhere is this message clearer than the realm of romance. Marriage is portrayed as negative. Fantasy sex is portrayed as quick and positive. And love is confused with sex. Sex and love are greatly distorted from God's original purpose.

The values of our culture are diametrically opposed to God's values. These messages completely contradict the biblical teaching that love requires commitment. Only the Bible can offer a clear picture of marriage and family. The influence of Hollywood's values on our culture has been devastating. People are bound together on the basis of humanistic experiences or a rootless romanticism based on feelings. The result is that most marriages begin with each mate loaded with expectations that few spouses could ever fulfill.

During stage one, partners regard a good marriage as romance and often good sex as good marriage. The stage of romance typifies the first year of marriage, although this stage may last the first three years. Everything is bright and rosy; neither spouse is overly tired. (After all, there are no children, at least for the first nine months.) Romantic feelings prevail, and the pressures of job and home don't dominate.

This cultural worldview has set them up for disappointment and hurt. Since so many relationships are not grounded in the Word of God, the crash is swift and painful.

STAGE TWO:
THE DAYS OF REALITY

The second stage usually occurs within the first three to five years of marriage, but may begin in the very first year. Sometimes the myths about sex and romance are destroyed before the honeymoon is over. Sooner or later, reality sets in. If there has been sex before marriage with one or more partners, sex within marriage just doesn't measure up.

Often reality is a harsh reminder of simply running out of time, as seen in the lives of Julie and Jim. Julie gets up by six, gets dressed, cooks, and is quickly off to work. After a hectic day at the office, she arrives home by six, fixes supper, eats, and finishes the dishes by eight. Washing clothes or house details may keep her busy until ten o'clock. By that time Julie is already thinking about getting up early the next morning, and she has had no real time for herself. Her husband Jim, oblivious to her workload, has been watching television all evening. By 10 PM, he has fully relaxed after his busy workday; now he's ready for romance.

And Julie? Emotionally, Julie is unable to respond. Jim wonders what's wrong with her!

Perhaps she is waiting for the day she can have children so she can stay at home. But when that day comes she will discover even greater pressure and responsibility. After several years, instead of experiencing marriage as a sexy honeymoon, Julie finds herself fighting for enough strength and personal time just to hold herself together.

The euphoria of romance is quickly replaced by the harsh realities of life. . . . Romance gives way to mediocrity.

Jim was idealistic when they married, a true believer in the romanticism of marriage. Deep in fantasy love, Jim loved to hold his sweetheart, and he thought his job was great. Before long, however he became frustrated and unsure about his future. Changing jobs was not an option since he would likely have to return to a starting salary. Now he feels pressure from Julie, who doesn't want to feel trapped by financial circumstances, and he doesn't want to upset her even more.

So the euphoria of romance is quickly replaced by the harsh realities of life. Fantasy love gives way to job pressures and money problems. As children come along, they demand an even greater commitment. Romance gives way to mediocrity.

During this sobering stage, feelings begin to wane. Depression overtakes joy and contentment. Romantic zeal fades. This can be catastrophic since the fantasy feelings were the primary basis for the marriage. Frequent expressions of love disappear, followed by an unwillingness to serve the other. Left unchecked, a scary feeling settles into the pit of Jim and Julie's stomachs that they may have made a mistake by marrying each other.

STAGE THREE:
THE DAYS OF RESENTMENT

When feelings have changed and creative, sacrificial acts disappear, marriage partners begin to deeply resent each other. Blaming begins with statements like "You never talk to me anymore," or "We *never* have sex anymore," or "You *always* . . ." It becomes obvious when one partner has reached the point of feeling "stuck" with his or her mate. The one who feels stuck resents the other's inadequacies and may even resent God for allowing the marriage to occur. The other mate feels judged, rejected, and misunderstood, which quickly degenerates into anger. Thus the cycle of resentment has begun.

When couples reach this point of deep resentment, they begin to lose hope. If they don't get help, they typically move in one of two directions. First, they may tragically move toward divorce. Since there is so little stigma in divorce today, many couples just give up and get out! But divorce is rarely the answer. All too often it only leads to more frustration, depression, and financial hardship. And then these couples usually remarry, only to carry with them emotional baggage and the extremely difficult adjustments of blending families.

The second direction is the *compromised marriage.* A large segment of marriages today fit into this category. A compromised marriage is one in which people don't really deal with their mistakes, attitudes, weaknesses, and differences. Instead, each goes his or her own way and purposely avoids the volatile areas of the marriage. It's a pretend marriage. On the surface, they appear to be all right, but inside they harbor deep resentment. Occasionally the pressure may build until the couple explode in anger. Several days of frustration will end with a statement similar to this: "Well, I wish things were different. But I am not going to end the relationship because of what it would do to the children. So, I'll just put up with the problems." Try as they will, compromised couples cannot prosper over the long haul.

Many supposedly successful marriages are really just two people going their own independent ways, being careful not to step on each other's toes.

Sexual dysfunction often appears in a compromised marriage. The wife may be so disillusioned that she simply has no sexual appetite. For instance, Matt is aware that his wife, Brenda, is aloof, even cold to him. He tries to ignore her passivity at first, but on a particular night, he observes Brenda undressing and his attraction cannot be restrained. Tired and resentful of Matt's lack of attention earlier in the evening, she refuses his advances. Matt explodes. Brenda feels angry and guilty at the same time. They fall asleep on opposite sides of the bed and awaken the next morning to "no comment."

Or consider the wife who is raising the children with a husband who is never home or remains uninvolved. Sharon sees personality or discipline problems developing in her children daily, and she cannot bear the burdens alone. Since she knows her husband resents her for saying anything, she tries to ignore the problems. One night John, who hasn't spent meaningful time with the children in weeks, gets angry with them, yells, and even spanks them. Unable to stand it, Sharon explodes, and the gap in the marriage widens.

Sadly, many supposedly successful marriages are really just two people going their own independent ways, being careful not to step on each other's toes. The husband loses himself in his work to compensate for the lack of respect at home. The wife becomes consumed with the children to compensate for the lack of intimacy within the marriage.

Compromised marriages often rock along until the partners reach their late forties or early fifties, and the children leave home. The true measure of their relationship comes when all they have is each other. Ultimately, most compromised relationships lead to deeper and deeper resentment. If not checked, resentment will destroy a person's life like a cancer.

STAGE FOUR:
THE DAYS OF REBELLION

Unresolved resentment impacts men and women differently. Women typically become critical, and then fearful. Men become hardened and uncaring. For a season, resentment may simmer behind the illusion of a healthy marriage, fueled by unmet needs. Sooner or later, however, the compounding resentment explodes into overt acts of rebellion against the spouse.

Paula entered marriage with deep romantic feelings for Steve. She viewed him with trust, placing him high on a pedestal. She dreamed of a model home and children. Her body was young and her self-image was at a peak.

But after several years of marriage, her dreams had turned to nightmares. She and Steve had failed to cope with reality in their marriage, and resentment consumed each of them. Her feelings for Steve were distant history. She not only didn't trust Steve, but she criticized his every move. Along with bearing children, the stress of the marriage had taken a toll on her once attractive figure. She didn't even like herself anymore. Her days often seemed burdensome, long, and introspective. The soured marriage was constantly on her mind. Rather than facing the future with confidence, Paula greeted each day with a fear of failure and an increasingly critical attitude toward Steve.

The soured marriage was constantly on her mind. . . . Paula greeted each day with a fear of failure and an increasingly critical attitude toward Steve.

What a sad picture. With two children, ages seven and four, Paula knows the tremendous personal responsibility they will demand over the next fifteen years. By then she will be forty-five and her youthful years will be long gone. All that will be left is a husband for whom she has lost her enthusiasm.

Paula has subconsciously become *fearful* and *depressed.* Fearful, hurting people sometimes take desperate actions to regain a sense of control in their lives. Often that action comes in the form of rebellion against God and the mate. Often in counseling wives say something like, "Life is no fun anymore," or "I don't enjoy people like I used to," or "So-and-so (another man) makes me feel so alive and appreciated." God created women and men in such a way that they require hope. Without it, rebellion can erupt into all kinds of behavior that will deliver the final blow to the marriage.

Steve, like most men, responded to his unresolved resentment differently. He hardened his feelings toward others, including his mate. He had become more *insensitive* and *self-centered* in their relationship. How different from when they first married. During the first months, Steve would have literally died for Paula. But as she became more aware of Steve's weaknesses, Paula increasingly criticized his actions. Steve's sense of self-confidence as the spiritual leader in his home plummeted. Feelings of failure replaced courage and creativity. Faced with Paula's growing criticism, Steve retreated. His respect for her was soon replaced with disgust and avoidance. How far can the stage of rebellion lead a man in his calloused disregard for his wife? Some years ago Carl showed me just how far.

After Carl entered my office for counseling, I quickly learned he and Alice had been married twenty years. As I listened, I was impressed with how romantic the early years of marriage were for this couple. With the passing of time, however, Alice's domineering personality made her critical of his every move. She frequently humiliated him by correcting him in public. Increasingly she sowed seeds of disrespect. At the time Carl came to my office, the two had separated.

As Carl's story unfolded, I could tell he had layers of resentment and bitterness deep inside. Over the next few weeks, Alice and Carl alternated with counseling appointments, but they never came together.

Not long after our first few appointments, Alice called me from the hospital to say that she was having emergency cancer surgery. She was terribly frightened, and asked if I would call Carl and ask him to visit her.

When I finally reached Carl, he was preparing to leave town on a deep-sea fishing trip. After I explained Alice's medical emergency, he replied, "That woman has been controlling my life for twenty years. I don't care if she dies and goes to hell; she isn't going to ruin my fishing trip!" And he hung up. Here was a man who worshiped his wife early in marriage, but now had become hardened against her. For Carl, rebellion took the shape of breaking her heart and spirit at a time when she most needed him.

But remember: Carl's heart didn't become calloused overnight. If not corrected, the patterns of fearfulness for women and hardness for men will deteriorate until both mates begin to think that the *best of life was missed because of their spouse.* The cancer of bitterness is predictable, progressive, and will become overwhelming. Don't play around with unresolved bitterness and resentment. You may think you have it under control today; tomorrow it may blow up in your face. *The spark of love and commitment fades one incident at a time.* Has bitterness taken root in your heart and marriage?

THE ULTIMATE SOLUTION

How can we as couples avoid moving to stages three and four? Sadly, even Christians can move into these later stages when God is not the center of their lives. But it need not be that way. Although all couples will experience the first two stages of romanticism and reality, stages three and four—resentment and rebellion—are not automatic. In fact, as the disillusionment of the reality stage sets in, every couple will arrive at a critical crossroads in their relationship: turn to God in faith, or begin the slippery slide into resentment and rebellion.

Submitting to Christ's love will allow you to have dominion over your self-centeredness and sin. As Christians, your mate and you can now find oneness in marriage and a new beginning by drawing closer to Christ.

What if you are not a Christian? Then the ultimate solution to stages three and four is to come to Christ in faith. Breaking the cycle of bitterness and resentment rooted deep within the human heart has only one cure: literally being saved by the Lord Jesus Christ. When you turn to Christ in faith, you literally access divine resources to keep your love fresh for one another.

Receiving the life and power of the Lord Jesus Christ . . . is the only true hope for restoring a marriage.

A man once asked, "Don, is it necessary to mention God when discussing my marriage problems?" We had just spent several hours discussing the four stages of a declining marriage. I answered his question with a question of my own.

"Mike, as we have talked about you and Judy, your struggles, conflicts, and rejection of each other, you said you could not seem to control your actions. Why?"

"I don't know," Mike replied.

"Two people who are egocentric and self-centered will naturally struggle," I explained. "When their feelings fade, they have no natural basis upon which to build a relationship. Frankly, only Jesus Christ can provide a lasting basis for your relationship, Mike."

"Yes, but I've heard all that before. Being a Christian didn't stop our friends Bill and Joyce from getting a divorce."

"Mike," I replied, "don't reject Christ's love and power because of some hypocrisy or downfall you've seen in someone else. God continues to love us even when we reject Him. Christ died for your sins so you could have eternal life. If you and Judy establish a relationship with Him, He will provide you with a foundation for your marriage, as well as the power to break out of these negative behaviors. Lasting relationships occur best when couples become 'one' in Christ. If you turn to Christ in humility, He will make you a child of God."

So it is for everyone. Receiving the life and power of the Lord Jesus Christ—the Bible calls it being "born again"—is the only true hope for restoring a marriage. Here's what the Bible tells you to do in order to accept Christ as Lord and Savior in your life.

1. Acknowledge that God has a wonderful plan for your life. God Himself has said that. "'For I know the plans that I have for you,' declares the Lord, 'plans for welfare and not for calamity to give you a future and a hope'" (Jeremiah 29:11).

2. Confess to God that you have missed His plan by living without Him. The Bible calls this sin. "For all have sinned and fall short of the glory of God" (Romans 3:23).

3. Accept the biblical truth that as the eternal Son of God, Jesus Christ died on a cross for your sins, was buried, and resurrected from the dead. "For I delivered to you as of first importance what I also received, that Christ died for our sins according to the Scriptures, and that He was buried, and that He was raised on the third day according to the Scriptures" (1 Corinthians 15:3–4).

4. On the basis of Christ's work on the cross, ask God to forgive you of all your sins. "If we confess our sins, He is faithful and righteous to forgive us our sins and to cleanse us from all unrighteousness" (1 John 1:9). This means you want Him to save you from your selfishness.

5. By faith, receive Jesus Christ into your life. "But as many as received Him, to them He gave the right to become children of God, even to those who believe in His name" (John 1:12).

"That if you confess with your mouth Jesus as Lord, and believe in your heart that God raised Him from the dead, you will be saved" (Romans 10:9).

If you have never taken the step of committing your life to Christ, we encourage you to do so right now. In the quietness of your heart, pray something like, "Lord Jesus, I need You. Please come into my heart and life right now and forgive my sin. Thank You for dying on the cross for me. Teach me how to live the Christian life. Help me to become a godly husband/wife. Thank You for coming into my life. In Jesus' name, amen."

If you believe these biblical truths and have sincerely prayed the prayer above, you are now a child of God. Jesus has come to live in your life for all time and eternity. God says, "And the testimony is this, that God has given us eternal life, and this life is in His Son. He who has the Son has the life; he who does not have the Son of God does not have the life" (1 John 5:11–12).

Submitting to Christ's love will allow you to have dominion over your self-centeredness and sin. You and your mate can now find oneness in marriage and a new beginning in life through Christ.

The balance of this book is designed to train you how to draw close to God in faith, apply principles from His Word to your marriage, and avoid the descent into resentment and rebellion.

IN SUMMARY

No spouse wants to move to stages three and four, resentment and rebellion. Yet after the stage of reality sets in, many couples (either one or both partners) respond with resentment, moving to stage three. They want their partner to give his or her 50 percent of responsibilities. This quickly turns into a critical inspection of the spouse; and a short list of observed failures begins to grow.

Soon each partner feels stuck with the other, which simply heightens the hurt and rejection. Once all alternatives have been exhausted, the couple admits there is a problem.

In addition to the sometimes painful realities that dash our romantic expectations, couples typically have to deal with a constant barrage of trials. Instead of standing unified, trials become just an other occasion to assign blame for more failures in our mates. Couples soon arrive at a point where they can't remember why they married in the first place.

In just a few short years, a couple can slide from marital bliss to the shocking reality of rejection. Without a godly solution, long-term struggles settle into a compromised marriage where both partners agree to disagree. But since compromise doesn't solve the problems, resentment and bitterness grow into rebellion. The dissolution of the marriage is just around the corner.

To desire to love is natural. To really love is supernatural. If God designed marriage, can He make it work? Parts 2 and 3 will demonstrate that God can and does make marriage work.

NOTE

1. Richard A. Swenson, Margin: *Restoring Emotional, Physical, Financial, and Time Reserves to Overloaded Lives* (Colorado Springs: Navpress, 1995) 85, 150.

part two

HOW TO MAKE LASTING COMMITMENTS IN MARRIAGE

CHAPTER FOUR

God's Plan, Man's Hope

◈ SUPPOSE YOU BECOME SICK AT WORK ONE DAY WITH a variety of symptoms: nausea, fever, aches and pains, red rashes, and profuse sweating. Alarmed, you go straight to the doctor, where he performs a variety of tests. After a thorough examination, the doctor makes the diagnosis and prescribes several prescription drugs. But once at home, you line up the prescription bottles on the kitchen counter and leave them there without taking the first pill.

What good did it do to visit the doctor if you don't follow his directions to regain your health? What good is it to submit to medical tests? Why bother to have prescriptions filled if you won't take the medication? None of these steps can help you regain your health unless you're willing to do what the doctor says.

Reading books about marriage won't automatically change your marriage. Neither will attending seminars or completing workbooks. If you want your marriage to improve, you must *apply* the principles you learn from God's Word. After more than three decades of marriage counseling, one thing has become very clear to us: *There is usually very little difference between Christian marriages and non-Christian marriages.* Christians may start out with the best of intentions for themselves and their mates. But unless they are willing to *apply*—that is, commit to obeying—the principles they hear, not much will change.

A successful marriage is not guaranteed by a good beginning; it can occur only *when two people daily apply God's Word to their marriage.* Marital oneness requires two people who each possess a supernatural mind-set, a perspective granted from God. As these two people obey the Lord and His Word, their faith will be rewarded with the blessing of oneness.

Marital oneness requires first *knowing* something, then *acting* on what one knows, followed by *persevering* through faith. In part 2 we will learn what God wants us to *know* about how and why He created marriage. In part 3 we will learn how to *apply* what we know to various practical areas of marriage.

SIN AND HUMAN RELATIONSHIPS

Before we discuss three reasons why God created mankind and marriage, it is essential to properly set the biblical context. The early chapters of Genesis describe the original marriage and how sin marred Adam and Eve's relationship with God, thus affecting all humans. Studying Genesis 1–3, we can make several fundamental observations before we can fully appreciate God's plan for marriage.

- Genesis 1–2 describe a time when sin and self-centeredness did not exist. Both Adam and Eve were perfect and pure when God spoke these words. As we read those two chapters, we conclude that God's perfect intent for mankind and marriage are clearly stated.

- Genesis 3 introduces mankind's rebellion against God. Because of sin, every relationship became distorted: relationships between God and mankind, all human relationships, mankind and nature, and even a person's relationship to himself. According to Isaiah 14:12–17 and Ezekiel 28:2–5; 12–19, God's authority was challenged by a fallen angel named Lucifer (Satan), who planned to make himself like God. In the verses above, Lucifer declared that he didn't need God to experience life. He set himself up as God and became independent from God. This reality is important because part of God's purpose in creating mankind and the resulting marriages was to demonstrate that only *dependence* on God can bring fulfillment and success in life. Satan is still in the business of enticing people into independence *from* God.

- Marriage was the first social institution God created, preceding even His relationship with Israel and the church. In marriage, Adam and Eve were blessed with a responsibility to carry out God's great purposes (described in the next section). If you are married, then you are also blessed with those same awesome responsibilities before God. Thus, your marriage is not an accident or afterthought of God. Instead, it is the basic foundation of all social structure on earth. Adam and Eve, and every couple that has followed, have a tremendous stake in God's plan of the ages.

- To fulfill these God-given purposes, it is essential that every couple become completely dependent on God Himself. Adam and Eve's dependence on God, as opposed to Satan's independence, was vital!

Yet through the ages, Satan still uses the same tactics: His desire is to lead rebellion and independence against God. Our purpose is to help you stand firm against this lie. As we consider God's plan, we must recognize the important part our marriages play in that plan. Let's see what our responsibility is.

GOD'S THREE PURPOSES
FOR MEN AND WOMEN

With this background, let's look specifically at why God created men and women and the institution of marriage. Genesis 1 describes all of creation. Verses 1–25 describe the creation of the heavens, the earth, vegetation, and animals; our focus will be on verses 26–31, which describe the creation of mankind. Here God's Word indicates three great purposes for men and women, to: (1) reflect God's image, (2) reproduce after their kind, and (3) reign over the creation.

The first reason God created marriage was for men and women to reflect His image together as a couple. That becomes clear in reading verses 26–27: "Then God said, 'Let Us make man in *Our image*, according to *Our likeness;* and let them rule over the fish of the sea and over the birds of the sky and over the cattle and over all the earth, and over every creeping thing that creeps on the earth.' God created man in His own *image*, in the *image of God* He created him; male and female He created them" (italics added).

Three times God uses the word "image" and once "likeness" to stress that *He wants mankind to reflect His image.* From the plural pronouns "Us" and "Our" used in verse 26, it is clear that God intended mankind to reflect the wholeness of the Trinity: the Father, Son, and Holy Spirit. Each person of the Trinity is unique in function, yet one in nature and purpose. The concept of reflecting God's light to a lost world is common in Scripture and can be found in passages such as Matthew 5:13–16 and Isaiah 60:1–5. What a privilege that God would choose to reveal Himself to the world through your marriage relationship!

Verse 27 contains a very important delineation about mankind: God mentions that "male and female He created them." Even though God made Adam and Eve to individually reflect His image, it is also true that together, in a profound and mysterious way, they would be able to reflect the *unity* or the *oneness* of God (see John 17:20–21 and Ephesians 5:31–32).

(So what about singles? Singles can reflect the image of God and can also best express as they join in oneness with the church or the body of Christ.

However, since this book is about marriage, we won't explore God's plan for singles, even though they too are called to reflect God's image in His church, made up of men and women.)

In marriage, couples best reflect God's image by *becoming one.* By creating Adam and Eve as the parents of humanity, God desired for them to model oneness to all who would follow. When couples reflect oneness, God is truly glorified. On the other hand, when strife replaces unity in marriage, the couple miss their greatest opportunity to reflect a loving God. Nothing in life is more tragic than being married and failing to reflect the unity of God's image. Incredibly, most couples are not even aware of God's plan for them to reflect Him!

A second tragedy in our generation is society's distortion of maleness and femaleness. The distinction between the two genders is under severe attack as the drive for a politically correct "unisex" society increases. Men and women desire to be like one another. Dress and roles have become blurred between the two. Each gender is in an identity crisis, resulting in unthinkable confusion and suffering. This is not the kind of unity God desires. As a result, even the ability to reflect God's image has suffered. Did He make a mistake? Certainly not! Each gender is vital. God is honored when a man and a woman unite to reveal His likeness and unity. God's plan is for masculinity and femininity to be distinct.

Oneness is essential if we want to reflect the image of God as a couple.

Men and women, God is instructing you from the Genesis passage that oneness in your marriage is not optional. If you hope to please God, then you must reflect His image. His reflection can be uniquely expressed between husband and wife, male and female. If God has indeed called you out of singleness into marriage, you and your mate must understand and experience God's eternal purpose.

Today many people seem uncertain about these ideas, either trying to decide whether to marry or if married, whether to divorce. Most are not aware that God has a plan for their marriage. Because Sally and I are committed to reflecting God's image through our marriage, divorce is not an option. I would be incomplete without my wife. Since I have learned God's purpose of reflecting Him in marriage, Sally's importance to me has multiplied in innumerable ways. Oneness is essential if we want to reflect the image of God as a couple.

The second purpose for mankind and marriage is to reproduce after our kind. Genesis 1:28 records: "God blessed them [Adam and Eve]; and God said to them, 'Be fruitful and multiply, and fill the earth.'"

No question here. God designed marriage to produce children, whom God regards as a blessing second only to the marriage relationship itself. The word *blessing* refutes any notion that God created marital sexual expression in a negative light. He blessed Adam and Eve's sexual union as another way of reflecting His unity in marriage.

With more than six billion people on the earth, you may think this purpose for marriage has been met. But look again. God's plan was not only for marriages to reflect His image and produce children. He also desires for our children to reproduce after our kind; that is, *to reflect His image.*

This purpose could also be stated, *"Reproduce a godly heritage* that will also reflect God's image." First, God told Adam and Eve to reflect His image. Next, God told them to increase that reflection through godly offspring. Adam and Eve together were to produce one small light on this huge earth. By reproducing godly children (who love, honor, and obey God), God desired that Adam and Eve's reflection be increased—eventually exceeding six billion lights. They were intended to be people just like you and me, who would reflect the truth that only dependence on God brings real life.

In this way, God has made marriage a strategic element in seeing the fulfillment of the Great Commission spoken by Jesus in Matthew 28:19–20: "Go therefore and *make disciples* of all the nations, baptizing them in the name of the Father and the Son and the Holy Spirit, teaching them to observe all that I commanded you; and lo, I am with you always, even to the end of the age" (italics added). And marriage becomes a model as well: In the same way we nurture children at home, we are to nurture and train disciples of Jesus to further God's kingdom here on earth.

God's third purpose for mankind is stated in the second half of Genesis 1:28, to "subdue [the earth]; and rule over . . . every living thing." God intended for Adam and Eve to rule or have dominion over the earth and its creatures. God makes it clear throughout Scripture that He wants married couples to take charge of everything that He has given them dominion over, including property, each mate's spiritual gifts, their children, financial income and assets, as well as social and political influences. All earthly resources are to be used as God's Spirit directs in order to bring honor to God.

God's charge to "subdue and rule" the earth includes not only the physical domain but the spiritual realm as well. Throughout the Old and New Testaments, the Holy Spirit exhorts believers to "be strong and courageous" (e.g., Joshua 1:6, 7, 9), "put on the full armor of God," and to "stand firm against the schemes of the devil" (Ephesians 6:11). God is honored as we exhibit victories in the spiritual realm for the sake of Christ. *Oneness in marriage is essential if we want to reign on planet Earth and bring glory to God.*

APPLYING GOD'S PURPOSES

In summary, God's plan for your marriage requires each of you to be dependent upon Him. You are called to (1) reflect His image, (2) raise godly children, and (3) reign over the earth. Your faith in God demonstrates to all creation that the only way to experiencing a fulfilled life now, as well as eternal life in the future, is through complete dependence upon Him.

In marriage, you will not accomplish these three goals unless each of you has a personal relationship with Jesus Christ as Savior. Every day couples marry with the intention of finding fulfillment apart from God, and the results are evident. As we noted in chapter 3, the ultimate solution is Jesus Christ within; He meets our deepest needs for spiritual intimacy and purpose in our marriages. No one can reflect the image of God and fulfill His purposes for marriage without God's help.

For Christians, goal one, *reflecting God's image* in a marriage, requires oneness with our spouse, and that, in turn, requires the ongoing work of Jesus Christ. Will non-Christians really be attracted to God through your example if you are divided as a couple? Absolutely not!

Similarly, *we can reproduce healthy, successful, and godly children* only by being one with our mates. When questioned, children consistently say that the most important aspect of family life is the way Mom and Dad love each other. When divided parents attempt to discipline children, without realizing it, they create opposite poles in their children. It's no wonder children take the opposite position from their parents at a later stage in life. Couples are shocked to learn that their lack of oneness in marriage has modeled division. Apart from oneness, child rearing is like grasping the wind.

Finally, we can attain *the third goal of reigning* over the physical earth when as a couple we are one. This is part of God's plan for couples: to effectively rule their unified resources for God's honor and to stand together in spiritual battle. Why should God increase your influence in the culture if you haven't faithfully managed what He has already given you? (See, for instance, Luke 16:10–11.)

You may have great plans, but they will be frustrated by division in your marriage. Can you handle the tremendous pressures of life without another to lean on? (Note Ecclesiastes 4:9–10). Maybe you can manage momentary pressure, but a lifetime of handling pressure alone will take a huge toll. Our outlook on life becomes warped under the incessant pressures of life. To adequately handle this battle, we need our spouses holding us up through prayer and spiritual encouragement.

When Sally and I married, we had not discovered God's purposes for marriage. Therefore the Holy Spirit could not call upon these Scriptures to convict us of our division, and we suffered terribly as a result. God's image, poorly reflected by us, suffered as well.

Since our discovering God's plans for marriage, the Holy Spirit can now instantly remind us when we falter in our oneness. Sally and I simply cannot reflect, reproduce, or reign without oneness in our marriage first. We literally shudder at the thought of not being one with each other.

What we fear most, though, is the thought of displeasing the heart of God—the same One who created us and sent Christ to die for us; the God who loves us to the end, in spite of how undeserving we are. If we are not one—unified— we are blocking His plan and missing the opportunity to reflect Him to others.

God is unchanging: "Jesus Christ is the same yesterday and today and forever" (Hebrews 13:8). Therefore, His plan for marriage is the same today as it was for Adam and Eve. We are either going to believe it, or we won't. We will either follow His plan and experience abundant life, or we won't. *Oneness in marriage is not an option.* It's essential.

CHAPTER FIVE

The Magna Carta
of Marriage

◈ AS WE SAW IN GENESIS 1:26–28, GOD VIEWED THE first couple as one. He refers to the male and female as "them," ("let them rule" and "God blessed them"); the pronoun indicates that God regarded them as one, as illustrated by the Godhead described in the plural pronouns "Us" and "Our" of Genesis 1:26. In fact, as a couple their ability to reflect God, reproduce, and reign was dependent on their oneness. If oneness is a prerequisite to success in marriage, then how can we accomplish such unity?

The answer to that question is found in Genesis 2, where God reveals the creation of mankind with Adam and Eve. They were the world's first couple as well as history's first marriage. Through them, God intended to show every couple who would follow what it meant to *become one.* Apart from verses that teach salvation and the ministry of the Holy Spirit, Genesis 2 has had more impact on our life and marriage than any other single passage of Scripture. Don't miss what God has for you in this key chapter. Genesis 2 is the Magna Carta of Marriage; it is God's blueprint for marriage.

In Genesis 2 we read the directions for marriage written by the Creator of marriage. The point of Genesis 1 is that married people can best fulfill God's purposes for creation (reflect, reproduce, reign) by being one with their mate. Genesis 2 is crucial because it tells us how to experience it.

In Genesis 2:18, God reveals a principle that is critical for experiencing oneness in marriage: God insures unity in the marriage by creating each person with needs that He meets through the life of the mate. God has created me with needs that He meets through Sally. Sally has needs that God meets in her life through me. Importantly, only as we each submit to God can He direct us in meeting one another's needs.

Experiencing this principle in real life involves recognizing four specific steps in how God provides for our personal needs. Those four steps, found in

Genesis 2 and depicted in figure 3, are discussed in the next section.

GOD CREATES A NEED

At the time of creation, Adam was different from you and me in several ways. First, he had no sin. Adam also lived in a *perfect physical environment*. Finally, and most importantly, Adam had a *perfect relationship* with the living God. Adam could actually experience God with two of his five senses. He could see the Shekinah glory of God as Moses would later see, and he could actually *hear* God speak. Scripture says that Adam walked and talked with God. Everything seemed to be just right for Adam.

Yet in verse 18, for the first time in all creation, God observes that something was "not good." "Then the Lord God said, 'It is not good for the man to be alone; I will make him a helper suitable for him'" (Genesis 2:18). It was not good for Adam to be alone. Notice that Adam did not complain to God about being alone. The thought never occurred to him; *God indicated* that Adam was alone. In calling attention to Adam's aloneness, God emphasized very clearly that man was not yet complete. In other words, God was not finished with His creation.

Adam was unable to reflect God's image by himself. Man was not created to stand alone, then or now. By God's wise design, He chose to create a need in mankind for human relationships in addition to fellowship with God. Thus, from the beginning of human history, *relationships are not an option*. The pattern, established by God, has not changed because of time or culture.

This need for human relationship in no way lessens our need for and

Figure 3
Four Steps in God's Meeting of Our Needs

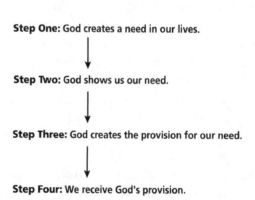

Step One: God creates a need in our lives.

Step Two: God shows us our need.

Step Three: God creates the provision for our need.

Step Four: We receive God's provision.

dependence upon God. Everything that God creates is designed to increase our dependence upon Him. God could have created Eve simultaneously with Adam. But to insure dependence upon Himself, God clearly showed Adam his need *first* so he would trust God for the fulfillment of that need. Thus Adam began a life of total trust in the perfect plan of the Most High.

He [God] chose to create a need in mankind for human relationships in addition to fellowship with God.

The word *suitable* means "to complete or to correspond to." This was God's way of saying that Adam was incomplete. In Genesis 1, God continually referred to human beings as "they" and "them." It is clear that God saw Adam and Eve as a *single unit of two*. Don't overlook this key insight!

After God observed that Adam was alone, you would expect to see God create Eve, right? *Wrong!* Instead, God assigned Adam a project that would clearly reveal the man's need for a helper: "Out of the ground the Lord God formed every beast of the field and every bird of the sky, and brought them to the man to see what he would call them; and whatever the man called a living creature, that was its name. The man gave names to all the cattle, and to the birds of the sky, and to every beast of the field, but for Adam there was not found a helper suitable for him" (Genesis 2:19–20).

GOD SHOWS US OUR NEED

What a shock! Instead of Eve, God brought all the animals to Adam. Why? The answer is found in the last part of verse 20: "but for Adam there was not found a helper suitable for him." God rarely gives us anything without first showing us our need. Remember that everything in creation is designed by God to increase our dependence upon Him.

Adam, however, initially didn't know what aloneness was. From his perspective, everything was perfect. As a result, he could not have fully appreciated Eve at this point. So how did Adam discover his need through naming animals?

To begin with, animals don't talk! He named the first and proceeded to the next. Same response. None of them spoke. Was he beginning to see a need? Animal after animal was named, yet not one could communicate with him. And surely he noticed that there were two of every animal, yet each was made differently. The animals were paired off—animal families, if you will. Most importantly, Adam learned there was no creature suitable for (similar to, corresponding to) him. There was no one to talk to, no one to eat with, and no one to complete him as a companion. The point is, *we must see our need before we can appreciate the provision for that need.*

I remember being so excited when my son, Todd, was born. I bought a football and took it to him while he was still in the hospital. Of course, he didn't appreciate it, since he had no need for a football as a newborn!

Well, I'm a slow learner. On Todd's fourth Christmas, I decided it was time for him to learn to ride a bicycle. I had always pictured Todd on a bike. Christmas Day found Todd excited about the bike, but it only lasted about two hours. In the months that followed, the bike sat unused in the garage. *He didn't have a need for a bike.*

When Todd was six, we moved to Little Rock, and he soon observed a neighbor boy riding a very special bike—a sporty black bike, without training wheels and with mud tires. Todd excitedly ran in, exclaiming, "Daddy, I've got to have a bike like Brent's!" Even though I was a slow learner, I was beginning to catch on.

"Todd," I said, "Daddy would love for you to have a bike like Brent's, but if you remember, you haven't ridden the other bike very much, and bikes cost a lot of money."

So Todd rode his bike without training wheels for four months, praying daily to the Lord for a "big bike like Brent's." Not one night passed in four months that Todd didn't pray for that bike. We were amazed at the fact that Todd didn't want to go to bed without praying. Before this, we encouraged him to pray, but he could never think of anything to say.

As Christmas neared, we were short of money. Sally told Todd that he would need to pray for our finances, especially to make our house payment. So Todd prayed earnestly for the house payment *and the bike.* As parents, we learned a lot about prayer from the faith of a child.

About a week before Christmas, a large, unexpected check arrived. Todd was not at all surprised. He *expected* God to answer. On Christmas morning, Todd found his big black and yellow bike with mud tires under the tree! How real God was becoming to him. His thrill with the bike didn't wane in two months or even the next two years. Todd cleaned and polished that bike and put it in the garage every night. It was very special to him because it was *God's provision* for a need that he had.

Do you see your need for your mate? Maybe you realized that fact when you were single, but do you realize how your mate fills your needs now? And are you sure how your mate needs you? God showed Adam his need *before* giving Eve to him so that he could fully appreciate, care for, and cherish God's gift. Certainly a worthy goal for every couple during the engagement period is to clearly understand their need for one another. Interestingly, married couples report they see more and more their need for each other as the years progress.

GOD CREATES THE PROVISION FOR OUR NEED

Now we're getting to the exciting part. Having first created Adam with a need for a relationship, and then having shown him his need, God now creates Eve to meet Adam's need. Genesis 2:21–22 records that "the Lord God caused a deep sleep to fall upon the man, and he slept; then He took one of his ribs and closed up the flesh at that place. The Lord God fashioned into a woman the rib which He had taken from the man, and brought her to the man."

God caused Adam to sleep while He created Eve. This is a beautiful picture of God's part—meeting our needs—and man's part—resting in God's promises. Most of us couples are not resting in God. Rather, we are actively looking, inspecting the assembly line of "Eves" and "Adams"—hoping to find the perfect one. Yet it is God who provides for our needs, both before and during marriage.

We've heard it said that God chose a rib to signify the perfect picture of the husband-wife relationship. The woman is under the protection of the man's arm but protects the man's most vital part— his heart. Eve was not taken from his head to rule over him, nor from his feet to be beneath him, but was formed alongside him to complete him, and vice versa. Husbands and wives are to be "fellow heir[s] of the grace of life" (1 Peter 3:7) as companions, lovers, friends, and parents.

The most strategic statement in the passage seems odd at first. God "*brought*" her to [Adam]." It seems God would have created Eve right next to Adam. Why did He bring her to Adam? God wanted Adam to know that just as it was God who had created her, it was also God *alone* who would *present* her to him as the greatest gift. For the unmarried, we believe God asks today, "Will you trust Me to bring your mate to you?" For the married, He asks, "Will you thank Me for the mate I have given you?" God desires complete dependence on Him for all our needs, be that before or after marriage.

WE RECEIVE GOD'S PROVISION

Such a great gift—our spouse—we should receive gladly. Notice how Adam embraced God's provision: "This is now bone of my bones, and flesh of my flesh; she shall be called Woman, because she was taken out of Man" (Genesis

2:23). The English text does not fully communicate Adam's excitement. A better translation of the Hebrew would be, "Great! Fantastic! Thank You, Lord! I'll take her!" Adam was 100 percent excited about her. Adam totally received Eve.

Was it Adam's ability to inspect Eve that caused him to *totally* receive her? Certainly not! Don't misunderstand me. I am sure Eve was very attractive to Adam. But since Adam had never seen a woman, he couldn't compare her with anyone else. What, then, was Adam's *basis* for receiving Eve? On what basis was he confident that she was "right" for him? Adam's acceptance of Eve was *based on who God was to him*, not Adam's ability to inspect Eve. God was the One who had created him. *God* created his need. *God* showed Adam his need. And God met his need with Eve. *Because Adam trusted God*, he received Eve by faith. He displayed great excitement because of God's *faithfulness*, not because of Eve's performance or lack of performance.

The point is that only God can meet your needs. He has created a need in you for relationships, which He meets primarily through a mate, but also through the church, family, and friends. He put this need in you to teach you dependence upon Him and to equip you to reflect His image to an imperfect world. You can then reproduce a godly heritage and reign on the earth. He will meet your aloneness need through someone who is also alone and imperfect. Beware of inspecting with your eyes, however. That is the same strategy Satan used to deceive Adam and Eve in Genesis 3.

Adam's acceptance of Eve was based on who God was to him.

We are at a key point in God's plan. God sought to protect man from Satan's sin of self-dependence by insuring that he would have to trust God to meet his aloneness needs. Therefore, God *requires that man receive his mate from Him*. If you are single, remember that God desires to provide your needs for a spouse. Wait on Him. God went out of His way to demonstrate the *pattern* of how He would work in history.

HOW TO VIEW
WEAKNESS IN YOUR MATE

Though God meets our needs in His provision of a mate, our mate will not be humanly perfect. Your mate may let you down; at times, your spouse will not meet your expectations. Every spouse certainly has weaknesses. But there is a healthy way to view those weaknesses.

Years ago I viewed Sally's weaknesses as a limitation to me with little hope of ever changing them. The notion of God's meeting my needs through her weaknesses simply made no sense. But God faithfully continued to teach me through His Word, and I began to realize that His perfect provision for my life was Sally—strengths *and* weaknesses. I began asking God for faith to stop seeing her weaknesses as a limitation and instead, to see how those same weaknesses could become a blessing.

With that prayer, I immediately began to experience a new freedom and hope in my marriage. I had relinquished the idea of changing her and simply accepted her by faith as a gift from God. I began to share this truth with others, and as time passed, I realized how great our marriage had become. What changed? God certainly didn't. But as my faith in God grew stronger, my perception of His gift to me in my wife dramatically changed.

What began as a tough step of faith years ago has continued to grow into one of the most blessed realities in my life. Sally might as well be perfect, because God has graciously allowed me to be totally satisfied with her. These truths have released Sally and me to experience hope and enjoyment in our marriage. God continues to reinforce that He has created us specifically for one another. The very things I would have changed in Sally in the beginning have turned out to be the very things I needed to help me mature in Christ.

What you view as a weakness in your mate today may indeed become a great blessing later in marriage.

For example, early in marriage I observed that Sally wasn't very goal-oriented. I'm the opposite. I have always had a five-year plan and a purpose to every plan. On occasion I'd ask, "Don't you have any goals?" She would give me a puzzled look and say, "I don't know. I guess I need to think about that." Sally was, and still is, the type of woman who wakes up every day, and whatever happens, happens.

One of my goals was to prepare for retirement, and at the time, my plan included buying and selling houses. So, during the same time that Sally had our four children in six years, we moved into six different houses. She *never* complained. We just packed up the boxes and moved.

While in the sixth house, it dawned on me what I had been doing to her. The Holy Spirit revealed that the very thing I had been most critical of in her early in our marriage had become a blessing to me. I was now glad she had not changed. The lights went on for me, and I began to thank God for this special woman in my life. *A goal-oriented wife would have never put up with my plans!* Sally made every move fun for the whole family. The friends we have established in every city through her have remained lifelong friends. She is God's gift to me —a fact God continues to reinforce in me each year. In faith, my challenge all along was to simply receive the gift God had prepared for me. Through her I have learned to be more flexible. She, on the other hand, enjoys my goals.

Taking this step of faith opened our eyes to the right way of viewing weaknesses in each other. You will find these five truths helpful in regarding your spouse's weaknesses.

1. God will meet your aloneness needs in spite of your mate's weaknesses.

2. God's only agent for changing your mate with promised results is unconditional love. That is also true for any relationship.

3. God actually uses your mate's weaknesses as a tool to perfect your character.

4. Your mate's weaknesses are an opportunity for you to be needed in his or her life.

5. What you view as a weakness in your mate today may indeed become a great blessing later in marriage.

Can you trust God to accomplish this work in your life now through your mate? If you're not yet married, can you trust Him for your future mate? If you can't, don't get married. If you are married and inspecting instead of believing God, then your mate is certainly living under a yoke of performance. Ask God to forgive you. In faith receive your mate from God just as he or she is, and thank Him for meeting your needs through this special person.

You can see how essential having a Christ-centered marriage is. Accepting the weaknesses of your mate in faith only makes sense if you are first able to trust God. Rejecting your mate after marriage is simply doubting God and His provision in your life. Doubt calls God's motives into question, leaving you unable to reflect His glory, reproduce a godly heritage, or reign victoriously in life.

I believe that God gave my wife to me, not because she is perfect, but because God is. Will you by faith receive your mate from God as His perfect provision for you?

A FORMULA FOR MARITAL ONENESS:
LEAVE PLUS CLEAVE EQUALS ONE FLESH

God concluded the Genesis 2 passage by stating another principle for every married couple. This principle reveals the formula for marital oneness. For those who follow it, God promises blessings. The formula is found in verses 24–25: "Therefore shall a man leave his father and his mother, and shall cleave unto his wife: and they shall be one flesh. And they were both naked, the man and his wife, and were not ashamed" (KJV).

Because neither Adam nor Eve had a literal father and mother, we know God introduced in these verses a principle intended for every married couple. The first part of this formula is *leave*. The word *leave* means to "abandon" or "break dependence upon." While no one should dishonor his or her parents, becoming married means breaking one's dependence on them. In fact, this principle would include severing any lingering strings to a former lifestyle: being single, sports, a job, finances, and so on. Countless couples get off to a rocky start due to an unwillingness to assume total responsibility for their new household. Obviously these aspects of life continue after marriage, but they must become secondary to the most important human relationship on earth: the marriage.

The second element in God's formula for marital oneness is found in the word *cleave*. "and shall cleave unto his wife." The word *cleave* means to "stick like glue." This same imagery was used in biblical days to describe melting metals together to form a stronger alloy. Faith in God is required to cleave. Our part is to leave, and God's part is to cleave us together. To the extent that both mates trust God for the outcome of their marriage, both will have the faith to "stick like glue."

Every marriage problem stems from either a failure to leave or a failure to cleave.

Jesus Christ reinforced the application of this principle to all marriages when He said, "Have ye not read, that he which made them at the beginning made them male and female, and said, For this cause shall a man leave father and mother, and shall cleave to his wife; and [the two] shall be one flesh? Wherefore they are no more [two], but one flesh. What therefore God hath joined together, let no man put asunder" (Matthew 19:4–6 KJV).

Clearly, God has established this principle as the basis of marriage. To experience marriage successfully, each mate must 100 percent leave his or her former state and then 100 percent cleave to the mate. We have found in counseling that every marriage problem stems from either a failure to *leave* or a failure to *cleave*. The only way you can 100 percent commit to your mate is to trust God for the outcome. Before marital oneness can occur, both mates must exhibit faith, a step that eliminates the concept of a fifty-fifty relationship.

The third aspect of God's formula for marital oneness is *becoming one flesh*. Here is a wonderful result and blessing of oneness: "They shall be one flesh" (Genesis 2:24 KJV). Loving one's mate by faith, instead of pressing the person to perform, releases amazing blessing and transparency. When God's Word says, "And the man and his wife were both naked and were not ashamed," (verse 25), the word *naked* implies being totally exposed, yet without threat: physically, emotionally, spiritually, or intellectually. Adam and Eve experienced total openness and transparency, with no masks. They were able to become one spiritually, emotionally, and physically. Oneness (one flesh) is the result of marital faith.

With the advent of sin, natural oneness was destroyed. It can be recaptured only through faith in God, and by applying His principles of marriage. Every person has the need to be loved unconditionally. However, that will not happen here on earth unless someone chooses to love you by faith.

If you were formerly divorced or not a Christian when you married, or just aren't positive you're married to the right person, the principle of oneness still works for you. Scripture tells us that God hates divorce (Malachi 2:16), and He desires for you to remain married. Therefore, the principles of leaving, cleaving, and becoming one flesh still represent God's desire for your marriage. If you will leave and cleave by faith, God indicates that oneness will result!

We also know that God forgives past failures when they are confessed to Him (1 John 1:9). He gives us a new beginning and tells us not to look back. Regardless of your past, God's plan for marriage still works today. Don't let Satan confuse you or rob you of a wonderfully satisfying marriage. Become one, and move ahead to reflect God, reproduce, and reign by His power. God is honored each time a couple commits to His plan for marriage.

The couple who believes that God brought them together, and that He will meet their needs in spite of their mate's weaknesses, will experience oneness. We must choose to follow Adam's example of receiving Eve in faith.

CHAPTER SIX

Power in Oneness Through the Holy Spirit

◈ APART FROM RECEIVING JESUS CHRIST AS SAVIOR, no other more practical issue exists than understanding the role of the Holy Spirit in marriage. Yet most believers do not understand the ministry and the power of the Holy Spirit: who He is, what He does, or how to release His power in their lives. The result is much confusion concerning His work in our lives.

Power to live the Christian life comes from the Holy Spirit. According to Jesus Himself, the Holy Spirit brings unity between individuals and leads us to love one another in order to honor the Father and the Son, (John 13:34–35; 16:13–14). The Spirit is the key source of oneness in marriage. It's one thing to know the right thing to do —to seek harmony in marriage; it's another matter for husband and wife to do it.

The apostle Paul prayed for believers that God "would grant you, according to the riches of His glory, to be strengthened with power through His Spirit in the inner man" (Ephesians 3:16). Nothing is more important to your marital peace, to the harmony be between your spouse and you, than releasing God's power in your marriage. To remain uninformed about the Holy Spirit is equivalent to choosing to fail. For that reason, we need to understand the identity of the Holy Spirit, His attributes, and how He ministers in our lives. By asking the questions "Who?" "What?" and "How?", we can learn much about the Holy Spirit.

WHO IS THE HOLY SPIRIT?

Who exactly is the Holy Spirit? Notice that He is a *who*, not a *what*. Above all, the Holy Spirit is God. The Holy Spirit is the third person of the Trinity: the Father, the Son, and the Holy Spirit. The Scripture itself refers to the Holy

Spirit as God (2 Corinthians 3:17– 18).

Since He is God, the Holy Spirit possesses divine attributes: He is eternal, all-knowing, all-powerful, and is present everywhere (1 Corinthians 2:10–11; Genesis 1:2; Psalm 139:7–8). Yet the Holy Spirit is distinct from the Father and the Son. Scripture reveals that the only unpardonable sin occurs against the Holy Spirit: rejecting His convictions regarding the work of Christ at the Cross. Clearly, the Holy Spirit is God.

In addition to His divine attributes, the Holy Spirit possesses a personality that includes emotions. Scripture actually portrays a vital relationship between the Holy Spirit and mankind—including you and me—in which we can obey or disobey Him (Acts 5:3). We are warned, "Do not grieve the Holy Spirit of God, by whom you were sealed for the day of redemption" (Ephesians 4:30), and "Do not quench the Spirit" (1 Thessalonians 5:19). Act 7:51 reveals that people can resist the work of the Holy Spirit. Yet, the Holy Spirit desires an intimate relationship with each of us.

At the close of his second letter to the Corinthians, Paul signed off this way, "The grace of the Lord Jesus Christ, and the love of God, and the fellowship of the Holy Spirit, be with you all" (2 Corinthians 13:14). The Holy Spirit deeply desires to be involved in your marriage. Do you desire fellowship with Him? Do you know what that means and what fellowship with Him is like? He has many roles in helping you to experience life to the fullest, both personally and with your spouse.

WHAT DOES THE HOLY SPIRIT DO?

The many roles of the Spirit in our lives and marriages are so important that Jesus emphasized the Spirit's significance and many roles while on earth. In His final discourse (John 14–16), Christ repeatedly drew attention to the Holy Spirit's vital role in living the Christian life after His departure.

> *If you love Me, you will keep My commandments. I will ask the Father, and He will give you another Helper, that He may be with you forever; that is the Spirit of truth, whom the world cannot receive, because it does not see Him or know Him, but you know Him because He abides with you and will be in you. I will not leave you as orphans; I will come to you (John 14:15–18).*
>
> *But I tell you the truth, it is to your advantage that I go away; for if I do not go away, the Helper will not come to you; but if I go, I will send Him to you. But when He, the Spirit of truth, comes, He will guide you*

into all the truth; for He will not speak on His own initiative, but whatever He hears, He will speak; and He will disclose to you what is to come. He will glorify Me; for He will take of Mine and will disclose it to you (John 16:7,13–14).

These statements were made at a key transition point in God's eternal plan. Christ was preparing momentarily to finish His role as Savior. Jesus made it clear that after His death, the Holy Spirit would be God's provision for living the Christian life.

Among the Spirit's many roles, let's look at six.

First, the Holy Spirit *convicts and sustains us*. Clearly, the Holy Spirit's influence in our lives begins before we become Christians. While we were yet lost, the Holy Spirit convicted us of sin. Jesus told His disciples, "And He, when He comes, will convict the world concerning sin and righteousness and judgment" (John 16:8). The Holy Spirit enlightens us with the story of Christ, then regenerates our soul with new life in Christ (Titus 3:4–6). Finally, God puts His seal on us for all eternity (Ephesians 1:13, 4:30). Is that important to you and your marriage? Absolutely! The Holy Spirit continues to convict and enlighten us throughout our lives. Marital oneness is dependent on His continued renewal in these vital ministries.

> *Faith is trusting God to accomplish what He says in spite of our mate's weaknesses.*

Second, the Holy Spirit *helps us*. In Scripture, He is called *the Helper*. Two points stand out. Notice that Christ said the Father "will give you another Helper, that He may be with you forever" (John 14:16). Some translations use the word "Comforter." The word means to "come alongside and strengthen." Christ was signifying that the Holy Spirit would fill His own place, doing for the disciples what He had done for them while He was on earth.

How important is the Holy Spirit's help to us? Christ indicated that "it is to your advantage that I go away; for if I do not go away, the Helper will not come to you" (John 16:7). Christ recognized that His leaving would bring salvation and the vital ministry of the Holy Spirit. The coming of the Holy Spirit was second in importance only to Christ's glorious and completed work at the Cross. Therefore, just as believers honor the work of Christ, they should also honor the work of the Holy Spirit. Because the Holy Spirit is God, He is worthy to be sought after, worshiped, and praised. The Holy Spirit brings honor to God the Father and God the Son.

If we desire to succeed in the Christian life, then Christ tells us that His Helper should become a major part of our lives. To become one in marriage, both mates must understand and accept the work of the Holy Spirit. They must cooperate with His plan through daily fellowship with Him.

Third, the Holy Spirit *teaches us.* Christ said it this way: "But the Helper, the Holy Spirit, whom the Father will send in My name, He will teach you all things, and bring to your remembrance all that I said to you" (John 14:26).

As our teacher, the Holy Spirit gives us spiritual knowledge and faith through the Word of God. In the initial chapters of this book, we have talked about developing a faith relationship in marriage instead of a performance-based relationship. A faith relationship can be defined as one in which the participants look beyond their mate's performance to God's sovereignty and promises. Instead of focusing on our mate's weaknesses, which is natural, we instead believe God's Word concerning our marriage. Faith is trusting God to accomplish what He says in spite of our mate's weaknesses. Scripture tells us where faith comes from: "So faith comes from hearing, and hearing by the word of Christ" (Romans 10:17). Where do we find the words of Christ? The Bible, of course.

One of the greatest indications that I am not depending on the Holy Spirit is the absence of power in my life.

If you want to be one in your marriage, faith will be required. Faith requires your involvement in studying the Word of Christ. The One who illuminates the Word is the Holy Spirit. "For to us God revealed them through the Spirit; for the Spirit searches all things, even the depths of God. For who among men knows the thoughts of a man except the spirit of the man which is in him? Even so the thoughts of God no one knows except the Spirit of God" (1 Corinthians 2:10–11).

You may have wondered why we have included so many Scripture texts in this book. It's because Sally and I felt both hope and conviction when we read passages like Genesis 1:26–28 and 2:18–25. If your life and marriage are touched by them, it will be the Holy Spirit teaching you. Sally or Don Meredith cannot do that. The Holy Spirit is our instructor, imparting spiritual knowledge and faith through the Word of God.

Fourth, the Holy Spirit *provides us with power.* He grants power to witness, overcome sin, and serve Him, as well as the power to be one in marriage. When Christ commissioned the disciples, He said, "But you will receive power when the Holy Spirit has come upon you; and you shall be My witnesses both in Jerusalem, and in all Judea and Samaria, and even to the remotest part of the earth" (Acts 1:8).

If you do not experience much power in your life and marriage, faith is the missing ingredient. Why? Because Christ left this earth in order for the Holy Spirit to indwell believers. All we have to do is call upon His power. One of the greatest indications that I am not depending on the Holy Spirit is the absence of power in my life. I cannot overcome my critical spirit in my marriage without His power. I cannot be a testimony to my wife, or anyone else for that matter, if I don't have His power. As a couple, you must be energized by His power to be a witness for Christ in marriage.

Fifth, the Holy Spirit *leads us,* guiding our decisions. Nearly sixty years on Earth has taught Sally and me that life has many twists and turns. Sometimes we anguish in our desires to follow God's leading. As we respond to Him, we draw tremendous comfort from yet another ministry of the Holy Spirit. He promises to provide guidance in life. The apostle Paul wrote, "So then, brethren, we are under obligation, not to the flesh, to live according to the flesh—for if you are living according to the flesh, you must die; but if by the Spirit you are putting to death the deeds of the body, you will live. For all who are being led by the Spirit of God, these are sons of God" (Romans 8:12–14). Clearly, Paul exhorts us to be led by the Spirit.

We love the way Ezekiel describes this leading of the Holy Spirit toward the nation of Israel. "Moreover, I will give you a new heart and put a new spirit within you; and I will remove the heart of stone from your flesh and give you a heart of flesh. I will put My Spirit within you and cause you to walk in My statutes, and you will be careful to observe My ordinances" (Ezekiel 36:26–27). That's precisely what we need in our marriages—the Holy Spirit to take away our stubborn and hardened hearts and cause us to be soft and pliable in His hands. Marital oneness will never happen unless both mates earnestly beseech the Holy Spirit to lead them. "But when He, the Spirit of truth, comes, He will guide you into all the truth" (John 16:13). His will be done, not ours. We will never be one by our wills, but only through seeking and following His will.

The final ministry of the Holy Spirit is one many of us desperately need. The Holy Spirit *comforts us.* Four times Jesus referred to the Holy Spirit as the Comforter. While mentioning suffering, Paul said this: "Blessed be the God and Father of our Lord Jesus Christ, the Father of mercies and God of all comfort; who comforts us in all our affliction, so that we will be able to comfort those who are in any affliction with the comfort with which we ourselves are comforted by God" (2 Corinthians 1:3–4).

Life is full of disappointments and afflictions. Sometimes our dreams shatter and our visions go unfulfilled. I, personally, have been burdened with deep discouragement at times. I thank God for the Holy Spirit's comfort. Many times He comforts me through my wife, and vice versa. The Holy Spirit replenishes our souls and reminds us of truth that may not be immediately evident. In His divine power, He replaces fear with hope. He imparts peace instead of despair. At times, this ministry alone sustains us.

What does the Holy Spirit do? He is our sustainer in life. As we release our will to His, He gives perspective and hope. As the psalmist said, "Come, let us worship and bow down, let us kneel before the Lord our Maker" (Psalm 95:6). Often, just kneeling down before the Lord as husband and wife, acknowledging Him as Lord and Creator, brings hope to weary souls. God, the Holy Spirit, brings comfort in the passages of life and marriage.

HOW DO WE RELEASE THE HOLY SPIRIT'S POWER IN OUR LIVES?

Experiencing the full power of the Holy Spirit is not something we necessarily do. Rather, releasing His power is a deliberate act that we ask *Him* to do in and through us. Allowing Him free reign in our lives can be measured by the fruit He produces in our lives. The Holy Spirit supplies the power; we simply act on His power by faith. The Scripture calls this faith-interaction with the Holy Spirit "fellowship," a time to "walk by the Spirit" (2 Corinthians 13:14; Galatians 5:16).

In order to adequately release the power of the Holy Spirit, we must acknowledge that our lives belong to Him. This includes our past, our present, and our future. All things must be given to Him to use as He desires. The apostle Paul called Christians to make a total sacrifice of their selves:

> *Therefore I urge you, brethren, by the mercies of God, to present your bodies a living and holy sacrifice, acceptable to God, which is your spiritual service of worship. And do not be conformed to this world, but be transformed by the renewing of your mind, so that you may prove what the will of God is, that which is good and acceptable and perfect (Romans 12:1–2).*

If God created us, He also knows what is best for us at all times. Therefore, it is our *reasonable* service to give Him not only our lives, but everything He entrusts to us. He then will show us that His will is good (for us), acceptable (to us), and perfect (in us).

Are you willing to give up your rights, pride, and willfulness? Can you trust God and His Word? To experience His power requires our total trust in Him.

Releasing the Holy Spirit's power in our lives comes by a faith interaction that leads to fellowship. How do we experience this fellowship? The first epistle of John introduces us to the two prerequisites for enjoying fellowship with the Holy Spirit: *confession* and *walking by the Spirit*. The apostle wrote:

This is the message we have heard from Him and announce to you, that God is Light, and in Him there is no darkness at all. If we say that we have fellowship with Him and yet walk in the darkness, we lie and do not practice the truth; but if we walk in the Light as He Himself is in the Light, we have fellowship with one another, and the blood of Jesus His Son cleanses us from all sin. . . . If we confess our sins, He is faithful and righteous to forgive us our sins and to cleanse us from all unrighteousness (1 John 1:5–7, 9).

John said that we must submit to God's perspective, or will, if we want to walk in fellowship with Him. He uses light as a metaphor for God's holiness and purity.

Apart from the cross of Christ, no one can claim to be holy. Instead, by faith we must enter into the grace and forgiveness of God shown at the Cross, and thus submit our wills to His control. If we submit to following Him, the Holy Spirit graciously fellowships with us while continually cleansing us from our sin through the blood of the Cross.

The two prerequisites to enjoying fellowship with the Holy Spirit [are] confession and walking by the Spirit.

Releasing the Holy Spirit's power in our lives includes turning from our selfish attitudes. Confession of sin means agreeing with God that what we did was indeed sin. We then turn from our sin (repent) and ask for God's forgiveness. His power is released as we ask the Holy Spirit to live in us, love through us, and forgive others through us. The Spirit does what is *natural* to Him—living the Christian life. But, now *He lives His life through us.*

This is critical to understand, since we are not "trying" to live the Christian life in our power. Instead, we relinquish our will to the Holy Spirit and trust Him to live through us. This process of trusting, not struggling, should be continual and lifelong. This means a sacrificial life, a cleansed life, and a life filled with power. What a freeing experience!

Paul called this leading of the Holy Spirit "walking by the Spirit," and this second prerequisite for fellowship prevents us from following our selfish desires. As the apostle wrote to the Galatian church,

Walk by the Spirit, and you will not carry out the desire of the flesh. For the flesh sets its desire against the Spirit, and the Spirit against the flesh; for these are in opposition to one another, so that you may not do the things that you please. But if you are led by the Spirit, you are not under the Law (Galatians 5:16–18).

Notice that Paul referred to a struggle that occurs in believers' lives: "For the flesh sets its desire against the Spirit, and the Spirit against the flesh; for these are in opposition to one another." *The flesh* is a term describing the natural self-centeredness present in all people, including Christians. These old patterns and tendencies constantly contend with the Holy Spirit for control. When we become Christians, we don't lose our flesh with its desires. The Holy Spirit is the only One who can *control* the flesh—self-centeredness, insensitivity to others, pride, greed, and so on. Under the control of His Spirit, Scripture tells us that the flesh is dead, or powerless.

THE FLESH VERSUS THE SPIRIT

The fruit evident in our lives reveals whether the flesh or the Holy Spirit is in control of our lives. Paul identifies the fruit of the flesh by saying, "Now the deeds of the flesh are evident, which are: immorality, impurity, sensuality, idolatry, sorcery, enmities, strife, jealousy, outbursts of anger, disputes, dissentions, factions, envying, drunkenness, carousing, and things like these, of which I forewarn you, just as I have forewarned you, that those who practice such things will not inherit the kingdom of God" (Galatians 5:19–21).

Couples controlled by the Holy Spirit naturally produce the fruit of the Holy Spirit. Oneness is a natural by-product.

The first thing we check when couples enter our counseling room is their fruit. If their fruit reveals arguing, jealousy, outbursts of anger, and so on, we know they are not in fellowship with the Holy Spirit. Oneness in marriage is impossible in the flesh.

The fruit of the Holy Spirit contrasts sharply with the fruit of the flesh. "The fruit of the Spirit is love, joy, peace, patience, kindness, goodness, faithfulness, gentleness, self-control" (Galatians 5:22–23). Notice, this is the fruit of His Spirit, not something we create on our own. Christians do not possess these wonderful virtues in and of themselves. We exhibit them because Christ lives in us. Couples controlled by the Holy Spirit naturally produce the fruit of the Holy Spirit. Oneness is a natural by-product. Peace reigns in their homes. The unity exhibited in marriage is an example to others of their submission to God's Holy Spirit.

Paul reveals that each of us can *choose* who controls our lives. "Now those who belong to Christ Jesus have crucified the flesh with its passions and desires. If we live by the Spirit, let us also walk by the Spirit. Let us not become boastful, challenging one another, envying one another" (Galatians 5:24–26). Because we have become Christians, we no longer are bound by our selfish tendencies. We can choose, by faith, to let the Holy Spirit take over.

THE ROLE OF FAITH

Releasing the Holy Spirit in your life and marriage involves faith and will; and, the apostle Paul says, it involves the power of Christ Himself: "I have been crucified with Christ; and it is no longer I who live, but Christ lives in me; and the life which I now live in the flesh I live by faith in the Son of God, who loved me and gave Himself up for me" (Galatians 2:20).

Walking in the Spirit simply means seeking a deeper, closer walk with the Spirit. The more He has of your life, the more fruit the Spirit can manifest through you. Walking in the Spirit starts with believing that Christ crucified the power of sin in your life by His death on the Cross. *That takes faith.* Next, believe the Holy Spirit will do what the Scriptures say: "If by the Spirit you are putting to death the deeds of the body, you will live. For all who are being led by the Spirit of God, these are sons of God" (Romans 8:13–14).

In the same way—by faith—Christ called His disciples to activate the Holy Spirit. "But you will receive power when the Holy Spirit has come upon you; and you shall be My witnesses both in Jerusalem, and in all Judea and Samaria, and even to the remotest part of the earth" (Acts 1:8). The disciples waited many days, until Pentecost, for the Spirit to come, but they waited in faith. (See Acts 1:12–14; 2:1–4.) Christ asks you to also show faith. It's true that you need help even to believe, but helping is a ministry of the Holy Spirit. He is your Helper, and He will lead you into incredible works for God if you will let Him. The question is, will you take Him at His word? If so, the Holy Spirit's power will be released in your life and marriage. As He convicts you of sin, agree with Him that the behavior or attitude is wrong. Following His lead, ask for forgiveness, and seek His will. Then He is free to exhibit the fruit of the Spirit through your life.

The Holy Spirit gives you the power to be one in marriage, to reflect God's image to a lost world, to reproduce His image through children and disciples, and to rule this world to His glory. The message is clear; the challenge is precise. What you allow the Holy Spirit to do through you will determine the health of your marriage.

CHAPTER SEVEN

How to Change Your Mate

⬚ TAKE THIS QUICK QUIZ. GOD CHOOSES TO USE TWO of the following three forces to change behavior in marriage. Which one of the following three approaches does God not honor?

1. Loving your spouse unconditionally
2. Giving kindness when you want to retaliate
3. Actively seeking to change your spouse through pouting, intimidation, or manipulation

Obviously the third choice fails to bring about healthy change in marriage, although it's the choice used frequently by most couples. *Nowhere in Scripture are we told to change people.* Only God changes people. He has not ordained you as judge, jury, and executioner over your spouse. Yet one of the most common complaints we hear in counseling is the inability to make a partner change to meet one's expectations. The truth is that God uses the *active force* of agape love (see Ephesians 5:22–33), combined with the *reactive force* of blessing (see 1 Peter 3:8–9), to refine people into His image . . . not ours. Since adjustments of expectations and behavior are such a hotbed of conflict in marriage, this chapter will explore how two people *actually change to become one* in a civil and godly manner.

LOVE: THE ACTIVE FORCE

Few things are as aggravating in life as trying to complete a job without having the right tools. Guys, try cutting down a tree with a bow saw instead of a chain saw, or changing the oil in your car without the correct wrenches. Ladies, try vacuuming the carpet with a handheld Dustbuster instead of a vacuum cleaner. Layer upon layer of frustration builds instead of efficiently getting the job done.

In the same way, God mandates that we use His methods to build oneness in marriage. His primary tool is *agape* love. *Agape* is the Greek word for love, specifically an unconditional love. (We will explore its nature in greater depth shortly.) Most husbands and wives, however, build their marriages using a self-centered, "fleshly" love that inevitably leads to frustration. This kind of love says, "I will be nice to you if you do what I want." Unfortunately, if the other person doesn't do what you want, that river of love evaporates into a tiny trickle of effort.

Conditional love disappears when circumstances change. If spouses change from rich to poor, sexy to unsexy, young to old, social to antisocial, athletic to nonathletic, healthy to unhealthy, or any number of other variables, most mates lose what they define as love. Are you building your marriage on this type of shallow, conditional love? Or are you willing to sell out for "the real thing"—loving your spouse with the powerful love of God? To clarify, let's compare and contrast three different levels of love.

THREE LEVELS OF LOVE

The Greek language used in the New Testament describes three specific levels of love.[1] The first level is *eros,* a love that is completely self-centered or self-absorbed. This kind of love accentuates the emotional and physical, with sexual attraction as the primary focus. Eros says, "Me first. I will love you in order to get what I want." Many couples today get married with eros love as their focal point, and do not even realize it! Why are so many marriages ending in divorce? It is because eros love is selfish, not sacrificial and giving. When the spouse's performance lowers, and feelings subside, eros love evaporates.

The second level of love is *philos.* This love involves mutual, tender affection between two people. It implies a "brotherly love," one we often experience in our family of origin, including our brothers and sisters. While eros love is self-centered, philos love is mutually satisfying. It appreciates and respects the other person. It says, "Yes, I love what you do for me, but I also sincerely respect you."

This level of love involves more sacrificial commitment than eros. The overwhelming majority of marriages in America are based on either eros or philos love. The problem with philos love is that when respect is lost, couples tend to revert to eros love, which by itself is undependable.

The third level of love is *agape.* Far superior to either of the other two kinds of love, *agape* is known as God's love. Scripture describes agape as the love that

God expressed through His Son Jesus Christ to mankind. This kind of love is the opposite of eros in that it is totally sacrificial. *Agape* love can only be measured by the sacrificial action of the giver. Unlike eros or philos, agape love does not depend on the attractiveness of the object loved. Rather, it is defined by the commitment of the giver. The lover is acting in obedience to God's commandment; therefore this level of love is God directed. It is first an issue between God and man, not between two people, and it does not always run with the natural inclination of feelings. This love is responsible and does not change as feelings change. This is the kind of love verbalized when we say our marriage vows—a never-ending commitment. There are no conditions or performance required for the spouse to receive this ongoing, committed love.

Agape love can only be measured by the sacrificial action of the giver.

If you are a Christian considering marriage and tell your future mate you love him or her, do you mean eros, philos, or *agape* love? God never called anyone to marriage apart from *agape* love. Marital oneness is impossible without it. Since God teaches dependence on Himself in marriage, it is absolutely necessary to trust Him first for this kind of love; then look toward such love developing in you. *Agape* love is first an issue between God and you. His love will then enable you to love your mate unconditionally by faith.

The Holy Spirit instructs husbands in Ephesians 5:25 to love as Christ loved. How did Christ love? The apostle Peter told us that Christ loved us at the Cross by "entrusting Himself to [His Father]"; this enabled Christ to have the faith to sacrifice for us. Christ remains the ultimate example to us of sacrificial love.

A LIFESTYLE OF LOVE

Biblical (*agape*) love is best described in 1 Corinthians 13 where the dimensions of love are clearly seen. Those qualities can transform your marriage relationship. Open your Bible and study how five elements of such love can apply to your marriage:

1. *Love is patient.* Genuine *agape* love will endure an offense even though a tide of emotion is welling up within you demanding retaliation. *Application:* First, such love enables you to have divine patience that waits and prays for the reformation of your mate rather than exhibiting resentment. Second, when you love while suffering patiently, you learn to handle insults and neglect from your mate until God can work

through His Word.

2. *Love is not provoked.* Love will not become bitter or resentful as a result of continuous irritation or offenses, or respond to them with touchiness or anger. *Application:* A weakness or offense in your mate will not produce bitterness or anger from you.

3. *Love bears all things.* Love will endure offenses from your mate and throw a cloak of silence over your suffering so that your mate's offenses are not divulged to the world. *Application:* If you have a non-Christian or nonspiritual spouse, be careful not to build a self-righteous attitude in the eyes of others. While godly church leaders or a few close friends may know your situation, don't make this common knowledge. Indeed, complaining about a spouse to sympathetic ears often becomes the fertile grounds for many affairs. Your mate needs to be able to trust you.

4. *Love believes all things.* Love will choose to believe the best about your mate; it always assumes his or her motives and intentions have integrity. *Application:* Often people become what we convince them they are. If we indicate that we suspect them, they will tend to be untrustworthy. Trusting your mate gives him or her a feeling of self-worth and acceptance, a key to effecting change in your mate.

5. *Love endures all things.* Love has the power to enable you to endure any trial with confidence and patience. Trials produce perseverance and blessings from God. *Application:* Divorce is an indication that you don't endure all things. *Agape* love doesn't quit when things get tough; it demonstrates permanent commitment.

Studying 1 Corinthians 13:4–8 can be an encouraging marital (or premarital) project. All the verbs in this passage are in the present tense, indicating that these characteristics of love are to be habitual. Because a person does not manifest one of these qualities in every instance, however, does not necessarily signal non-commitment. The apostle Paul is referring to a "lifestyle" of love.

God's love leaves no place for the statement, "I don't love you anymore." It does, however, hold some absolute promises for us. For example, "There is no fear in love; but perfect love casts out fear, because fear involves punishment, and the one who fears is not perfected in love" (1 John 4:18). The word used for love here is *agape.* The verse says two things will result from *agape* love: (1) Fear will be driven out and (2) love will perfect, or complete, your spouse. Fear is the opposite of faith and hope. If love for your mate depends on performance, he or she will be fearful and insecure. On the other hand, if you love by faith as Christ did, and overlook your mate's weaknesses, your *agape* love will drive the fear from your mate because there is no retribution. Your mate's peace and satisfaction will then provoke your spouse toward more faith and hope. Usually, your mate will then return the faith love to you.

In addition, God implies that agape love helps perfect the object of your love—your mate. That is, His agape love demonstrated through you will produce faith in your spouse, both toward God and you. How do you change your mate? *You "agape" him or her, and allow God to do the changing.*

If husbands will follow Christ's pattern of love, they too will . . . have the promise of participating with Christ in changing their mates.

Another example of the power of *commitment love* occurs in a passage where God ties the promise of Christ's love to marriage. In Ephesians 5:25–33, the husband is charged with the same role in marriage as Christ Himself has with the church. Like Christ, the husband also inherits several promises that Christ received. The Scripture commands husbands to love their wives as Christ loved the church (verse 25), and it reveals (in verses 26–27) two results of Christ's love. First, His love sanctifies us, the church. Second, because of Christ's love, we will be presented back to Him in a perfected state. If husbands will follow Christ's pattern of love, they too will benefit from the same effects that Christ received. They too will have the promise of participating with Christ in changing their mates. Consider these results:

1. When you love your mate as Christ loved, you will sanctify, or set him or her apart by your special commitment. In other words, a woman who is loved unconditionally is set apart from other women who are not loved in this way. A woman who is loved unconditionally is free from marital anxiety and fear and is better able to live a contented life with her spouse and family.
2. A husband who loves with agape love will have the hope of seeing change in his mate. She will be presented back to him, "having no spot or wrinkle or any such thing; but that she would be holy and blameless" (Ephesians 5:27). One day, Christ will show husbands who exhibit such love to their wives how their faith was used to help accomplish these spiritual results. In my life, I have seen God do these things in Sally's life right before my eyes.

In all my years of counseling, I have never seen any other active approach gain these kinds of results. It is not unusual to hear complaints about having to love God's way. *But nothing else works.* Neither manipulation, verbal assault, bribes, nor subtle lying will work like agape love.

Don't experience a poor counterfeit of God's love. Experience *agape* love toward your mate, and trust God for the outcome. The fearlessness, transparency, and peace of such a relationship are what married life was meant to be. Bless your mate by giving your partner the assurance that he or she will never hear you say, "I don't love you anymore."

BLESSING: THE REACTIVE FORCE OF LOVE

"In the three years since my husband started his new business, the children and I have not had a vacation. We have done without a lot of things so Bob could succeed. Then two weeks ago his real appreciation for us came through loud and clear." Vicki's voice showed anger, and her eyes flashed as she told me her story. "First of all, I got the Master Card bill and discovered that Bob had purchased a used motorboat to the tune of $5,000. When I called him at the office, he exploded and told me that he and some of his buddies were planning to go fishing for ten days in Mexico and needed a boat! I was so furious I hardly spoke to him for the next two weeks.

"The day he left to fish, I took the Visa card and the children and flew home to Mom's for ten days of fun, to the tune of $5,250."

Vicki had done the human thing. She retaliated and "really showed him." But how did it help her? Did it change Bob? Did two wrongs make a right? Was Bob more in love with her than before? Did it serve any useful purpose to have two people insulted instead of one? Three months later Vicki returned for counseling with Bob at her side. The hurt, bitterness, and ruin were still flaming.

Couples today are not prepared for the consequences that result from the insult cycle in their marriages. Yet, many end up as victims. As time passes, these cycles become vicious whirlwinds. Scripture tells us that we can stop these insult cycles by returning a blessing when wronged or insulted.

Our human nature does not want to offer a blessing after receiving an insult. Our instinct is to follow Vicki's example: "I'll show him. He hasn't seen anything yet! I've just begun to fight." In our rights-oriented society, God's way seems ridiculous and painfully slow. We don't think it will work. Rather, we want change instantly because we live in an instant society. Remember, God's ways are not always our ways and His timing is not ours either. What's happening in your marriage? Are you ready to listen to God?

To better understand what God means when He says to return a blessing when insulted, we need to define what the Scripture refers to as an insult and a blessing. There are many examples of each, and we will look at several.

Concerning *insults,* the Scriptures give many exhortations. Seven are particularly relevant to marriage:

1. Name-calling. God admonishes us not to belittle others. Name-calling is always a threat to marital love and causes fear in the one receiving the insult. Any consistent negative reference to someone is demoralizing and destroys self-confidence. (See Matthew 5:22.) Imagine hearing words like *dummy, stupid, moron,* or *idiot* or worse.
2. Sarcasm and ridicule. Dwelling on intellectual, social, or physical ineptness certainly hampers marital oneness. Examples: "You burned the food again!" "Why are you so quiet when we're with our friends? I wish you'd just speak up!" "You can't do anything right!" (See Proverbs 18:6; Ephesians 4:29.)
3. A nagging wife. Scripture is bold in its condemnation of a woman who doesn't trust or respect her husband enough to stop nagging on any given subject. "How many times do I have to tell you?" or "You *never* do this for me," or "You *always* come home late!" (See Proverbs 21:9; 27:15–16.)
4. A contentious man. Scripture speaks just as forcefully of a quarrelsome man who is always picking a fight. This kind of macho man thinks he is always right, refuses to back down, bullies his wife, and is too arrogant to ask for forgiveness (Proverbs 26:21).
5. An unbridled tongue. Scripture speaks of the powerfully negative effect of the tongue when it is not controlled. We can poison and destroy another person by using profanity, cutting remarks that put down each other, and always citing the negative in any situation. Sometimes the effects can scar our mate or child for life. (See James 3:5–10.)
6. Lying to your spouse. Scripture speaks of the serious consequences of not telling the full truth, covering the truth, or using little white lies. This results in a lack of trust and openness between spouses and causes disunity. "Lying lips are an abomination to the Lord" (Proverbs 12:22).
7. Insult and abuse in general. Immorality (which would include adultery, homosexuality, and pornography), sorcery, enmities (including profanity), strife, dissensions, drunkenness, and unrighteousness of all types are grouped in this last category. (See Galatians 5:19–21.)

When you are wronged, God says to bless a person instead of insulting him. An insult is usually the natural human response, while blessing a person requires a decision of the will and empowerment by the Holy Spirit. Consider the following uses of blessing in Scripture, and apply them to your marriage.

1. Giving praise to God. (See Luke 1:64; 6:28; and 2 Timothy 1:3–6.) Concerning your mate, ask yourself, *What positive qualities about my mate can I use to verbally praise him or her?*
2. Giving thanks to God for His gifts and favor. (See Luke 1:64; 2:28–32; and Mark 6:41.) Concerning your mate, ask yourself, *What qualities about my mate am I thankful for, and how can I communicate this to him or her?*
3. Calling down God's favor. (See 1 Samuel 12:23.) Concerning your mate, ask yourself, *What specific areas of my mate's life should I pray that the Lord will bless?*
4. Benefits bestowed. (See Mark 6:41 and Luke 11:13.) Consider benefits (such as gifts, acts of service) that you can bestow upon your mate.
5. Seeking counsel. (See Proverbs 27:9.) Honor your spouse by seeking his or her advice.
6. Encouragement and fellowship. (See Philippians 2:1–4.) Consider areas of your spouse's life where you can encourage him or her. Ask yourself, *Am I spending enough quality time so I know what is really on his or her heart?*

You know what blesses and what insults your mate. If you don't, simply ask your mate. These examples from Scripture are mentioned to broaden your perspective. Become an expert on how to bless your spouse, and then practice giving blessings. Remember, "Give, and it will be given to you. They will pour into your lap a good measure—pressed down, shaken together, and running over. For by your standard of measure it will be measured to you in return" (Luke 6:38, italics added). If you are always critical, criticism will come back to you. If you are an encourager, encouragement will come back to you. It is your choice. Give agape love and it will be returned.

As figure 4 shows, the blessing cycle is as rewarding and ongoing as the insult cycle is damaging and ongoing. And the results could not be more different. The couple caught in the insult cycle find themselves (1) unable to be one in their marriage; (2) unable to reflect, reproduce, and reign; and (3) unable to receive a blessing. In contrast, the couple who enter the blessing cycle find their relationship blessed with (1) oneness; (2) the ability to reflect, reproduce, and reign; and (3) more blessings.

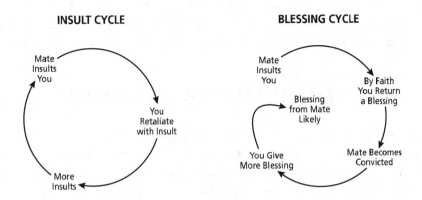

Figure 4
The Cycles of Insults and Blessings

INSULT CYCLE

Mate
Insults
You

You
Retaliate
with Insult

More
Insults

BLESSING CYCLE

Mate
Insults
You

By Faith
You Return
a Blessing

Blessing
from Mate
Likely

Mate Becomes
Convicted

You Give
More Blessing

With such great rewards from blessing each other, why do marriages turn into insult battlefields instead of blessings, as God intended? The answer takes us right back to a key biblical theme found throughout Scripture and highlighted in Galatians 5:16–26. If you are a Christian, two forces are operating in your life. One is your self-centered will (the flesh). The other is your "new spiritual creation" given to you at the point you received Christ as Savior (note 2 Corinthians 5:17). These two are in conflict with one another. Your will follows the natural impulses of the flesh, while your new spiritual creation heeds God's will, as revealed by the Holy Spirit. The Spirit uses Scripture to reveal God's will. These two forces approach life from entirely different perspectives.

The chart on page 85 compares this divergent thought. As you study it, you may be amazed at the difference between God's perspective and man's. God says it this way, "For My thoughts are not your thoughts, neither are your ways My ways" (Isaiah 55:8). The insights on the following page demonstrate the conflicts between the way men and women naturally think compared to God's perspective.

I don't know about you, but when I read through the chart, the Holy Spirit nudges me. "Don, wake up to My ways." The term "faith relationship" demands dependence on God's perspective, not my own. Humanly speaking, it does not make sense for me to bless when I have been wronged. Yet, as the Holy Spirit applies God's perspective through His Word, I begin to think, "Wait a minute, maybe God has a better way!"

The next question we must ask is, "Does God ever give you the right to retaliate?" No, He does not. He does tell us to seek wise counsel. He does give specific instruction concerning church discipline. He does tell us not to be drawn into sin. But He never gives us the right to retaliate. Instead, the New Testament asks that we seek to return good for evil done to us: "Bless those who curse you, pray for those who mistreat you," Jesus said (Luke 6:28); "See that no one repays another with evil for evil, but always seek after that which is good for one another and for all people," Paul added (1 Thessalonians 5:15).

WHY RETURN A BLESSING?

No question about it, God condemns revenge—all the time! With that established, it is wise to look at God's better way. After instructing husbands and wives concerning the marriage relationship (1 Peter 3:1–7), Peter explained why it's better to return a blessing rather than an insult when wronged.

> To sum up, all of you be harmonious, sympathetic, brotherly, kindhearted, and humble in spirit; not returning evil for evil, or insult for insult, but giving a blessing instead; for you were called for the very purpose that you might inherit a blessing. For The one who desires life, to love and see good days, must keep his tongue from evil and his lips from speaking deceit. He must turn away from evil and do good; he must seek peace and pursue it. For the eyes of the Lord are toward the righteous, and His ears attend to their prayer, but the face of the Lord is against those who do evil (1 Peter 3:8–12).

The apostle offered four reasons to give a blessing to those who wrong us. First, Peter said, "for you were called for the very purpose that you might inherit a blessing." In other words, a *blessing beget a blessing.* And a blessing is what God desires for you. He doesn't want you to insult, because He knows that will result in a returned insult, leading to more frustration.

Second, God implies that blessing one another will result in "good days," or a long life. Certainly, that is true. Stress destroys, while *blessing prospers and benefits.*

Why return a blessing? Because it works!

Third, when you bless, you have the hope of pleasing God, and that "His ears attend to [your] prayers." That is a significant promise. When we are in God's will, "all authority in heaven and earth" is available. *Returning a blessing allows God to bless us through answered prayer.*

Finally, God further releases you from the need to return an insult by saying in effect, "If your mate is really wrong, I will take care of it." The Scripture declares, "The face of the Lord is against those who do evil." *God can better deal with your mate* because of His great love and forgiveness that tempers His justice. When God

MAN'S PERSPECTIVE VERSUS GOD'S PERSPECTIVE

MAN'S PERSPECTIVE (THE WORLD'S SYSTEM)	GOD'S PERSPECTIVE
1. People are my problem.	"Seek first His kingdom and His righteousness, and all these things will be added to you" (Matthew 6:33).
2. Success is the first priority.	"For our struggle is not against flesh and blood, but against the . . . powers, against the . . . spiritual forces of wickedness in the heavenly places" (Ephesians 6:12).
3. Hold on to what you've got at all costs or you will lose everything.	"Give, and it will be given to you. They will pour into your lap a good measure—pressed down, shaken together, and running over" (Luke 6:38).
4. Material possessions will bring more happiness.	"Blessed are those who hunger and thirst for righteousness, for they shall be satisfied" (Matthew 5:6).
5. Most of my problems are caused by the one in authority.	"Every person is to be in subjection to the governing authorities. For there is no authority except from God, and those which exist are established by God. For rulers are not a cause of fear for good behavior, but for evil" (Romans 13:1, 3).
6. Love your friends, but get your enemies before they get you.	"But I say to you, love your enemies and pray for those who persecute you" (Matthew 5:44).
7. If only I had married someone more gifted I would be happier.	"But one and the same Spirit works all these things, distributing to each one individually just as He wills" (1 Corinthians 12:11).
8. In this life, you've got to take care of Old Number One.	"If anyone wants to be first, he shall be last of all and servant of all" (Mark 9:35).
9. My mate can't do anything. If only I had married someone God can use.	"I planted, Apollos watered, but God was causing the growth. So then neither the one who plants nor the one who waters is anything, but God who causes the growth" (1 Corinthians 3:6–7).
10. I'll teach him or her not to cross me.	"Never take your own revenge, beloved, but leave room for the wrath of God, for it is written, "Vengeance is Mine, I will repay," says the Lord" (Romans 12:19).
11. I'm going to the top and I don't care whom I have to step on to get there.	"Humble yourselves under the mighty hand of God, that He may exalt you at the proper time" (1 Peter 5:6).

disciplines, He redeems. When you try to play God in your mate's life, you destroy.

Which makes sense to you now, returning a blessing or an insult? His Word indicates that returning a blessing is God's will. It opens the door to blessing, life, good days, and God's favor. So why return a blessing? Because it works!

The next question is, "How do we give a blessing?" Christ's own life provides an excellent example as described in 1 Peter 2:21–25. The context is suffering in trials, yet a wonderful picture emerges showing how Christ responded to insults. Think back to Vicki's response to Bob and compare her actions to our Lord's response. Do you see the difference?

HOW TO RESPOND TO INSULTS

Our model for how to respond to insults is the Master Himself, the Lord Jesus Christ. Peter has described how the Lord Jesus responded to insults.

> *For you have been called for this purpose, since Christ also suffered for you, leaving you an example for you to follow in His steps, who committed no sin, nor was any deceit found in His mouth; and while being reviled, He did not revile in return; while suffering, He uttered no threats, but kept entrusting Himself to Him who judges righteously; and He Himself bore our sins in His body on the cross, so that we might die to sin and live to righteousness; for by His wounds you were healed (1 Peter 2:21–24).*

The first thing we are to do is *remove any sin in our own lives.* Note that Christ was innocent—He had committed no sin! When your mate insults you, first ask yourself, "Did I do anything to provoke my mate?" If you did, confess your sin, first to God, and then to your mate. Usually we bear some fault too. Perhaps 90 percent of the time when Sally insults me, I did something to provoke her. My first step —your first step—in responding to your mate's insult is to determine your role in her response. "Sweetheart, I know I must have done something to provoke your response. How have I hurt you? Can we talk about it?"

After understanding the issue, you may need to ask your mate's forgiveness. Only when you confess *your* failure will God be able to work in your mate's life, either to bring conviction or restoration.

The second step in responding to an insult is to return a blessing. Christ died to heal the very people who had ignored Him, wounded Him, and crucified Him. The implication is clear: Christ not only refused to insult them, but He blessed them. Each mate must make a *willful* decision to return a blessing in spite of the hurt just experienced. Your will must be submitted to God's will. Look beneath the insult to the reason for the behavior or words. Look for ways to bless your mate. Look for ways to praise your mate and communicate your love deliberately. Do something specific to build up his or her spirit.

Most people insult others because they are hurting inside, and have tremendous emotional needs themselves. Insulting can be a release mechanism. You can interrupt this tendency with kindness. Jesus uttered no threats when insults were thrown at Him. He had every "right" to threaten the people who were sending Him to the cross. But Jesus knew that insults and threats do not work. They only cause more hatred. By not returning an insult, you humble yourself and allow God's principle of blessing to work.

The third step is just as important: *Commit yourself and your situation to the Lord.* Jesus turned to His Father for hope, insight, and strength. Humanly, Christ did not want to suffer, but He kept His Father's perspective. He knew that even though it was momentarily tough, in the long run His Father's will was best. You must yield to God's will and perspective also.

As you yield to the Holy Spirit, He will change your perspective. You will begin to say, "God gave me this person, and therefore *my struggle is not against my mate,* but Satan, who deceives me into thinking that my mate is the problem." That is the source of all spiritual problems, according to Ephesians 6:12. As you catch God's perspective, you can thank Him for the situation. As you yield the situation to the Lord, it can be used to make you more like Christ. Only the Lord can convict and adequately deal with your mate's offense.

The last step is: *Be willing to suffer in order that God can heal your offender.* Jesus *purposed* to die on a cross so that you might be healed (1 Peter 2:24–25). God never says the momentary cost of returning a blessing will be small. In fact, He implies that at times it will be very tough. (Remember, the Crucifixion was an ugly event.) Yet, God guarantees a blessing for your efforts and peace in your heart. It may not be just what you expect, but God will bless you in ways you have never dreamed.

Determine to stop the insult cycle and return a blessing instead through the power of the Holy Spirit. The more you learn to bless, the more blessings you will receive in return.

How do you change your mate? You apply the active force of agape love. When wronged, apply the reactive force of love which is the act of blessing. Both of these go against our human nature. That is why faith is necessary. Faith occurs when you override your human instinct by acting on God's Word, through the power of the Holy Spirit.

NOTE

1. These definitions of love are found in William E. Vine, *Vine's Expository Dictionary of New Testament Words* (Uhrichsville, Ohio: Barbour, 1985).

CHAPTER EIGHT

God's Order for Marital Oneness (Love and Respect)

◈ FROM ITS FOUNDING IN 1776, IN A WAR OF independence against England, America and its people have always valued independence and self-reliance. And now, at the start of the twenty-first century, the thought of yielding a measure of autonomy or space in order to submit to anyone still contradicts every cultural message Americans hear. Many husbands and wives feel the same way: "I don't want to lose my independence to my spouse." Yet in the Bible's call to serve each other, the Scriptures teach husbands and wives to practice submission to each other.

Years ago, a deeply agitated woman came to us with her concerns regarding her role as wife. She thought she knew what God intended for women, but told us, "I have struggled with guilt feelings lately because I've begun to question the issue of submission in marriage for a woman. I am confused about what submission means and if it applies to women anymore."

Men are equally confused. Some see a wife's role as the opportunity to become a macho, rude dictator, bellowing out commands. Christian couples with marital problems often admit they're confused about biblical roles. When Sally and I began to analyze this frustration over the issue of "headship and submission," we found several questions at the crux of the debate:

- Did God create men and women equally?
- Did God intend for men and women to have different roles in the family?
- Do men have an advantage over women from God's perspective?
- What does it mean for the husband to love the wife?
- Why did God give a different command to women: one of respect?

These issues have reached great magnitude because of our cultural emphasis on the "oppressed" wife. To answer these questions, let's begin with the scriptural job descriptions of men and women in marriage. The man's responsibility is stated in Ephesians 5:25–33 and 1 Peter 3:7, and the woman's responsibility is found in 1 Peter 3:1–6. Both responsibilities, however, are summed up in Ephesians 5:21: "Be subject to one another in the fear of Christ."

As you approach these Scriptures and consider these points, be careful. You may soon begin thinking, *Oh, not that again! If I hear these points one more time, I'll scream!* If these issues are not placed in the larger context of God's whole plan for marriage, they can become legalistic. From God's perspective, however, love and respect should not be a source of struggle nor a task to accomplish. Rather, understanding each role can be the evidence of a loving relationship.

God's Perspective on Love and Submission (Respect)

	HUSBAND	WIFE
KEY VERSE (Ephesians 5:21)	"Be subject to one another in the fear of Christ."	"Be subject to one another in the fear of Christ."
ROLE	Love	Submission
ABSOLUTE COMMAND	*Love* without conditions	*Submit* without a word
SUPPORTING SCRIPTURES	Ephesians 5:25–33; 1 Peter 3:7	1 Peter 2:13; 3:1–6
PROMISES	1. Sanctify her 2. Present her 3. Have prayers answered	1. Silence foolishness 2. May win husband to Christ 3. Have no fear 4. Have a spirit precious to God
PICTURES	1. Love her as own body 2. Nourish her 3. Cherish her 4. Honor/understand her 5. Exemplify Christ	1. Gentle and quiet spirit 2. Respect husband 3. Holy women who hoped in God 4. The example of Sarah

We will define biblically what love and submission mean. The accompanying chart on God's perspective on these words summarizes well the differences in the husbands' and wives' roles.

Although the roles of husband and wife differ, a careful review of Ephesians 5:25–33 and 1 Peter 2:13; 3:1–7 demonstrates that *there is no favoritism on God's part toward either the man or the woman.* In fact, the two passages are parallel in several important ways. (See chart above.) As we look at the Ephesians and 1 Peter passages, one fundamental truth becomes clear: God made men and women to be equal but different in role and function.

God made men and women to be equal but different in role and function.

Each passage begins with a command that is very strong in the original language. They leave little doubt about the responsibilities of both the husband and wife. Each passage lists a number of exciting promises that result from following the commands. These promises motivate, soften, and become the hope of the commands. The passages also include illustrations to clarify our understanding of each role and to provide a hint as to how you can fulfill them successfully.

We also need to consider the similar contexts in which these two passages are written. In Ephesians 1–3, Paul wrote that Christians are to walk in a manner worthy of His calling because of Christ's suffering at the Cross. In Ephesians 5:15–21, he added that as we walk in the Spirit of God, four things will result.

1. We will speak to one another with psalms and hymns (understanding God's motivation).
2. We will sing and make melody with our hearts to the Lord (praise Him for that motivation).
3. We will be able to give thanks for all things in His name (because we understand His will).
4. We'll make ourselves subject to one another in the fear of the Lord (because we understand God's provisions for relationships).

For a husband, he will understand Christ's challenge only when he understands how to walk in the power of the Holy Spirit and seeks the mind of Christ. Without that perspective, a man will never fulfill his role. With that perspective, a husband can understand what it means to submit to his wife, and what it means to love his wife. He will learn, for instance, that both love and submission mean listening to her heart, respecting her opinions, and honoring her thoughts.

In like manner, before teaching the importance of a wife's submission in

1 Peter 3, Peter drew the readers' minds back to Christ's suffering on the cross. There Jesus submitted Himself to unjust suffering, and "kept entrusting Himself to Him [God the Father] who judges righteously" (2:23). Peter was saying, "Women, before you can properly understand your responsibility to your husbands, you too must have the perspective of Christ." So, the contexts of both passages are parallel in that both focus on Christ's suffering prior to the call to obedience.

THE COMMANDS

As you compare the two passages, look at the command to each mate. First, read the command to the man: "Husbands, love your wives, just as Christ also loved the church and gave Himself up for her" (Ephesians 5:25). The word for *love* used in this command is the word *agape*, which you will recall is a God-given and God-directed love that does not exist apart from God. We called it "commitment love" in the previous chapter. That is why it is illustrated by Christ's love for the church.

What was the church doing when Christ came and died for her? She was nonexistent. (The few followers, called "disciples," were in despair and disarray after Jesus' arrest.) People were rebelling against God and ultimately crucified Jesus Christ! By Christ's example, we learn that God's love was initiated totally by the Giver; it did not take into account the actions of the one loved (Romans 5:8). The same must be true as husbands love their wives. Husbands are to love sacrificially while setting aside their rights, pleasing God the Father just as Christ did.

Now men, read the command of Ephesians 5:25 again. Talk about 100 percent responsibility! There are no exception clauses here. There are no excuses. Should God ask you one day, "How did you love your wife?" you might be tempted to say, "Well, Lord, You know I loved her in certain areas. But it was hard to love her completely. She didn't always deserve it. And remember, Lord, she had an affair, and she was untrustworthy. I just couldn't love her unconditionally." You might try to prove she didn't deserve your love.

But the Lord will say, "I didn't ask you about your mate's weaknesses. I asked you, 'How did you respond to My command to love her as I loved you?'"

There are no exceptions! God knows your mate's weaknesses, be because He created her. He even knows her sins, because Christ died for her. He wants you to love her, no matter what she does or does not do. That is your 100 percent responsibility! Hard? Indeed, it's impossible on your own. But by His Spirit working in and through you, you can love your wife as Jesus Christ loved us and gave Himself up for us. The wife's number one need is to be loved unconditionally and told often. God never told a wife to love her husband. Wives do that intuitively, because that is her biggest need. But He did tell husbands to love because that's the thing they take for granted in the relationship. A wife cannot hear enough, "I love you because..."

The wife, on the other hand, is given an equally firm command. "In the same way, you wives, be submissive to your own husbands so that even if any of them are disobedient to the word, they may be won without a word by the behavior of their wives, as they observe your chaste and respectful behavior" (1 Peter 3:1-2).

Let's stop here to define the word submission. Many women think submission means to be walked on, to not express an opinion, just do whatever the husband wants. That could not be further from the truth. The word submission means to fall into line with your husband in order that oneness can take place. It means loving your husband enough to tell him you respect him for the things he does for you and your children. The words "submit" and "respect" will be interchangeable from here on out. It is one and the same meaning.

Why is a wife told to respect her husband? Because that is his greatest need. You will never hear a husband say about the work place, "I wish people would just tell me they loved me." No, you will hear him say, though, "I just need a little respect." A wife can raise her husband's self image several notches every time she says, "Honey, I really respect you for..." Respect is what a husband wants and needs more than anything, therefore God gives that command to the wife.

So, submission in marriage means respecting your husband enough to follow his leadership in the home, Eph. 5:33 says, "The wife must respect her husband."

A husband serves his wife by loving her above all others, devoting himself to her, seeking her opinions, and valuing her as a person. He speaks love and demonstrates love. A wife serves her husband by treating him with respect, seeking his opinions, and valuing him as a person. She speaks respect and demonstrates respect.

Women are to submit themselves to their husbands as they entrust themselves to God. Again, the wife, like the husband, will have to answer the Lord when He asks, "How did you respond with respect to your husband?" No matter how strong the proof of her husband's weaknesses, there are no exception clauses in God's command to her. Peter made this clear by stating, "even if any of them are

Submission means that you place yourself under another. . . . It is never the right of the husband to make his wife submit.

disobedient to the word." Then Peter sealed the strength of the command by saying a wife must submit to her husband's leadership with a respectful attitude. It takes tremendous spiritual perspective to submit as Christ did, yet He requires it of godly wives. Certainly it's easier to follow a man who loves the Lord and is being obedient to love his wife unconditionally.

We see no favoritism in these parallel commands to the husband or wife. Both are overwhelming commands. Both require complete submission to Jesus Christ. Both husband and wife must willingly obey under the loving care of a mighty God! Be careful not to inject your cultural thinking at this point. When you submit to your mate, you are submitting to God. He is not talking about winners and losers. Instead, God outlines His will for marriage that results in oneness. Trust Him that when He commands us to love and submit, He intends only blessing and unity.

PROMISES TO HUSBANDS ABOUT WIVES

The Lord is gracious to quickly draw our eyes from these strong commands to the associated promises. Our obedience brings positive outcomes. First, the husband draws encouragement from the results of showing love similar to Christ's: "That He might sanctify her, having cleansed her by the washing of water with the word, that He might present to Himself the church in all her glory, having no spot or wrinkle or any such thing; but that she should be holy and blameless" (Ephesians 5:26–27).

The promise to the husband is twofold: (1) that he might sanctify his wife and (2) that he might present his wife spotless. A husband cannot accomplish these things in the eternal sense as God does, but this kind of love on the man's part will produce results similar to those coming from Christ's love.

The word *sanctify* should encourage us. *Sanctify* means to "set apart from the rest." You're set apart in Christ in that you're free from death because of His death and resurrection. A wife is set apart by her husband because his love is not based on her performance, and she is therefore free to be "more than ordinary."

Just as the Spirit reminds us daily of our forgiveness by washing us with the Word of God, so a wife, through experience, must be able to trust her husband's commitment to love her. And, men, this seemingly impossible command to love is not so hard when you realize the results will be a receptive and appreciative wife! A woman who is loved with agape love is a pleasant and beautiful woman indeed!

Next, God promises the husband that if he loves his wife sacrificially, she will be perfected by this love. When Paul speaks of having "no spot or wrinkle," the word *spot* means "moral stain," and the word *wrinkle* means to be "filled with inner struggles." Using these words implies the outward and inner results of Christ's work. Christ's work results in eternal perfection, but Paul implies the similar, temporal result of the husband's sacrificial love. Christ's love is so freeing and creative in your life that you're able to experience both outward joy and inward peace. The face and countenance of a Christian should not show the signs of inward stress and pressure that an unbeliever may have.

During my married life, God has graciously demonstrated the "no spot or wrinkle" promise to me. Sally has always desired to please God with all her heart. But I also believe Sally has become a godly wife and mother, partially because I have dared to love her unconditionally by faith. When I place her under performance, fear results. Yet, when I love her as Christ loved the church, hope and faith are the results. Sacrificial love produces a more beautiful wife, internally as well as externally.

Husbands, I am not saying that God will make our wives "beauties" right before our eyes. But our wives will find inner joy by having loving relationships with us. Sally does not spend even minutes a day being distressed over our relationship. My commitment love has freed her to become characterized by an outward glow and an inner joy that makes her very attractive. I am convinced that one day God will show me that my faith was used by Him to make her more internally peaceful, which showed on her countenance. Added to that is a change that she has expressed to others and me. Sally actually loves God more, and understands the unconditional love of God better, because God's love has had "arms" through me.

God promises husbands that if they can keep Christ's perspective in loving their wives, He will actually use husbands as instruments of redemption in the lives of their mates. Her peace and joy will be noticeable. People will say, "What a joy it is to know your wife. Her life really motivates me."

God gives another powerful promise to husbands: "You husbands in the same way, live with your wives in an understanding way, as with someone weaker, since she is a woman; and show her honor as a fellow heir of the grace of life, so that your prayers will not be hindered"(1 Peter 3:7). If husbands will honor their wives as joint heirs with them in the grace of life, God will answer their prayers. Understanding her will involve a great deal of time and energy. It involves asking her how she feels on any given subject and not always trying to solve her problems. Sometimes she doesn't need a solution, just a listening ear. She needs to feel that you *want* to understand her.

What does it mean to honor your wife? It simply means to consider your wife's needs above your own. Honoring means listening to her and communicating with her. It involves giving her quality time and attention. If you value

Our [wives will] actually love God more . . . because God's love has had "arms" through [us].

your wife's insights concerning life, marriage, raising children, friendships, careers, church, decision making, how your gifts differ, and so on, she will truly be a joint heir with you. There will be harmony, not discord. Sin will not be obstructing your relationship with God, and God promises answers to your prayers!

Husbands, you cannot demand respect from your wife; you can only earn it. You do this through tenderly and patiently understanding and honoring her. This is what it means to be "subject to one another in the fear of Christ" (Ephesians 5:21).

PROMISES TO WIVES ABOUT HUSBANDS

Likewise, the woman also has been given promises that result from her submission to her husband. Respectful submission is always voluntary on her part. It requires faith in God's perspective and plan. Peter described the promises in his first epistle:

> For such is the will of God that by doing right you may silence the igno-
> rance of foolish men. . . . Your adornment must not be merely external—
> braiding the hair, and wearing gold jewelry, or putting on dresses; but let
> it be the hidden person of the heart, with the imperishable quality of a
> gentle and quiet spirit, which is precious in the sight of God. For in this
> way in former times the holy women also, who hoped in God, used to
> adorn themselves, being submissive to their own husbands; just as Sarah
> obeyed Abraham, calling him lord, and you have become her children if you
> do what is right without being frightened by any fear (1 Peter 2:15; 3:3–6).

God instructs women to submit to their husbands, not because of their perfection, but because of God's faithfulness. A woman should never regard submission as being to her husband, but as being to the Lord. God's faithfulness is your hope, just as it was the hope of Christ as He went to the Cross.

The first promise occurs in 1 Peter 2:15. While not yet speaking directly of marriage, Peter mentions a result of submission that occurs from a relationship other than marriage. Peter tells us that if we do what is right, we can "silence the ignorance of foolish men." That is powerful.

This is followed closely by a second promise, indicated in 1 Peter 3:1. Wives who submit themselves as unto the Lord may win their husbands by their behavior without nagging. Again, God shows the wife that she can be an instrument of the Lord, effecting change in his attitude toward God. Notice, there is no other way to effect change in a husband. Nagging is neither a way of making peace nor of making a husband do what is right. The woman who struggles with submission has never really believed God that her respect is the key to his response. Her resistance only leads to frustration for both of them.

Wives, we're not talking about poor communication here. Throughout Scripture you find instruction on how and when to communicate. However, this passage deals with weakness on the part of the husband. When a wife nears the point of nagging or preaching, she must get out of the way so that God can work in her husband's life. This is a tough decision requiring faith and complete dependence on God.

I have grown to so respect my wife that when I am wrong and she is gracious toward me, I feel overwhelmed and confess my mistakes. She may say something like, "Don, I have expressed my opinion on that subject, but I want you to pray about it. Before the Lord, whatever you decide, I will respect that." As a man, I can bear witness to the power God releases in my life through her gracious attitude. When she does that, I want to do right! I always pray about decisions, especially when she has first expressed her feelings. I listen to her much more effectively when I feel that she is not judging me or mistrusting me. I have often found that her intuition has kept me from making a mistake that I would have made if I hadn't consulted her.

A wife's gracious attitude frees the husband to go to the Lord and seek His will. The couple can then pray about it together, and God will always show them what to do.

Finally, God promises that the woman who keeps His perspective and trusts Him more than human devices (trickery, manipulative words, or physical charms) will be precious to God. What a promise! God places a very high value on a woman who esteems her husband. He says her trust will cause her to have a "gentle and quiet spirit." *Gentle* means not causing her husband to be frustrated or ruffled. *Quiet* means causing her husband to be soothed when he is upset or frustrated. A mother is naturally good at this with children but not always with her husband.

To the woman who seeks God's heart, it means a great deal to be precious in His sight. Peter wrote that respectful wives would be like Sarah, who had no fear. Most women are paralyzed with fears: fears of growing old, losing love, appreciation, or wealth, facing death, and more. Most would love to be fearless. God chose Sarah to illustrate His promise. Her husband Abraham was far from perfect. Yet Sarah submitted herself and was not afraid. A very wealthy man, Abraham was called by God to leave his home in search of a new place. God promised to lead him. Abraham went by faith, taking Sarah and all their servants. During the

A wife's gracious attitude frees the husband to go to the Lord and seek His will.

trip, Abraham came upon a very harsh kingdom. Rather than trusting God that he wouldn't be killed, he told Sarah to pretend to be his sister. She would find favor with the king and thus spare Abraham's life. And Sarah remained silent!

Let me ask you: Has your husband ever told you to do anything so ridiculous—to pretend you are his sister? Abraham pulled this trick, not once, but twice! Sarah's hope was not in Abraham at this point, but in God, who judges righteously. God protected her both times. And God can protect you from your husband's mistakes even when you are affected by them. If you are faithful, God will give you peace and richly bless your path.

Considering both the commands and promises to the husband and wife, there is no advantage to either role. Both commands call for total faith. On the other hand, God's promises to both husbands and wives take the sting out of the commands and give hope.

HIS TO CHERISH, HERS TO TRUST

The New Testament explains how these roles are implemented. Husbands are to cherish; wives are to trust. The husband receives two practical word pictures of his role: the words *cherish* and *nourish*. Here's how the apostle Paul pictured the husband loving his wife: "So husbands ought also to love their own wives as their own bodies. He who loves his own wife loves himself; for no one ever hated his own flesh, but nourishes and cherishes it, just as Christ also does the church, because we are members of His body" (Ephesians 5:28–30).

A woman who puts her hope in God instead of in human schemes exhibits a gentle and quiet spirit toward her husband.

Husbands are to love their wives as they love their own bodies. Most men are instinctively aware of the value of their own bodies; they do not have to consciously think about loving them. If anyone, or anything, hurts or threatens it, they respond with corrective action. God is telling us men how important our wives should be. You and I are to be so sensitive to our wives that if anything hurt or threatened them, we would take immediate corrective action to protect them.

You are to *nourish* and *cherish* your wife. These two words are beautiful ways of describing the love God is talking about. *Nourish*, used only twice in the New Testament, literally means "to keep warm at the perfect temperature." It was used to describe a mother bird keeping her chicks under her wing at perfect body temperature. Husbands are to be so involved in their wives' care that they know from moment to moment what her needs are in order to meet them.

Even more descriptive is the word *cherish*. The only other place this word is used in Scripture is 1 Thessalonians 2:7: "But we proved to be gentle among you, as a nursing mother tenderlycares for her own children." Have you ever noticed that mothers are almost perfect in responding to the needs of their newborn? Even women who normally struggle when serving others usually have a natural desire to give joyfully to their babies without resentment. An infant makes selfish demands with little capacity to appreciate its mother's sacrifice. Yet a good mother will reshape her life for her baby with very little struggle. She does it because she feels blessed, and she senses her absolute responsibility. She has an innate desire to do what has to be done.

Think of that picture of a loving mother: In spite of her burden, a mother instinctively knows that her baby is a blessing from God.

This illustration opened my eyes to God's perspective. God was telling me that if I really understood how important Sally was to my creation purpose, I would gladly treat her as a mother would treat a nursing newborn. The lights went on. What God said in Genesis 1 and 2 took on an even more beautiful meaning. Like naming the animals for Adam, this passage registered for me. Sally's meaning as a gift and provision deepened tremendously. She became valuable and precious to me.

Men, our culture does not teach us to view marriage this way. Such care and concern for wives are not found in the average American home. Yet this is God's pattern. Do you love your wife as much as you do your own body? Do you know her needs? Are you sensitive to her? Have you altered your lifestyle in order that she might be set apart and glorified? Do you treat her with dignity and honor her? Do you take this responsibility from the Lord as completely as Christ took His responsibility for you, regardless of performance? Are you totally committed to her?

God illustrates submission to wives by talking about their "respectful behavior," their "gentle and quiet spirit," and their "hope in God." Each of these perspectives is dependent upon knowing and trusting God. First, the wife begins by demonstrating a respectful attitude toward her husband. God says, "Love him into right behavior." When your husband is wrong, your first response is usually to tell him so. God says there is a better way—a way that will win him without condemning words. The only way a woman can act respectfully when her husband falters is to view God as the guarantor of her needs. When a wife understands how God made her husband, she will discover from Scripture how to wisely influence him to submit to God.

A woman who puts her hope in God instead of in human schemes exhibits a gentle and quiet spirit toward her husband. Remember, 1 Peter 3 contrasts her outer and inner beauty. Peter wrote that women should not ignore their physical appearance, but to concentrate on the inner qualities. Wives, you do need to look good for your husbands. But your primary efforts are to be in developing your spiritual walk with the Lord, so that Christlike qualities will come through to your husband.

Jesus loves your husband and died for him. Your life should exemplify that. A gentle and quiet spirit will soothe the soul of your husband like nothing else in the world. He will enjoy coming home to you.

The woman who places her hope in God will be able to call her husband "lord." This means she is able to esteem him above what he deserves, because she views him from God's perspective. Her loving spirit toward him then will free him to submit to the Lord and grow spiritually. With proper love and submission, there will be oneness in marriage. The cycle of loving and esteeming is a blessing cycle indeed!

UNDERSTANDING MEN'S AND WOMEN'S ROLES:
THE LEGALISTIC LEVEL

In working with Christians, I have discovered three basic levels of understanding of the husband's and wife's roles and responsibilities. These levels are as different as night and day. Evaluate them and decide where you are—and where you need to be.

Many church people live at *the legalistic level.* As husbands and wives, they understand that God commands them to be lovers or submitters.

Some wives . . . think the word submit means "to be walked on," . . . The concept . . . [has] no basis whatsoever in Scripture.

They know these two commands but feel they are impossible to obey. After a talk on "headship and submission," these spouses always try to find a way out. The wife may say, "Please pray for me as I try to submit to this monster that I married." The husband may say, "I'm the head, but she won't do anything I tell her to do." They've both missed the point altogether.

Down through the centuries, men have used the issue of "headship" as a club over their wives' heads. Completely missing their responsibility to love, they hear only the command for their wives to submit. They feel right in "lording it over" their wives. No wonder wives resent their husbands!

An equally unfortunate response shown by some wives who object to God's command to submit is to deny the command altogether. Their need to defend their rights reveals a basic legalistic fear that God is going to deny them something. Perhaps they fear that they will not be fulfilled as a person. They think the word *submit* means "to be walked on," or "to become a doormat." These women have missed the bigger picture of Christ's commands. The concepts of "lording it over" and "being walked on" have no basis whatsoever in Scripture. Fear and rebellion result from these misunderstandings.

There is very little hope for the legalistic man and woman. Either defensive or defeated, they run from one book to the next, trying to find the key. One week they might try a new plan and for several weeks their hopes are high. Soon, however, the newness of the project wears off. Things happen to discourage them. Once again, they begin to search for another book or marriage seminar. Books and seminars are fine, but rightly understanding the Word of God, mixed with faith, is what endures!

UNDERSTANDING ROLES:
THE PROMISE LEVEL

The next level of understanding is significantly better. *The promise level* exists when couples look beyond God's command to love and submit to His promise of blessing. Many successful marriages are at this level of understanding because they focus on God's promises. They live with joyful expectancy of God working in their marriages. They believe and act upon God's Word that produces results in their lives and reinforces their efforts. Their marriages grow in hope based on the certainty of God's Word. In and through God's promises, they are assured of everything needed to make life successful.

The potential of a marriage focused on God's promises is clear: "His divine power has granted to us everything pertaining to life and godliness, through the true knowledge of Him who called us by His own glory and excellence. For by these He has granted to us His precious and magnificent promises, so that by them you may become partakers of the divine nature" (2 Peter 1:3–4).

Beyond leaning on God's promises, what could possibly add to your understanding of love and submission? The answer is: seeing life from God's perspective. When we trust that God's perspective on marriage roles is right, we are moving to the wisdom level about our marriages.

UNDERSTANDING ROLES:
THE WISDOM LEVEL

Wisdom is the final level of understanding. Wisdom involves living and seeing life from God's perspective. Only through God's wisdom, made known through the Holy Spirit, can you come to fully accept and embrace love and submission. Each mate must individually come to the point of totally rejoicing in his or her roles because they are from God's loving hand. It takes wisdom to do that.

Wisdom is essential. Without it you are still vulnerable. More important, wisdom recognizes the integrity of God's character. Few Christians realize that their questioning of love and respect really questions the character of God. Ask yourself, "How did I come to question God in the first place concerning roles?" We believe the main reason Christians question their roles is that ultimately they do not trust God's good character. They doubt God's plan; they doubt that He designed the best way of relating in marriage. Godly wisdom says our roles were created by a loving God for our benefit.

Several things are vital if Christians desire wisdom. First, you must ask the Holy Spirit to teach you. Second, you need to understand who caused marriage and relational problems in the first place. Originally, who was the author of sin? Satan. How did he deceive Adam and Eve? He lied to them. Who do you think is the source of the world's rejection of God's order in marriage? Yes, Satan. The Father of Lies is still at work. In the next chapter, Satan's schemes will be revealed.

Finally, wisdom flourishes in an atmosphere of mutual submission where each partner serves the other. Servanthood marked the ministry of Christ, and accordingly, God's Word directs husbands and wives to be subject to one another (Ephesians 5:21). A man serves a woman by providing her greatest need: love. A woman serves a man by providing his greatest need: respect.

After understanding Satan and how he deceives people, you must embrace God and His Word. When you establish your trust in Him, and ignore Satan's lies, then you can step out in faith. Wisdom will allow you to set aside your fear (of limitations) in assuming the roles of love and submission. Rightly understanding the Word, revealed to you through the Holy Spirit, releases you from being deceived again. God's promises can be understood and enacted upon more freely. Oneness is then possible, to the praise and honor of God.

CHAPTER NINE

Wisdom or Deceit

◈ SOMETIMES A HUSBAND BECOMES FRUSTRATED OVER God's command to love his wife no matter what—even if she has disappointed him a thousand times. At times, he may recoil with, "I don't have to put up with this. She's driving me crazy!" Similarly, a wife may cry "unfair" when she learns that her scriptural responsibility to submit applies even when her husband is insensitive and irresponsible. "It's not fair!" she may say. "I can't respect a man like that."

How can we handle these situations wisely? Love and respect sound great, but regrettably, they are tough issues in real life. In this chapter you will discover why men and women struggle with their marriage roles.

Thus far, you have seen that God is the author of relationships. It was God who created the need in you for relationships, and God who chose to make Adam and Eve His example for marriage. Since God is ultimately responsible to meet our needs, we know that He will not allow anything to prevent Him from meeting these responsibilities. Therefore, God guarantees the outcome of relationships that are directed by Him.

As we learned in the previous chapter, God does not consider either role in marriage as better. God did not create the husband and wife roles to be issues of performance, importance, success, or even superiority. Both are vital to marital blessing. When God told couples to love and respect, He did not intend strife to be the result. Love and submission are simply God's basis for marital oneness. Without love and submission, there can be no oneness. If couples reject God's order, they cannot fulfill His or their purposes in their marriages.

The apostle Paul emphasized the importance of God's order; it applies equally to the Trinity as it does to a married couple: "But I want you to understand that Christ is the head of every man, and the man is the head of a woman, and God is the head of Christ" (1 Corinthians 11:3). Obviously God has created an order for successful relationships. His intention for marriage compares to His relationship with the Trinity. That's good news, for God

When God tells us to love and submit, He intends only . . . blessing.

intends no less for marriage than for Himself. In fact, Christ was both lover and submitter, and saw no threat in either role. He knew that His role, compared to His Father's, had nothing to do with winning or losing. Is Christ any less God than the Father? Any less glorified? Certainly not!

When God tells us to love and submit, He intends only order, blessing, and oneness—not struggle. The problem, then, is not that God made a mistake providing roles, but rather that people have been deceived. A person who sees life from God's perspective, and who understands God's purpose concerning relationships, will not question His order. Husbands and wives controlled by self-centeredness will question any differences between the roles as being unfair.

DECEPTION IN THE GARDEN

Couples must realize that Satan is the source of their confusion concerning love and submission. Satan wants you to see your mate as the problem rather than himself. Yet the Scriptures plainly teach that such marital struggles are spiritual in nature. "For our struggle is not against flesh and blood [people], but against the rulers, against the powers, against the world forces of this darkness, against the spiritual forces of wickedness in the heavenly places" (Ephesians 6:12).

Satan delights in destroying marriages because oneness in marriage is a threat to his purposes. If he can destroy marriages, he can also limit God's purposes for that couple. And his strategy is to feed us lies—lies about our partner and about God's plan. Recall what Jesus said about Satan: "He was a murderer from the beginning, and does not stand in the truth because there is no truth in him. Whenever he speaks a lie, he speaks from his own nature, for he is a liar and the father of lies" (John 8:44). Satan knows that if his lies are successful, he can end oneness on earth.

Look at the example of Satan's deceit in the Garden of Eden in Genesis 3. God created a perfect environment; every need had been met. Adam and Eve had no desire for other things, no longings, no dreams of things being better. Since God desired this perfect relationship to last for eternity, He placed the tree of life within the garden. If Adam and Eve ate from this tree first, they would live for all eternity in a perfect state.

The only threat to this eternal perfection was another tree, the tree of the knowledge of good and evil. God told Adam and Eve not to eat of that tree saying, "If you eat of it, you will surely die." Since they had no sinful nature, and since they were perfectly dependent on the Lord, they did not even consider the tree to be a struggle. Adam and Eve trusted God. They knew that not eating from that tree was totally for their good!

However, Satan distorted the purpose of the tree. He disputed God's purpose by calling His Word into question. (See Genesis 3:1–7.) He said they would not die if they ate of the tree, and implied that the real reason God did not want them to eat of the tree was because they would become like God. His message was: "God is really trying to limit you. He is trying to keep you from being like Him." Satan subtly changed God's purpose from one of protection to one of limitation. Satan appealed to their eyes, appetites, and pride in tempting them. They believed a lie, and they sinned.

Satan is still in the business of deceiving. He uses the same tactics today. When God originally instructed you to love and submit, what was His purpose? It was to allow you to experience relationships, accomplish His plan of the ages, meet your needs, and to equip you to reflect, reproduce, and reign. God knew that without love and submission, there would be no satisfying relationships and no oneness.

Satan has distorted God's purpose by suggesting that love and submission present a limitation, by telling husbands to resist being lovers, and wives to resent submitting. "Why should I love her? She doesn't deserve it." Or "Why should I submit to him? He's no better than I am. I'm smarter, more talented, and more successful." Like in the garden, Satan deceives people into seeing love and submission as limits to rights and freedom in marriage.

GOD'S REDEMPTIVE SOLUTIONS

After Adam and Eve had sinned, God inquired into what they had done. "The man said, 'The woman whom You gave to be with me, she gave me from the tree, and I ate.' Then the Lord God said to the woman, 'What is this you have done?' And the woman said, 'The serpent deceived me, and I ate'" (verses 12–13). What happened to their oneness? Adam immediately blamed Eve by failing to take responsibility. Ultimately, Adam blamed God for giving Eve to him. Adam believed a lie and then blamed God.

Who had changed? Not God! Both Adam and Eve were deceived and disobeyed God. This taste of rebellion gave birth to the self-centeredness of man. Oneness in marriage has suffered since that event.

In love, God has intervened in history to rescue humankind and to defeat

Satan's rebellion. First, God established a redemptive curse for Adam and Eve. The woman was given the burden of bearing children and rearing them in the home. "I will greatly multiply your pain in childbirth, in pain you shall bring forth children; yet your desire shall be for your husband, and he shall rule over you" (verse 16).

The man was given the mandate to toil in life for sustenance by hard work: "Cursed is the ground because of you; in toil you shall eat of it all the days of your life. Both thorns and thistles it shall grow for you; and you will eat the plants of the field" (verses 17–18). God greatly increased Adam and Eve's burden to protect them from their selfishness.

Yet God demonstrated His grace by removing Adam and Eve from the garden (verse 23) so that their struggle with sin and death would not be eternal, but temporary. The stage was thereby set for all people to receive new bodies for all eternity by the coming of Christ. God's ultimate act of love—sending His only Son to die on a cross so that men and women could again be in perfect union with Him—will one day bring those who receive the Savior into a perfect environment, with a perfected body and mind. God's response in the garden was a curse. But His gracious and redemptive solution to man's rebellion will someday restore us to the perfect state of Genesis 1 and 2.

If Christians do not submit themselves to each other in humility, they will become a threat, a discouragement . . . in the lives of their mates.

Genesis 3:16 contains a statement that has become the source of the current debate on love and submission. God said, "[The man] shall rule over [the woman]." Today, American culture rebels against this statement. However, the word rule means to lead and to make decisions. It doesn't imply dictatorship in any way.

Prior to the Fall, Adam and Eve's oneness with God and with each other functioned perfectly. Their submission to God was not in question. There was no mention of submission between Adam and Eve because both were totally submitted to God "as one." When sin occurred, Adam and Eve lost their oneness. To protect them from their self-centeredness, God ordained an order of relationships. This order is necessary for oneness and blessing in marriage. Even though men and women are now confused because of Satan's deceit, God's order remains the same. It takes both love and submission to experience oneness.

After the lie in the garden, Satan's second greatest lie concerns love and submission. When God said to love and submit, He intended only good. Without both love and respect, God cannot meet our aloneness needs. Without both, oneness is impossible. Only through oneness can God's purposes be accomplished. Satan does not want that! If Christians do not submit themselves to each other in humility, they will become a threat, a discouragement, and a source of rejection and judgment in the lives of their mates. Unless they love and serve unconditionally, they will never gain respect. There are no agape relationships without both love and submission.

Satan deceives us by appealing to our pride and self-centered nature. He convinces husbands that it is justifiable to demand their wives' obedience, while simultaneously whispering to wives that submission equals oppression. As was stated earlier, those thoughts are antibiblical. Each mate should ask God's forgiveness for doubting His creation of roles in marriage. By faith, accept God's forgiveness and power, and live according to His Word.

In the future, share these truths with others to insure they are renewed in your own life. Only as you renew your mind with Scripture can the Holy Spirit protect you from ignorance and Satan's deceit. Thank God for your new understanding of love and submission. Encourage your mate with your new insight and commitment.

WISDOM:
HAVING GOD'S VIEWPOINT

By trusting God the Father, Jesus could view love and submission not as limitations but as the greatest blessings in all eternity. Christ both loved the church and submitted to His Father. Consider His perspective and the result of both roles from the following passage.

> *Therefore if there is any encouragement in Christ, if there is any consolation of love, if there is any fellowship of the Spirit, if any affection and compassion, make my joy complete by being of the same mind, maintaining the same love, united in spirit, intent on one purpose. Do nothing from selfishness or empty conceit, but with humility of mind regard one another as more important than yourselves; do not merely look out for your own personal interests, but also for the interests of others. Have this attitude in yourselves which was also in Christ Jesus, who, although He existed in the form of God, did not regard equality with God a thing to be grasped. . . . He humbled Himself by becoming obedient to the point of death, even death on a cross. For this reason also, God highly exalted Him (Philippians 2:1–6; 8–9).*

The apostle Paul said that if we desire to experience encouragement in

Christ, love, fellowship of the Spirit, compassion, or affection in this life, we must be one with others and with God. He described oneness as "being of the same mind, maintaining the same love, united in spirit, intent on one purpose." The goals that Paul mentioned describe desires that are common to all people. Oneness is God's goal for all relationships, be they in the Trinity, the church, or in marriage.

His commands to love or submit become not limits but the door to relationships and blessings.

The key to finding oneness, Paul wrote, is having humility of mind toward others. Obviously selfishness has no place here. Many people fear that being humble means being spineless. However, humility is not an emotional cowering, but a mark of one with a strong awareness of God's sovereignty in any given situation. This perspective allows both husbands and wives to esteem each other above themselves. Without a humble attitude, there is no encouragement, love, fellowship, affection, or compassion. With Christ's attitude, however, you can serve your mate freely, without being resentful or feeling limited. Jesus displayed the perfect example while washing His disciples' feet.

Having loved his own who were in the world, he now showed them the full extent of his love. He poured water into a basin and began to wash his disciples' feet, drying them with the towel that was wrapped around him. "Do you understand what I have done for you?" he asked them. "You call me 'Teacher' and 'Lord,' and rightly so, for that is what I am. Now that I, your Lord and Teacher, have washed your feet, you also should wash one another's feet. I have set you an example that you should do as I have done for you (John 13:1, 5, 12–15 NIV).

Remember, God created you to be incomplete without relationships. He created you to be unable to accomplish your creation purposes of reflecting His image, reproducing a godly heritage, or reigning on earth without relationships. God cannot meet your needs without love and submission. As you keep God's perspective of relationships before you, His commands to love or submit become not limits but the door to relationships and blessings. Therefore, with a humble attitude, you can actually esteem others higher than yourself, even in tough situations. You can serve others in love. That is how Jesus Christ Himself lived.

The call for us, as husbands, is to graciously love and serve our wives, thereby allowing them to become beautiful women of God.

The call for us, as wives, is to graciously esteem our husbands by giving them respect, thereby encouraging them to follow Christ.

Every great marriage has two people who are free from the struggle of questioning God's Word. They recognize that Satan will try to deceive them; thus neither will regard the other mate as the problem. Nor does either mate succumb to Satan's lies. Each knows that he has already been defeated at the Cross. The two mates are victorious over Satan's schemes, claiming the victory that Jesus already won, "having disarmed the powers and authorities, . . . triumphing over them by the cross" (Colossians 2:15 NIV). The result of a couple's faith and obedience will be oneness and blessing in their personal lives and in their marriage.

FIVE VITAL COMMITMENTS

As we conclude part 2 of *Two Becoming One,* consider the faith principles of chapters 4–9 that can allow you to experience a supernatural faith relationship in your marriage. Each of these insights requires faith on your part. As you read through the following list of marriage commitments, ask yourself these two questions: (1) Do I understand what God is saying? (2) Am I applying faith concerning this issue right now?

Each of the following commitments is vital to a faith marriage.

1. Couples need to commit themselves to God's purposes of reflecting, reproducing, and reigning.
2. Couples must accept each other from God as His personal provision for their needs.
3. Couples must release God's power in their marriage by daily submitting to the Holy Spirit.
4. Couples must understand that they can only change their mate through the active force of agape love or the reactive force of blessing.
5. Couples must seek God's wisdom concerning marital roles.

These five commitments form the core of a faith relationship. Nothing is more practical to married life than these. Review these commitments often.

The call for oneness reaches into all relationships, and was part of Jesus' prayer to the Father just before He died: "I do not ask on behalf of these alone, but for those also who believe in Me through their word; that they may all be one; even as You, Father, are in Me and I in You, that they also may be in Us, so that the world may believe that You sent Me" (John 17:20–21). God's plan to reach a lost world would depend on oneness. So marriage success requires oneness.

At this point you may be thinking, "These are great principles, but how do I apply them to the practical areas of marriage, such as communication, money, sex, and so on?" Let me say that these five major commitments are the basis or foundation for the practical areas. If you don't understand the faith concepts just covered, you will not be able to apply faith to the practical areas of marriage. Biblical faith is defined as follows. "Now faith is the assurance of things hoped for, the conviction of things not seen" (Hebrews 11:1).

Many times in marriage, your human instinct will override God's perspective. At those times, ideally, God will bring a Scripture verse to your mind, and faith will take over. Your marriage will then be characterized as one that acts supernaturally, based on the facts of God's Word, not on human ingenuity.

Now we can move on to part 3 and the everyday issues that occur in marriage such as male and female differences, communication, romance, finances, trials, and in-laws. As we keep God's perspective of the principles just covered, the daily areas developed in the next section will fall into place.

part three

APPLYING BIBLICAL PRINCIPLES TO YOUR MARRIAGE

A Man of Commitment

▣ WHAT IS THE MARK OF A GREAT HUSBAND? IS IT financial responsibility, social prominence, strength and vigor, or being a successful father? As important as these areas are, there is a much greater issue. The mark of a great husband is an absolute, unfailing commitment to his wife. A husband cannot bless his wife more than by loving her as a gift from God. Husbands who faithfully ask God for marital direction are rare indeed. As men, we often fail to recognize marriage as a covenant with our mate and with God.

THE MARRIAGE COVENANT

When a man marries, he makes a commitment, or covenant, with God and his wife to (1) oversee his family in order that they might reflect the image of God properly, (2) raise his children to love and follow the Lord, and (3) provide leadership in reigning over what God gives him. As God's man, the husband is to be responsible to God for his wife and family.

Our Lord Jesus talked plainly about a man's marriage covenant:

"So they are no longer two, but one flesh. What therefore God has joined together, let no man separate" (Matthew 19:6). I feel deep fear in my heart when I think of men, especially Christian men, who break this covenant. Divorce is not God's will. It's always a poor solution with tremendous negative ramifications. Below is a vivid description of how God feels about a husband's breaking that marriage vow through divorce.

The Lord has been a witness between you and the wife of your youth, against whom you have dealt treacherously, though she is your companion and your wife by covenant. But not one has done so who has a remnant of the Spirit. And what did that one do while he was seeking a godly offspring? Take heed then to your spirit, and let no one deal treacherously against the wife of your youth. "For I hate divorce," says the Lord, the God of Israel, "and him who covers his garment with wrong," says the Lord of hosts. "So take heed to your spirit, that you do not deal treacherously" (Malachi 2:14–16).

God Himself is a witness and a participant in the covenant a husband makes with his wife. No man can break that covenant and be led by the Spirit of God. God not only hates divorce, but He will judge the one who does the wrong in the divorce. God considers a man's responsibility toward his wife as a covenant with Him. He gave marriage to man as a blessing; therefore, the husband is responsible to be faithful to that covenant, no matter what the cost. It is much more difficult to raise up godly offspring when there has been a divorce. God not only hates divorce because oneness is destroyed, but because children are irreversibly affected. Oneness is broken in divorce, resulting in great pain to both the couple and the children.

God takes His covenants seriously, and marriage is a covenant. If you want to be characterized as a great husband, put away any thoughts about divorce or finding a better mate. Place your faith in God and commit yourself to sacrificial love that will, over time, soften even the hardest heart.

IF YOU HAVE TO "TOUGH IT OUT"

James offered several instructions about responding to tough trials in James 1:2–7. Later he described godly responses to disagreements.

This you know, my beloved brethren. But everyone must be quick to hear, slow to speak and slow to anger; for the anger of man does not achieve the righteousness of God. Therefore, putting aside all filthiness and all that remains of wickedness, in humility receive the word implanted, which is able to save your souls. But prove yourselves doers of the word, and not merely hearers who delude themselves (James 1:19–22).

Based on James's advice, here is a helpful list to remember during trying times in marriage. If there is a battle in your marriage, take note of the following:

1. Don't react, but listen to your wife.
2. Don't speak too quickly; wait for your emotions to subside.

3. Don't explode in anger; nothing good ever comes from outbursts of anger.
4. Stop your immoral involvement such as lying, cheating, bad language, pornography, and so on.
5. Seek counsel if any of the above points (1–4) have become negative behavior or habits.
6. Humbly study God's Word for the answers to your problems, seeking counsel when necessary.
7. Act on your faith, not on your feelings.
8. Boldly believe God, regardless of your wife's response. This may include renewing your covenant with your mate.

James 5:16 contains two final points of instruction: "Confess your sins to one another, and pray for one another." Thus, here are items nine and ten:

9. Confess your sins to your wife so both of you can be emotionally healed.
10. Pray earnestly. God has the ability and desire to change your life, motivate your wife, and remove your fears.

The sovereignty of God can motivate us as husbands. Just think: God is a partner with you in your marriage! That should inspire you to serve and please Him. Be aware that your marriage is part of God's eternal plan. You have entered into a marriage covenant, or agreement, and God is a partner with you.

RULE AND SERVE

As I search Scripture to discover God's will for husbands, here are two of the most salient duties: Husbands are to rule and serve.

In the Old Testament, God said, "[The man] shall rule over [the woman]" (Genesis 3:16). In the New Testament, God compared a husband's responsibility to his wife to that of Christ's responsibility to the church (Ephesians 5:25). These truths indicate two major principles in the practice of the husband's covenant to his wife. First, he is to rule. You are a benevolent ruler, not a dictator. Men are to take authority with the humility of a servant. Rather than demanding respect from your wife, you can only earn it. Demanding destroys a wife emotionally, and may eventually destroy the marriage. *Ruling means taking authority with a gracious, loving spirit* toward your wife and children. The goal is the second truth of the covenant: to serve them and encourage them to be all that God wants them to be.

Indeed, the husband moves beyond ruler to be a priest to his wife. The word *priest* means *minister,* emphasizing the role of servant and counselor. You are to be so aware of her needs that you go out of the way to meet them. Most men do not know the needs of their wives without asking them. Don't assume you know until she tells you. Communication is the most important aspect of serving. Serve her, be her loving administrator, and take authority for her life and needs in a way that supports and encourages her.

There must be a careful balance in both of these responsibilities to rule and to be a priest/servant. If the husband overemphasizes his authority, his wife will lose respect and trust. If the husband is only a servant, she will be insecure and lack direction. In searching both Scripture and common sense for what it means to rule (lead) and to be a servant in marriage, we have noticed several specific areas of responsibility for a man. As the husband, he should:

- Protect
- Provide
- Initiate love
- Pray
- Emphasize future hope
- Take authority in conflict
- Meet physical needs
- Support relationship development
- Share time struggles
- Help with children's discipline and instruction
- Communicate, communicate, communicate!

Three major commands are given in the New Testament to husbands describing how to fulfill the responsibilities listed above.

1. Understand Your Wife

Husbands ought to understand, or "know," their wives, wrote the apostle Peter: "You husbands in the same way, live with your wives in an understanding way, as with someone weaker, since she is a woman; and show her honor as a fellow heir of the grace of life, so that your prayers will not be hindered" (1 Peter 3:7). Peter is commanding you to be an expert about your wife.

In order to understand her, you must make it a point to ask your wife about her emotional, spiritual, physical, and intellectual needs. Seek your wife's opinion regularly. Knowing her is not an automatic thing. If you don't work at hearing her, you won't know when she is under stress, when she just needs some physical exercise, when she needs a day off, or a night out with you. To understand her also means to honor her, to lift her up, to treat her with utmost respect. The word "weaker vessel" means "fine china." Treat her like fine china, not everyday pottery. She is of great value to you.

Do you know what a perfect day is for your wife? A perfect date? What she really likes to do on vacations? If not, find out. Do you have good communication with her on a daily basis? Peter commanded a husband to know his wife, living with her "in an understanding way"; otherwise sin and struggle will prevail, and a man's prayers will not be answered. How can you be out of fellowship with your wife and expect God to answer when you pray?

How can you be out of fellowship with your wife and expect God to answer when you pray?

"Fellow heirs" means that all of life and all God's blessings are to be shared by the two of you. Decisions you make—raising the children, moving, changing jobs, church, trials, joys and frustrations, and many others—all are to be shared. *Never* make decisions concerning any of these things without complete communication and agreement with your wife.

2. Be Responsible to Your Wife

You must know your wife so completely that you can uniquely apply your responsibilities to fit her specific needs. The Scripture commands that husbands love their wives "just as Christ also loved the church and gave Himself up for her" (Ephesians 5:25). God's command to love includes the idea of giving up your life for her in the same way Christ gave Himself up for the church.

Although husbands do not expect God will require them literally to die, they should be willing. God expects us men to get involved in all issues that cause our wives to fear, physically or emotionally. Physical protection, financial protection, emotional protection, fear of failure, fear of aging, and meeting the spiritual and physical needs of children are good examples of issues where a husband might sacrifice for his wife. The husband shields her from the fear of facing issues alone that may cause her fear or frustration. So as you prepare to meet your wife's needs, first know her and sacrificially take responsibility for her fears and desires.

3. Love Your Wife as You Love Yourself

Paul commanded husbands "to love their own wives as their own bodies" by nourishing and cherishing them (Ephesians 5:28–29). These words connote comfort. Paul is saying to attend sensitively and selflessly to your wife's needs like a mother would a nursing child. Keep her warm by monitoring her intimate emotional and physical needs, just as you care daily for your own needs.

God commands you, in your covenant with Him, to give up your own selfishness by putting her first in priority after Him.

STRATEGIES FOR APPLYING THE COVENANT

Develop a strategy for your wife and family. After you determine the areas of importance in light of your wife's needs, then establish several objectives in each area. Develop a plan for each objective, set priorities, and then schedule their application. A little planning will improve your success significantly.

The following are some ideas from our marriage counseling. Let the Holy Spirit show you which of the following you need to apply to your wife and family.

Leadership

A good husband thrives on being a "shock absorber" for his wife by anticipating his wife's needs and fears. Here are three practical ways to provide leadership for your wife.

First, encourage self-worth. The factors that affect feelings of self-worth are usually obvious: intellect, appearance, productivity, success in relationships, and financial freedom, among others. Discover mutual areas of interest with your wife and work at communication in that area.

Some of the best ways to encourage your wife include seeking out her intellectual interests and finding one where she can teach you. Show interest in her appearance, and support her desire to have a sufficient wardrobe for career and social events. Become an expert on her abilities. If she has a hobby, encourage her. If she does something well in private, sensitively make her friends aware of those skills or qualities. Look for ways to involve her talents publicly. If she is a mother, help her develop in-home income, if she desires it. Assist with household chores and especially be involved in raising your children. Monitor her relationships and assist her in developing friends. Help her organize her schedule. Steps like these help to build her self-worth.

Second, provide comfort. Never allow your wife to experience pain without sharing it with her. A death in the family, a difficult child, frustration in her career, or a disappointment in relationships may require your help. Comfort her and take responsibility for helping her find a solution.

Third, facilitate spiritual maturity. Your hope for mutual faith in your marriage is related to your wife's maturity as well as yours. Do everything possible to assist her spiritual interest. Encourage her efforts to minister to others or attend church functions. As a couple, plan to be involved in leading small groups or teaching Sunday school. Plan activities with your children to free your wife. One of her greatest joys, however, will be watching you take spiritual leadership in your home and church. Many wives have expressed their joy in seeing their husbands excel spiritually.

Financial Security

Work at giving your wife financial hope for the future. A personal savings account for her is important if possible. Special needs like lingerie, hair styling, exercise classes, and hobbies are not all that expensive, and they mean a lot to her. Take family finances seriously. Study chapter 14, apply it to your own situation, and make a personal commitment to adjust according to God's will.

The Scripture strongly advocates that a husband provide for the welfare of his wife. "But if anyone does not provide for his own, and especially for those of his household, he has denied the faith and is worse than an unbeliever" (1 Timothy 5:8).

Romance

Romance in marriage is a man's shared responsibility; romantic moments are extremely important to a woman. Be a romantic lover to your mate. Women love small, inexpensive surprises, small jewelry, flowers purchased from a street vendor—and not just on birthdays or holidays. Unique gifts are great, too. An occasional love letter or card catches her off guard. Quantity is not so important as quality and consistency. (Chapter 13 will provide specific ideas for cultivating romance.)

Romance includes kindling and maintaining sexual interest. And the Scriptures tell a husband to enjoy sexual passion with his wife, and with her alone. "Let your fountain be blessed, and rejoice in the wife of your youth. As a loving hind and a graceful doe, let her breasts satisfy you at all times; be exhilarated always with her love" (Proverbs 5:18–19). Delighting yourself in your wife's physical charms will not only make her feel cherished but will focus your attention on her, where it should be.

Communication

Your wife must communicate with you to maintain her confidence and emotional stability. She cannot respond adequately without a total relationship. Romance will die without communication. If your wife says that you do not communicate with her enough, seek counsel to help define and correct the problem.

Men and women tend to define communication differently. If a man doesn't look at his wife and listen as she talks (sometimes up to thirty minutes) before giving his opinion, then she feels they have not communicated. Women *need* to talk to solve a problem. Men tend to want the bottom line with fewer words expressed. Men tend to think *before* they talk, and women think *as* they talk. Learn this well.

Husbands, never give your wives the silent treatment. Love requires regular communication. Instead of withholding yourself, open your life to her.

Give her words of encouragement. Don't withhold positive words that have the power to heal.

Communication includes talking about feelings of anger. Remember, anger is a common human emotion; you should recognize and deal with it quickly. "Do not let the sun go down on your anger," Paul warned (Ephesians 4:26). Why? Because God knows that when you accumulate anger, it keeps you from putting the past behind you. Only forgiveness heals the past while renewing your hope for the future.

Men tend to think before they talk, and women think as they talk.

Be very careful about accumulating unresolved conflict in your marriage. "Do not let any unwholesome talk come out of your mouths, but only what is helpful for building others up according to their needs, that it may benefit those who listen. . . . Be kind and compassionate to one another, forgiving each other, just as in Christ God forgave you" (Ephesians 4:29, 32 NIV).

Hurtful words tend to stay around a long time. Sometimes, after little verbal shots you take at your mate, you may spend a lot of time trying to undo them. Be quick to ask for forgiveness when hurtful things are said. Remember, "It is to a man's honor to avoid strife, but every fool is quick to quarrel" (Proverbs. 20:3 NIV).

Make daily communication with your spouse a priority. Ask her often how you are doing in this important area of marriage and be prepared to work a lifetime improving on this skill. Don't ever take for granted that you are communicating enough. Learn to communicate according to her definition.

Prayer

Pray for your wife daily. Ask God to give you love for her and to help you be sensitive to her needs. It's also important to pray for your children on a daily basis. Ask your wife and children how to pray for them. As the years pass, the children will come to you or call you with their prayer requests, even when they leave home.

Open prayer, perhaps more than any other thing, demonstrates your care for them and ultimately shows them God's love.

Authority During Decision Making

Decisions and conflicts constantly develop in the home. Men are to assume authority during such conflicts. Instead of being passive, they are to take responsibility and become involved in the decision making.

If the right decision is not obvious between you and your spouse, take responsibility to insure that the decision is made. If there is conflict between your children, help them resolve it. Husbands and wives need to set examples for their children in conflict resolution. A passive, uninvolved father is especially frustrating to children.

Time Management and Physical Activity

Time management is a major problem for most wives. A husband is in the best position to assist his wife in working out her schedule and priorities. Begin by working out a priority list with your wife. General categories that need to be considered are personal time with the Lord, marriage relationship, relationships with children, career, friendships, church ministry, recreation, and work.

Set a brief planning meeting, perhaps fifteen minutes each Sunday night, to agree on a week's schedule. Help her eliminate activities that leave her over-committed. After understanding her schedule, help her diversify activities. Arrange for her to be out of the home regularly if you have small children. When possible, commit to staying home to give her that freedom. Taking care of your children when your wife is away is not baby-sitting. It is your responsibility as a joint heir in the grace of life.

A balanced schedule includes specific time together alone, even if you have children. A date once a week will do wonders for both of you and will strengthen your communication. Take charge on Friday night and let her sleep in on Saturday morning. If she has preschoolers, relieve her from the five o'clock horror show at dinner and the bedtime scene by taking over with one or both duties. If your wife works outside the home, make sure that you share the chores and the responsibilities of the home with her. *Ask* her what needs to be done.

With your wife's and your busy schedules, take an active interest in your wife's and your health. Exercise together if possible, and make sure you both have physical checkups. Convince your wife that her body is attractive. Do not let her set unrealistic weight goals. A husband's sensitivity, coupled with realistic weight goals, will result in your wife's satisfaction with her body. Allow her to share her concerns about your physical situation, also. Don't reject her input.

Taking walks together frequently can also help your communication. If possible, discover a mutually enjoyable sport such as tennis, golf, fishing, bicycling, or running.

The Family's Identity and Hope

Help your wife and children understand that they are part of a uniquely developed family by God's choice. Develop this identity with activities that promote family togetherness, such as vacations, sports, church activities, youth activities, or family camps. If you promote family times as the children grow up, they will return for family outings even as adults. Make it a priority.

As part of securing your family's identity, always communicate your future vision and plans with your wife. Get her full input. Nothing affects a woman more than low expectations for your future, and that of your children. Don't expect your wife to understand your future vision without explaining it to her and making sure she comprehends it. If you plan to make a career change, she should not be the last one to find out about it.

Mutual Interests

Too many couples lose their desire to be together because they no longer have mutual interests. If you try, you can develop some mutual interests. Travel is a great possibility. Fun, sports, hobbies, and intellectual stimulation are all vital to a growing relationship.

Aging

Without spiritual interest, productivity, relationships, and responsibilities, people really suffer as they age. Protect yourselves from slow depression; develop spiritual interests and activities that can continue until death. If you do find depression developing, seek godly advice or medical help.

Typically, our wives will begin to dream about their future goals during their forties. The empty nest is right around the corner, and your wife will want to know that the rest of her life will be productive. Her early dreams are usually wrapped up in marriage and raising children. But, along about early midlife, she begins to ask questions about what she wants to accomplish as she ages. Help your wife fulfill her dreams. Many women begin second careers at this point.

When grandchildren appear, husbands should allow those youngsters to become part of their lives, even if the grandchildren seem to scramble your schedule and exhaust you. They can help you stay active and make you feel important.

Continue to work as long as possible before retiring and then use your talents part time. Earlier sacrifices of making time for ministry will pay off in your later years. As your work-related activities decrease, your service to the Lord and His people can continually increase. Most of all, maintain your commitment to your wife intellectually, emotionally, spiritually, and sexually.

CHILD REARING

For those couples who have children, a key strategy involves rearing children. By sharing the pressure of raising the children, husbands protect and honor their wives in a very practical way. The children's educational and emotional needs as well as their physical and spiritual development are vital to a mother's feeling of well-being. Husbands should seek to understand those concerns as they occur and to shoulder them with their wives.

Children long for an intimate relationship with their fathers. When that occurs, fathers will have deep, lasting respect from them and the children's mothers. Husbands, take first responsibility for the children in two areas: discipline and instruction. As Paul urged us, "Fathers, do not provoke your children to anger; but bring them up in the discipline and instruction of the Lord" (Ephesians 6:4).

Discipline

Discipline affects a child's character development. Stay involved in discipline and do not leave it primarily to your wife. Watch for power struggles between your wife and your children. Monitor your wife's emotional weariness. When it rises, check her struggle with the children. Take responsibility for special problems like tantrums or hyperactivity. Personally take care of discipline problems at school. Stay ahead by anticipating problems instead of always having to respond. Establish a relationship with each individual child and take each out alone at least once a month for an activity (or just to a restaurant) to build that relationship.

We believe spanking should be done only in the early years, and it will not be needed often if used correctly. Always explain why you are spanking, and love them tenderly afterward. As the child grows, there should be more talking and less spanking. James Dobson has written several books on the parent-child relationship that Sally and I recommend, including *Dare to Discipline* and *The Strong-Willed Child*. We also recommend *How to Really Love Your Child* and *How to Really Love Your Teenager*, both by Ross Campbell.

Instruction

Husbands, you are ultimately responsible for the spiritual development of your children. Biblical mandates are given to teach children and instruct them in the Lord, including the following key passage:

> *These commandments that I give you today are to be upon your hearts. Impress them on your children. Talk about them when you sit at home and when you walk along the road, when you lie down and when you get up* (Deuteronomy 6:6–7).

Spending even an hour a week putting your children to bed is a good start. Spending personal time with them on the weekends is invaluable. Communicate with your child to find out where he or she is spiritually. Help your children solve problems. As a father, take the lead in establishing rules concerning dating and behavior with the opposite sex. Work with your wife, but keep the responsibility on your shoulders.

When possible, involve your children in establishing the rules. Make sure to set the rules before a problem develops. Anticipation is everything in child rearing. For example, don't wait until your children are fifteen to tell them they cannot date until sixteen. That's too late. Stay ahead of the game. You need to tell them at age eleven or twelve, before the need arises. They won't question the rule at that age, and will have plenty of time to tell their friends and to think about it. Establish good communication early in their lives, and it will continue, even after they leave home.

A VISION FOR YOUR MARRIAGE

"Where there is no vision, the people perish" (Proverbs 29:18 KJV). Unfortunately, most men don't have much vision for their lives. Yet, a man who seeks the Lord for life will experience fullness and joy. He and his wife will be spiritually uplifted. Consider these areas of planning for your marriage. Doing so will give direction and hope for your family.

Spiritual Responsibility

In counseling with men, I (Don) have seen tremendous need in their lives for authority and respect. I believe that for growth in Christ, men need to be dealing with spiritual issues as part of their duties. There is tremendous joy for men in church leadership, especially in a church that regards elders 'or other lay leaders' roles as a real ministry. In fact, Paul called such ministry "a fine work" (1 Timothy 3:1). If your church does not encourage personal ministry, volunteer to begin a lay program to develop spiritual responsibility. Lead a men's group, or as a couple, lead a marriage class. Become an elder or deacon if asked. God desires that you find His perspective on life, and spiritual leadership is vital to doing so. No matter what your gifts or abilities, seek counsel on a plan that helps you develop spiritual responsibilities in the home, in your church, or in Christian organizations.

Are you being mentored by someone, and are you in the process of mentoring another man? Remember the call: "The things which you have heard from me in the presence of many witnesses, entrust these to faithful men who will be able to teach others also" (2 Timothy 2:2). Remember the axiom, "We only keep what we give away."

Accountability

As much as men like to be self-confident and independent, they have deep needs for counsel from others. Such counsel may include one or more people to whom a man is accountable and consults regularly. Men have a strong need in their lives for protection from wrong decisions, for wisdom in their marriage and in child rearing, and for encouragement in their jobs.

Several times in my life, I have had to make a significant decision that was difficult for me and somewhat threatening for my family. Finding myself suddenly under considerable emotional and professional pressure, and knowing I needed to provide firm, directional family leadership, I quickly realized I could become vulnerable to Satan's inevitable attack.

To protect myself and my family, Sally and I have always had an advisory group surrounding us to give wise counsel. We usually describe our situation to them and give a historical evaluation of Sally and myself. These men and women stand with us and always give honest feedback. More importantly, they rally to our support by helping us develop an aggressive plan for the future. I usually am totally remotivated, my wife trusts and respects my openness, and I have deepened my relationship with these people. The body of Christ demands our accountability to mature believers. God says, "Without consultation, plans are frustrated, but with many counselors they succeed" (Proverbs 15:22).

The most natural place for a man to find mentors or wise counselors should be his local church. Begin to observe older couples and church leaders. Gather information concerning each leader's expertise and areas of wisdom; then cross-check your observations with the pastoral staff. After confirming your observations, decide which leader best fits your needs and seems most approachable. Ask him for a brief appointment. Most older people love to share their life experiences. If your wife and you seek joint counsel or mentoring, approach a couple. If you pray, God will lead you to the right person or couple.

In addition to looking in your church, you may find God's choice at work, in the neighborhood, or in a Bible study group. Bigger decisions many times require several counselors for better perspective and for confirmation.

Work

In Genesis 3, God instructed Adam to toil and sweat. Many men never face this fact of life. Instead, they devise all kinds of ways to get out of work like changing jobs, get-rich-quick schemes, and looking for greener grass. The times when I was unsure of my vocation were among the most frustrating and depressing periods of my life. These were also times that drove me to my knees before God.

Statistics have shown that most men change jobs several times before they discover what they really enjoy doing. About 10 percent of the male population change jobs easily, while an even larger percent tend to stay in their present job whether or not they like it. Most research indicates that the men who usually succeed in the long run are those who demonstrate perseverance in their chosen field. If you feel frustrated and inconsistent in your working experience, seek counsel. Make yourself accountable to a wiser older brother. Develop a plan to gradually refocus your job. Pursue what you enjoy and do well.

Several organizations offer helpful career assessments and feedback on finding careers where you can best use your strengths. One of them is the Life Pathways division of Crown Financial Ministries. Their "Career Direct" assessment reveals strengths in the areas of personality, skills, vocational interests, and values. For more information, call Crown Financial Ministries at 1-800-722-1976.

A Woman of Wisdom

PROVERBS ENDS WITH VERSES EXALTING THE NOBLE wife. So honored is this woman that "her children rise up and bless her; her husband also, and he praises her, saying: 'Many daughters have done nobly, but you excel them all'" (31:28–29). Deep in her heart, every woman likes to be characterized as excellent. Hearing a husband say, "You excel them all" brings joy to any wife. If you are a wife, do you consider yourself a gift from the Lord to your husband? Would you be identified as a wise woman who is skillful at living?

"The wise woman builds her house," wrote Solomon, "but the foolish tears it down with her own hands" (Proverbs 14:1). Let's consider how wives can keep their homes and marriages strong. This chapter is for wives, to help them solidify some foundational issues and to increase in wisdom. I (Sally) hope the principles of Scripture contained here both comfort and challenge your life as a wife and daughter of God.

Over the years, Don and I have counseled and worked with many wives. We've experienced joy as their faith matured, but also cried as others missed God's perspective. Out of respect for those women and the Lord, we present the following insights.

Every woman must be able to answer four foundational questions before she can be released to enjoy life in the home:

1. Am I limited by my role as a wife?
2. What are the limits to submission?
3. Is the home my key to success as a wife?
4. How can I understand and help my husband?

If you get clear direction on these four issues, you'll have vision and wisdom in your marriage. As you read, ask God to reveal His perspective of how a woman can be fulfilled in marriage.

DOES MY ROLE AS WIFE LIMIT ME?

In the past few decades, our society has encouraged women to question and even doubt their need to have specific roles in marriage. Certainly society has challenged the scriptural calling for women. We believe, however, that the biblical role has been misunderstood: Men have seen it one way, and women the other. Considering the world's criticisms, women must have faith in God's Word and the God of the Word if they hope to maintain God's perspective. This battle must be taken seriously and approached aggressively. These truths, taken from the Word of God, are vital to experiencing God's best in marriage.

Wives, God did not stack the cards against you. On the contrary, God places special significance on a woman who is a wife or mother. As bad as society can be, without the woman' maintaining order, demonstrating love within the home, and acknowledging God's rightful place in the home, I'm not sure society would be as peaceful as it is. The issues may be tough and sometimes confusing, but God's Word remains our sure foundation.

Women are equal to men in every respect. . . . The issue is . . . determining how God intended most women to find expression.

Many women today, including Christian women, are asking, "Why must I be under a man's leadership? I deserve to be equal with a man. I am not less qualified, motivated, or capable. Yes, God, I do question your role for me."

Are women equal? Oh, yes, women are equal to men in every respect, with the single exception of physical strength. While women function differently in some ways, they too need equal expression of intellect, emotions, and physical attributes. Women should have equal opportunities publicly, as well as privately. God did not intend for women to lack expression in any way. The issue is not one of equality, but determining how God intended most women to find expression.

God's plan has never been for men and women to become more alike. God does not want the genders to become more competitive and rights oriented. Our hope lies in stepping out in faith to find fulfillment where God places us. His placement may vary with different stages of life.

I'm not talking about men and women in the workplace and marketplace. Women are not commanded to be under any man's leadership. She is perfectly capable to be in leadership in the workplace or in government. There are a few examples of these positions in the Bible. (Consider Deborah and Esther, for instance.) Rather, our focus, of course, is the *marriage relationship.*

In marriage, God has placed the man in the position of servant-leader, not because he is better or more qualified, but because people work better when they have structure. God knew that this was the very best structure to cause husbands and wives to function with as little discord as possible. He also knew it was the best method for raising children. In no way is God limiting either the man or the woman. Rather, He is giving them a method of fulfillment and oneness.

Women, can you trust God, knowing fully who He is? Is His plan for your life best, regardless of any momentary suffering? Admittedly, submission (or learning respect) is contrary to your human nature, and it is impossible to endure without faith. You cannot stand still in your understanding. You are either gaining or losing ground constantly.

In 1 Peter 1:12–21, Peter exhorted Christians to holiness and growth. In verse 12 he basically said, "Won't you realize that you are not serving yourselves, but God?" God's Holy Spirit gives these precious biblical promises to you. They are so great that they intrigue even angels! Remember, *submission* means to respect your husband enough to allow him leadership in your home. It is not just a trial or something you suffer. As you grow in your understanding of it through God's Word, it becomes a real blessing. You will never be more loved, appreciated, and cherished. Your needs will never be more fulfilled. You see, these are the precious promises of God Himself. Women long to be loved the way God says a husband should love.

The most important issue, then, is to become creative, not critical, in drawing out the best aspects of each one's personality.

Peter continued, "Therefore, prepare your minds for action, keep sober in spirit, fix your hope completely on the grace to be brought to you at the revelation of Jesus Christ" (verse 13). Your struggle is one of the mind. Don't allow Satan to deceive you into thinking you have a better plan than God. Decide that God can sufficiently carry you through tough situations. Often we have to put away our self-centered rights. Peter later noted that we should not trade our hope in God for a hope in temporary or perishable things, like silver and gold (verse 18). Similarly, your hope must be placed in the proper person— the perfect Lord Jesus Christ—rather than your husband.

You will occasionally suffer in your role as a wife, but Jesus called us to follow Him, and He was perfectly submitted to His Father. Was Jesus limited in the long run by His submission? No, and neither will you be as a wife.

WHAT ARE THE LIMITS TO SUBMISSION?

The question of limits is a valid one. Scripture clearly communicates that submission by men and women alike will be tested by suffering. We can accept such suffering when it comes from doing good, but not from evil (see 2 Peter 3:17). God's Word absolutely assures the greatest blessing to the one who submits, yet no one can use submission as an excuse for sinning. God will not absolve you from responsibility for sin just because someone told you to do it and you submitted to the sinful request.

On the other hand, a wise woman will use such a request as an opportunity to be creative in understanding her husband's real need. You must ask yourself, "What is the need in my husband's life behind the request he is making?" Next, try to meet that need without contradicting Scripture.

An example of submitting to the point of sin is Sapphira's response to her husband, recorded in Acts 5. Sapphira agreed to sin with Ananias, and, as a result, God took both of their lives. If your husband has asked you to do something you think is sin, seek counsel before you respond. A good advisor will give perspective and options that can honor your husband, yet not directly follow a request that violates Scripture. For most, the request will never go that far. As your husband sees your respectful attitude toward him, he will more than likely be more concerned with how you think and feel.

Submission is not simply keeping quiet. . . . That's lack of communication.

Another limit of submission in your role as a wife is not to submit to any physical or emotional abuse. God never intended that a husband be cruel to his wife. On the contrary, a husband is to love and serve her. If there is either physical or emotional abuse (consistently putting you down, calling you names, and so on), then counsel should be sought quickly. Many good counselors are available to deal with this devastating issue.

A word about what submission is *not* is in order. Submission is not simply keeping quiet and doing whatever your husband says. That's lack of communication. Throughout Scripture, God states that He is more interested in your heart than your actions. Let's talk about your attitudes in communication.

In an effort to help your understanding of this important area, begin by looking at the biblical command for your communication with Him:

> *Be anxious for nothing, but in everything by prayer and supplication with thanksgiving let your requests be made known to God. And the peace of God, which surpasses all comprehension, will guard your hearts and your minds in Christ Jesus (Philippians 4:6–7).*

God desires for you to express to Him not only your needs, but your very wants. He doesn't promise to give you your wants, although many times in His grace, He does. He does promise peace beyond your understanding. The key thought is that He wants you to tell Him your wants, to talk to Him. What is prayer but simply talking to God? Now if God wants you to talk with Him, would He ask that wives not talk to their husbands? Absolutely not! That would be a contradiction of Scripture.

What God is saying in this passage is, "Women, if your husband has an attitude of being disobedient to God's Word, then do not provoke him further by nagging or hitting him with Bible verses again and again." Instead, inwardly make a faith decision to trust God at that moment, so you can outwardly win your husband with your positive actions. You must place your hope in God, not your husband, and allow him to be wrong—even fail—so that the Lord can convict him. You simply love and encourage him by how you treat him. "Let your speech always be with grace, as though seasoned with salt, so that you will know how you should respond to each person" (Colossians 4:6).

Your hope should never be in your husband's ability . . . to change, but in the Lord, who does the changing.

Once you have told your husband you think he is wrong in some way, don't continue to harp on that issue. Turn it over to God and let Him deal with it. A wife should be able to express her opinions freely and lovingly; in fact, her husband will want her to do so.

However, your hope should never be in your husband's ability or willingness to change, but in the Lord, who does the changing. You want him to know how you feel about the matter. But you must assure him that you love him, no matter what, and that you will support him in prayer. Then wait for God to work in his life.

The balance to this freedom to communicate feelings is the strong warning God gives about the poison of our mouths. In Romans 3, Paul wrote that the mouth is "an open grave" (verse 13) capable of unbelievable destruction. James taught that we should be slow to anger and slow to speak, or we will lose God's blessing (James 1:19–20). A good thermometer of a respectful wife is how she uses her mouth. Proverbs 15 declares, "A gentle answer turns away wrath. . . . How delightful is a timely word!" (verses 1, 23).

If a woman has God's perspective, she will do the following:

1. Wait for the proper time to tell her husband her negative thoughts.
2. Talk to the Lord about it in the meantime.
3. Speak peaceably when the time comes—without anger, bitterness, resentment, or belittling.

4. Trust the Lord for the outcome even when no change is seen. When it comes to communication, remember that men and women are different. We never come at the same problem the same way. Both perspectives are needed to solve problems.

IS THE HOME THE KEY
TO MY SUCCESS AS A WIFE?

With all the negative publicity homemakers have been getting in recent years, along with the glamour attributed to the working woman, it's no surprise that wives question their vocation in the home. I constantly run into young wives who plan to have children at a late age or don't intend to have children at all.

While it is OK for women to have careers, it is best for mothers to stay at home with children once they arrive.

They say they cannot fully express themselves in the home. More and more wives are attributing their struggles in life to being captive to the house and the children. Again, the question must be asked, "Did God make a mistake by placing wives and mothers in the home?"

Because of the importance and diligence necessary in a homemaker's responsibilities, we must emphasize the value of the home. Close on the heels of Satan's deceit concerning submission is his deceit concerning the value of the home. With the help of our culture, Satan has convinced women that their existence in the home is a barrier to fulfillment. Once a woman's eyes focus on herself instead of God, she begins a lonely uphill battle. The many struggles of the home quickly wear her down and defeat her spirit of hope, resulting in fear—the enemy of faith.

Note the consistent pattern of Satan. He first catches a woman in a struggle (and a homemaker has plenty of them). At that point of conflict, the woman's consciousness of God's presence is low. Being deceived, she does not directly doubt God; instead, she places the blame on her husband or the home situation. The moment a woman sees a person or responsibility in the home as the problem, her commitment is broken. She then begins to subconsciously resent and rebel against the one she blames: her husband (but ultimately the Lord). Once she has begun to resent or rebel, her whole relationship with God and her family is affected.

Yes, the home is the key to a wife's success. While it is OK for women to have careers, it is best for mothers to stay at home with children once they arrive. Children are given to us by God to raise and nurture for only eighteen years. This is a very short but important time in our lives and theirs. During the formative years, it is vital that Mom remains in the home for many reasons: security, faith training, time spent with children, early education, love, and physical attention. There usually are some creative alternatives to working full time: working three days a week, getting home by three o'clock, computer work in the home, and so on.

Years ago the feminist movement rose to power by exhibiting proof of the plight of the average woman. I agree with the movement on issues of equal pay for equal work, but I disagree on two major issues: the cause of the homemaker's problems and the solutions offered. In essence, these women were saying that it is a mistake to have defined roles, either in or out of the home. While our country has rightly tried to give freedom of expression to women in the workplace, leaders have done a poor job of communicating the importance of being a wife and a mother. I am not downplaying the fact that many women work outside the home, some because of desire, others because of economic necessity, and still others without children at home. But far too often women mistakenly believe they cannot be fulfilled without working outside the home. Nothing could be farther from the truth.

Putting work outside the home on hold . . . will require an adjustment in the family finances, since there will only be one paycheck.

Many women make the mistake of thinking that they are no longer needed in the home when the child enters school and therefore reenter the workplace. Children still need Mom at home at every age. It is particularly important for mothers to stay at home during the teen years. Many temptations occur naturally for teens when Mom is not at home: sex, crime, pornography, and drugs. Add to this the fact that most other moms in the neighborhood work. Therefore, you may be one of the few moms to whom kids will come and talk after school. This certainly was true for all four of our children in their teen years. I was there to answer questions for them and for their friends. We opened our home for ministries such as Young Life and Fellowship of Christian Athletes, and kids were welcome in our home, day or night. The challenge as parents is to influence your children and their friends with religious and moral values.

This may mean putting work outside the home on hold. In *Women Leaving the Workplace*, author Larry Burkett points out that this will require an adjustment in the family finances, since there will only be one paycheck. The benefit will be having more time to make the home a genuine haven for the family. When your children leave home for college, you'll then be free to pursue a career, more education, a ministry to other women, or even to travel with your husband. You'll feel good about the time you spent with your children, and will not wish you could do it over.

The wise woman will search for God's perspective and His personal will for her life, using Scripture as the primary standard. This in no way limits her in the home or in the workplace. It is a matter of God's calling and timing in her life.

A GODLY PERSPECTIVE

Proverbs 31 describes a godly woman who is creative in and out of her home. Since no woman could ever accomplish all that she did, I believe this example is written for women of all eras to show the unlimited possibilities of a godly woman. Her mind held different values than we see the world teaching us today. Her mental freedom allowed her creativity to flow.

Listen to God's description of this woman's life, mentioned in the final two verses of Proverbs: "Charm is deceitful and beauty is vain, but a woman who fears the Lord, she shall be praised. Give her the product of her hands, and let her works praise her in the gates" (Proverbs 31:30–31).

The word *charm* describes a superficial graciousness, and the word used for *beauty* means "vaporous." God is saying that the woman who places her hope in her superficiality or temporary youthful attractiveness is headed for disaster. But the woman who fears the Lord shall find total expression and praise. The term fear means "reverential awe," meaning she doesn't question God's plan for her as a woman. She doesn't place her hope in the ideologies of the world, but instead commits her hope to the Lord and His view of life.

This woman is promised—and receives—praise. The product of her hands is her home and all that it contains. The gates are the public places. She is known by what her home (her husband and each child) turns out to be. God may call some women out of the home, but I believe that the home is the greatest place for most wives to find fulfillment. When people are asked about their mothers, they usually don't talk about what she does. Rather, most focus on her character—who she is.

Significantly, this godly woman is characterized by hope and by work: "Strength and dignity are her clothing, and she smiles at the future. She opens her mouth in wisdom, and the teaching of kindness is on her tongue. She looks well to the ways of her household, and does not eat the bread of idleness" (verses 25–27).

Here is a woman of stature! She is not defeated by a woe-is-me attitude. *Strength* and *dignity* indicate she is a confident woman whose compassion and love free her of future worry. Her faith brings her success, and hope fills her heart.

This woman is able to smile at the future. She does not fear it because she has prepared her household for it physically, emotionally, and spiritually. As she meets the needs of her husband and children, her needs are met. She teaches wisdom and skill in the art of living by teaching biblical truths to her children so that they too will follow the Lord. She leads them to salvation and instructs them in their walk with Him. In order to do this, she spends personal time with the Lord and views her work positively. Her role is so fulfilling and far-reaching that she thanks the Lord for the privilege of being a wife and mother.

The Proverbs 31 woman is emotionally and physically able to work hard and sacrificially, "and does not eat the bread of idleness." Idleness is destructive to a woman's self-image and her spiritual walk. Since the godly woman doesn't resent being needed, she is available to meet the needs of her household.

Note also (in verses 13–24) that this woman has a great diversity in her work that takes her in and out of the home. Women who suffer anxiety over their role in the home typically lack diversity in daily tasks, not overwork. Women need both tasks that involve people and stimulate their intellect, as well as give them authority. Work is vital to life. It takes hard work to raise children properly and to run a household well—tasks that are neither mindless nor trivial.

Many women believe the lie that God has limited their fulfillment in the home.

Finally, the godly wife is creative with her abilities and displays much energy. Among the many duties (see verses 13–16), she looks for clothing material (wool and flax), shops in far places, cooks, buys and sells property, tends to a garden (vineyard), and sews. She also works in community affairs with the poor and needy (verse 20), makes and sells clothes (verse 24), and teaches in the community (verse 26).

Any way you look at her, she is not limited privately or publicly. Few men have the freedom to be as far-reaching and diversified as this woman, and yet many women believe the lie that God has limited their fulfillment in the home. The truth is, men are motivated by these types of women and their positive attitudes toward the home. The Proverbs 31 woman is wise enough to believe God, and her family praises her for her steadfastness.

Many women say they want opportunities to do more things. If you plan to be active, you will need physical stamina. It is no little thing that God states, "She girds herself with strength and makes her arms strong" (verse 17). A godly woman seeks to maintain her energy level and usually succeeds.

In counseling, I am amazed at the number of women who are physically tired. If a woman says she is tired, it is hard to ask her to do more. Many women believe the way to restore lost energy is to rest more. That may be true in momentary cases of exhaustion, but with any long-term problem, the opposite is often true. Exercise will actually increase your energy level. Our friend in Proverbs 31 kept herself strong and her energy level high. If you are overly exhausted, see a doctor. Otherwise, staying active is good for both your physical and mental health.

The result of this wife's efforts is the praise of her husband and children. God structured the emotions of children and the desires of husbands to naturally seek her. Because self-worth and self-expression can only be measured by relating to people and to God, this was a gracious act of God. In our case, five people naturally run to me: Don and my four kids! Have you ever noticed that when big football players say "Hi" on TV, they usually say "Hi, Mom!" Very few say, "Hi, Dad!" or anyone else! Mothers are so loved and revered.

What a fantastic honor to be a wife and mother!

As mothers, we receive the awesome God-given privilege of bearing and raising children. Mothers get to spend the most time reproducing a godly heritage. A mother uniquely understands each child and his or her emotional makeup. She gets to answer the majority of their questions. She gets to guide them into most of the spiritual truth they learn. It's her heart they hear the most. As children grow, they run to Mom when hurt or when trouble confronts them. Often she is the first to hear about whom they love and want to marry. She gets to help plan their weddings. It is her skirts that cradle the new grandchildren. I can't think of a better and more rewarding job!

Mothers get to spend the most time reproducing a godly heritage.

Since this role has critical generational effects, don't sell your children and grandchildren short by not spending time with them. Together with your husband, practice the biblical mandates given to parents to teach and instruct children in the Lord. (See in particular Deuteronomy 6:6–7, 20; Psalm 78:5–8.)

So what are the keys to success for a married woman?

- Constantly seek God's perspective on life.
- Become a model by serving your husband and children.
- Allow God to meet your needs through your husband, children, and opportunities in your home.
- Remember that outside activities, including a career, can be fulfilling if the needs in your home have been met first.
- Find a woman's group or Bible study to help encourage your own spiritual growth. Your own spiritual health is vitally important to nurturing the family God has given you.

HOW CAN I UNDERSTAND
AND HELP MY HUSBAND?

A quick review of trends impacting American men will illustrate how women can be supportive of their husbands.

As women of this generation shout, "I am not going to take this oppression anymore," men are suffering unbearably themselves. The pressures on the job and in society affect men's health, including their mortality. After age twenty-four, 20 percent more men commit suicide than women. After age forty, men die at a quicker rate than women.[1]

Men are frustrated because they no longer experience natural authority over those in their care.

What is happening to American men? It is not a simple question. Since the culture seems to strike hardest at the role of men, try to understand some of their struggles.

Few men own a home without debt, and less own land. Almost all men work for someone else. With loan institutions or bosses in firm control, men typically feel helpless or fear a lack of dominion over their lives. Furthermore, men are frustrated because they no longer experience natural authority over those in their care. The authoritarian influence of the past has turned into the democratic home of the twentieth century. The father is often just another vote in the family. No wonder the lack of male leadership is one of the greatest problems in America, even among Christian men. Husbands experience anxiety and loss of personal dignity in their families, leading to a role identity crisis for many. In turn, this crisis tends to promote hostility toward or withdrawal from their wives.

Today, there is a lack of effective male role models for young men. With more than one-third of American children coming from broken homes, young men move through their developmental years without observing assertive, confident, and sensitive men of direction. Many young men have no concept of what a father is, does, and should be. Girls also lack the fatherly love so necessary to a healthy maturing process and, as a result, often have more difficulty in the sexual area because they crave male attention.

Help by Avoiding Comparison

To answer the question, "How can a wife help her husband?" begin by realizing that just as women must confront the superwoman image, men are affected deeply by the tremendous pressure of comparison with other fantasy supermen images. The mass media offer daily the powerful president, the wise senator, the handsome executive, or the stylish athlete. Husbands receive little incentive to develop a man's inner qualities, such as faithfulness and consistency. Instead, more emphasis is placed on outer qualities, such as athletic ability, wealth, and appearance. A man can, over time, become discouraged with the barrage of comparison and competition.

The godly woman must be realistic about who her husband is and also be able to envision what he can become. Without a plan or direction from God, the natural tendency would be to ignore these things. But a woman who desires to be a godly wife to her husband will look beyond his weaknesses, encouraging him toward total fulfillment.

Women, your highest calling as wives is to understand, love, and help your husbands to be fulfilled, motivated, and responsible men. Do not compare your husband to other men and find him wanting. Instead, envision his potential even as God does, and encourage him to pursue it.

Help by Showing Compassion

In the same way, a wife should not allow her dissatisfaction with her husband to overshadow her compassion for him. Compassion is a deep, unselfish concern for another. God knows that our husbands will discourage us at times as well, yet He desires that we experience the best. Therefore, as Christ does, we should show compassion for our husbands.

It's not uncommon for a wife to lose perspective concerning her husband's weaknesses. In fact, she can become so discouraged and distrustful of her mate that she can no longer believe God will work through him. The husband's failure causes her to nag. Proverbs speaks of such a woman: "A constant dripping on a day of steady rain and a contentious woman are alike; he who would restrain her restrains the wind, and grasps oil with his right hand" (Proverbs 27:15–16).

A wife who constantly nags her husband in a quarrelsome and strife-ridden way will soon be unwilling to follow his leadership. Reversing that process will be more difficult than stopping the wind or grasping oil in your hand, according to God's Word.

Often a wife will ask Don if he would lead her husband to Christ or convince him of some spiritual truth. She usually has made matters worse by asking several women's groups to pray for him. Instead, she needs to start by realizing that her attitude of spiritual superiority toward him has usually angered or discouraged him over a period of time. This man is really rejecting his wife's attitude, not Christ. If we can get her to ask her husband's forgiveness and love him for who he is, the husband is usually open to talking about a God powerful enough to get his wife to say she was wrong!

Wives also say, "If you could just get my husband to spend more time with the children, things would be fine." Unfortunately, a wife may have so covered their husbands with guilt and rejection that every time the children enter the room, the father subconsciously feels whipped. These feelings retard a man's natural aggressiveness, and make him want to shun his own children because they are a reminder of his failures. Hardly anyone is motivated like this. By trusting her children to God first, a wife can then ask a husband's forgiveness for judging him, and give him the freedom to spend time with the kids as he feels he should. This man is free to be convicted by the Lord without being sidetracked by feelings of anger and rejection.

I have seen men treat new cars better than their wives. Why? Because a car is their total, unabridged responsibility. God created men to sense and respond to real dependence. They naturally feel more responsible for a wife who's there for better or worse.

An attentive wife knows how to please her husband. Your husband has tremendous demands placed upon his life from all directions. Often you cannot control those outside demands, but you can control your attitudes of love and acceptance toward your husband. You can cause him to look forward to coming home.

Help Him by Knowing His Needs

Scripture teaches that your husband has certain God-given needs that must be fulfilled: needs to protect, to own, to have authority, to be productive, to love, and to reproduce his image. Let's look at eight of these needs. (Some are mentioned briefly, since they are covered in more detail elsewhere.) Consider the areas where you can specifically help him meet his needs.

FIRST, EVERY HUSBAND HAS A NEED TO TRUST. There are fragile areas of every spouse's life that he/she does not want or need the public to know. These intimacies should be shared just between the two of you and aren't meant for anyone else. He needs to confide in someone he can trust, and a wife has an opportunity to fulfill that role. Don't breach his trust in you. Of the noble wife it's said, "The heart of her husband trusts in her, and he will have no lack of gain. She does him good and not evil all the days of her life" (Proverbs 31:11–12).

SECOND, EVERY HUSBAND HAS VOCATIONAL NEEDS. Usually a man's work sets the pattern for the other areas of his life. A man satisfied with his work is a happy man. A wife is in an excellent position to study her husband to see what he enjoys doing. Watch him play as well as work, since many times what he does with his free time reveals what he really enjoys. Encourage and uplift your mate in his work. Many men enjoy what they are doing, but secretly feel others do not adequately respect them for it. Hearing that you are proud of him can make a tremendous difference to your husband since he deeply desires your respect.

Be willing to adjust your spending and standard of living to allow your husband to change his career, if necessary. Even if the change brings the family a lower salary and a lower living standard, be willing to accept the adjustments of a potential move or different work hours—after, of course, discussion and recognizing this is the leading of the Lord. Anything you do to stabilize and increase his happiness helps you, too. A man has an almost constant need in life to reevaluate his vocation. He needs the freedom of knowing his wife will support him in all his endeavors.

THIRD, EVERY HUSBAND HAS SPIRITUAL NEEDS. Scripture places significant importance on spiritual leadership in a man's life. Encourage any inclination your husband shows toward taking spiritual responsibility. Especially after age thirty, a man's feeling of importance can be increased if he is involved in church leadership or in a discipleship process. This may require you to have a Bible study in your home or to make friends with the spouses of your husband's friends.

He needs a refuge in his home, away from the business of his workday.

Whatever it takes, help all you can. If your husband is not gifted in public ministry, perhaps he can facilitate small groups in your church—an excellent way to develop his leadership skills.

However, don't push him. Pressuring him to lead a group won't be beneficial if his spiritual gifts lie in other areas such as service or helps. Remember, God does the motivating. Always encourage your husband in his spiritual leadership, reminding him of opportunities in the home. This includes leading in thankgiving at mealtime, directing family devotions, and praying with and for you and the family. A husband does not need to be outgoing to lead his family spiritually and to develop his own spiritual life.

FOURTH, EVERY HUSBAND HAS SEXUAL NEEDS. This need is very important to most men, and detailed information is contained in chapter 13. Recognizing the differing sexual needs between men and women is very helpful in understanding that your husband is very normal.

FIFTH, EVERY HUSBAND HAS A NEED FOR TIME ALONE. Recognize that often your husband may think and solve problems in his mind before he talks about them. The opposite is true of women. Sometimes he brings issues from the workplace home with him. He needs a refuge in his home, away from the business of his workday. Men usually bury themselves in the newspaper, TV, the home office, or bedroom to unwind. A wise wife gives him some down time before engaging in conversation or having him play with the children.

SIXTH, EVERY HUSBAND HAS RELATIONSHIP NEEDS. Many husbands are loners. If you add to those the large number of couples who do not develop mutual friends, the problem becomes staggering. Relationships are very important in a man's life. You receive benefits from your husband's relationships, including better communication, diversity of interests, and increased hope in life. Observe people your husband naturally likes and create social settings where he feels comfortable. When possible, pursue his interests with friends. The more you do sacrificially for him, the more he will return the blessing.

SEVENTH, EVERY HUSBAND HAS INTELLECTUAL NEEDS. Do what you can to recognize your husband's intellectual interests. Initiate a mutual discussion on an issue, and your husband will look forward to sharing his thoughts with you. A husband who feels his wife cares about his intellectual interests feels a special closeness with her. She becomes a real friend. In addition, if she listens to him in even one area, he can then listen to her in other areas without feeling she is preaching.

EIGHTH, EVERY HUSBAND HAS AUTHORITATIVE NEEDS. A wife who encourages her husband's leadership in her life is a protected woman. This sounds good, but how do you do it? Two ways to give your husband authority and revive his natural desire to protect you are to praise him and place your hope in God alone.

A wife who encourages her husband's leadership in her life is a protected woman.

The mother is a model to the children. If she doesn't respect him, neither will they. Give your children a blessing by insisting that they respect their father. Praise their dad to them for what he has done. Children can also have a powerful influence on the dad. If the wife is complimentary when not in his presence, the children will compliment him to his face.

Verbal praise is extremely vital to a man. When a wife praises her husband, it demonstrates her love for him. When she is critical, it shows she does not understand the faith perspective of marriage. "An anxious heart weighs a man down, but a kind word cheers him up" (Proverbs 12:25 NIV).

Remember, God gave the mandate for wives to submit, or respect, their husbands. Why? Because respect is the greatest need for men.

A wise woman releases her husband to take leadership in her life by placing her hope in God. She allows him to be fully mature—including letting him make mistakes without recriminations—because she views him as a gift from God with no limitation to her fulfillment. The Holy Spirit is then free to help her understand her husband in particular and the differences in men and women in general.

Let's become women whose "pleasant words are a honeycomb, sweet to the soul and healing to the bones" (Proverbs 16:24).

NOTE

1. *World Almanac and Book of Facts* (Mahwah, N.J.: Funk and Wagnalls, 1996).

CHAPTER TWELVE

Truths and Myths about Marriage Sexuality

⊞ S EX. WHAT A POWERFUL DRIVE GOD CREATED IN men and women! Anyone considering marriage, and those already married, should plan to fully pursue sexual expression within marriage. You might say, "What an unnecessary statement! Sure, I plan to do just that." Yet marriage counselors all over America report that couples mention the sexual relationship as one of their most difficult areas of struggle.

God has much to say about sexuality in Scripture, leaving no doubt about its importance to marital love. He also created sexual love to require faith. It should be no surprise that God wants you to depend on Him in this area. Once again, knowing Scripture will allow the Holy Spirit to both teach and convict you. Open your mind and heart to the Holy Spirit as you read God's directions.

This chapter will look at the myths of sexual expression and the biblical truths and guidelines that free husbands and wives to express their sexuality in healthy, loving ways. Our discussion of sexual expression in marriage is so important that we will conclude it in chapter 13 with a look at three key topics: (1) sexual differences between men and women, (2) advice to men and women, and (3) dealing with past or recent premarital sexual encounters.

Before we look at problems and myths in the sexual relationship, a word of encouragement. First and foremost for a successful sexual relationship, *remember that God created sexual expression.* He fully intended pleasure and blessing in its creation. Israel's King Solomon and his young wife from Shulim stated it best:

"How beautiful you are, my darling, how beautiful you are! Your eyes are like doves."

"How handsome you are, my beloved, and so pleasant! Indeed, our couch is luxuriant!" (Song of Solomon 1:15–16).

This is only one of many biblical passages that express the excitement and happiness God intended for marital love. Discerning God's intention for the physical relationship to be a blessing will go a long way toward mental and physical enjoyment of one another.

WHY PROBLEMS DEVELOP

Though God has intended blessing for marriages, many Christian couples develop problems in the marriage bed.

"I am angry and bitterly disappointed about my sexual experience," a Christian woman once told us. "I was so expectant and excited when I got married, only to find shock and mediocrity," she said. "It is not at all what I had thought it would be. What surprises me most is that I am probably more of a problem than my husband."

We never cease to be amazed at the number of men and women who say similar things three or four years into marriage. It is not necessary for this to happen.

There are three basic reasons why couples experience frustration in this most intimate of relationships. The primary cause of frustration is the cultural programming they have received. The film and television industries create false sexual images. The media subtly imply that only physically attractive people really succeed sexually and that great sexual compatability comes quickly and easily. Movies seldom depict sexual failure or growth! Reality is ignored and replaced with a fantasy image, which somehow escapes us in the reality of the bedroom. Meanwhile, the wholesale merchandising of sex by advertisers has contributed significantly to the growth of pornography. False comparison, false images, guilt, and disappointment reign in our culture as a result. These factors confuse us, leaving us unsure of what God really desires for us sexually.

The second major cause of sexual frustration today is the nature of human beings. As we have mentioned numerous times, men and women are self-centered beings.

Problems in the sexual relationship are a prime example. Self-centeredness in any area can devastate a marriage, but that is particularly true with sex and romance. Each partner brings to the bedroom different standards, desires, and inhibitions about sex. Each may carry a certain amount of scar tissue from the past. Pride is also involved. We want to be self-sufficient and, therefore, we don't want to admit we don't know it all. We have difficulty asking for help. We tend to blame our spouses when sex isn't as exciting as we dreamed it would be, or as Hollywood portrays it to be.

The third major cause of sexual problems results from the lack of quality

Christian teaching on sex. For the most part, Christian leadership has not responded well to people's needs in this area, and has not taught positive truths from God's Word concerning sex. When there were attempts in the past, the teaching was often legalistic: a bunch of no's, without answers to "why not?" questions.

Most couples we have worked with in counseling and seminars tell us they never have received specific instructions on sex from anyone with authority in their lives. Our culture, man's nature, and ineffective teaching have resulted in a sexually frustrated society.

CULTURAL AND RELIGIOUS MYTHS CONCERNING SEX

Over the centuries, human nature and the poor cultural models have produced sexual hang-ups in couples. Before couples can escape this entrapment, those patterns must be identified. Usually identifying them will help couples begin the process of overriding their effects. Occasionally, it may be necessary to seek help from a professional Christian counselor.

We have indicated that the film and television industries have contributed to sexual struggles in marriage by creating false sexual images. This certainly is true in the image of the so-called "all-American" male. The virile male typically is portrayed as a "Ready Freddie"—always ready to perform sexually. The man who is not instantaneously ready at all times may be suspected of being less of a man. Men and women alike subject themselves to this thinking. The result is that men may try to prove themselves on the one hand, or they may develop insecurity about their manhood, thinking they should be more aggressive and successful. Either of these can add real pressure to their sexual experience. Women who accept this image are often surprised and sometimes frustrated that their husband does not act like the infamous "Ready Freddie."

The virile male typically is portrayed as a "Ready Freddie"— always ready to perform sexually.

All things considered, a man's sexual motivation and function are not all that different from a woman's. He experiences times of low interest also, and may need sensitivity and motivation from his wife. Generally speaking, however, men think about sex more often than women at any given age. This is not abnormal, wives!

And what about the women's expectations? Unlike the men, most women who remain virgins before marriage need an adjustment period before becoming an aggressive lover after marriage. It is important to note that if a woman has a healthy relationship with her father and a healthy relationship with the Lord, she will have fewer problems adjusting to her sexual relationship.

Early experimentation with sex or having multiple sex partners before marriage may produce guilt and/or problems with desire on the part of the female. The same experiences by the male may make the man overly aggressive sexually toward his wife. Wise counsel may be needed to overcome past experiences. (This will be discussed more in the final section of the next chapter.)

Feelings and romance usually are the result of a healthy relationship, not its cause.

As your wife seeks God's perspective, you should exhibit tremendous sensitivity, patience, and acceptance. Your goal should be to motivate her sexually by loving her unconditionally.

The other prevalent myth about sexual expression concerns romance and sexual desire. Couples must realize that the media helped to create false images concerning sexual desire. These false images communicate, "If you really love me, you will naturally want to have sex." Certainly any agape marriage will experience romance and sexual desire, but feelings and romance usually are *the result* of a healthy relationship, *not its cause.* Throughout the marriage, a couple should dialogue often to discover new ways to sexual and romantic excitement.

Romance is not automatic. Time, effort, and creativity must be invested in the relationship before romance blossoms. Understanding God's Word, seeking counsel, and having open communication will cause the sexual union to succeed over time.

BIBLICAL TRUTHS ABOUT THE SEXUAL RELATIONSHIP

In Scripture, God has spoken boldly concerning sexual matters. To understand His perspective, begin by learning the Biblical absolutes concerning sexual love. The following eleven truths are of vital importance to a successful and healthy sexual relationship because they represent the guideposts for spiritual counsel on sexual matters.

Truth 1: Sexuality is God's Creation

It is important that every man and woman realize that God unquestionably created his or her sexuality. Genesis 1:27 says, "God created man in His own image, in the image of God He created him; male and female He created them." Physical anatomies represent one of the most significant differences in

God's creation of male and female. These differences affect all our being, from our moods and emotions to our perspectives.

Clearly, God created man and woman as different sexual entities with the opportunity to become "one flesh." The creation of sexual differences was no accident, but a deliberate part of God's unique plan. God designed you to accept your sexuality and to seek positive fulfillment in marriage. Hollywood did not create sex—God did! And since everything that He created was very good (Genesis 1:31), you are free to seek its fullness. Sex can be fun, creative, and very rewarding. Solomon and his Shulammite wife knew this.

Truth 2: Physical Love Is for Procreation and Pleasure

The second major reality from Scripture is that God intended sex and marriage to produce children and for pleasure. Sometimes we remember the first reason but ignore the second. But both are divine purposes of physical oneness.

There are exceptions, but the emphasis is clear. God created both sex and children to be a blessing. Therefore, sex and marriage give you a wonderful picture of God's love for you. The love you experience for your children gives you a small glimpse as to how much love God has for you.

Children give couples the opportunity to reproduce not only God's image, but their images as well (see, for example, Genesis 5:3). God created sex for procreation. He had commanded Adam and Eve to be fruitful and multiply and fill the earth (Genesis 1:28), and Solomon wrote, "Behold, children are a gift of the Lord; the fruit of the womb is a reward (Psalm 127:3).

Without a doubt, God associates pleasure and excitement with the sexual relationship.

The world promotes the concept that sex is a natural instinct. But God designed sex to be the result of total expression between a husband and wife. Sex was never meant to be shared apart from the unity of the marriage relationship. Children were to be a result of the unique and permanent relationship between the husband and wife.

Significantly, God refers to sexual relations in the opening chapters of Genesis in the context of *blessing*—a word that refers to a high state of joy and pleasure. God devotes a whole book of the Bible to describing this blessing and its associated joys: Song of Solomon. Here the Bible has said of sexual love, "Its flashes are flashes of fire, the very flame of the Lord" (8:6). Without a doubt, God associates pleasure and excitement with the sexual relationship. Solomon used romantic, sensuous language when he declared a wife to be "a loving doe, a graceful deer," and urged the husband, "May her breasts satisfy you always, may you ever be captivated by her love" (Proverbs 5:19 NIV).

Truth 3: Physical love is a picture of Christ and the Church

Paul says in Ephesians 5:31-32 "this mystery (of marriage) is great, but I speak of Christ and the Church."

God intended that the physical act of intimacy between a husband and wife be a beautiful earthly picture of His union with us. Physical intimacy is His picture of completeness - making two people one. It is His arms of love touching us in a physical way. The unity between a husband and wife, including the physical, is to be a reflection of His very character.

Paul went so far as to compare the love between a husband and wife as the very picture of Christ and His Bride, the Church.

As we invite Jesus Christ to come into our lives and to dwell there - that very act is a picture of the marriage union. From that time forward, we are to come together regularly. The regularity of physical intimacy reminds us that in the same way, our relationship with Christ should be regular and consistent, joyful and refreshing. We are to have time with our Lord in personal, private ways, as with no other. Physical intimacy is to be exclusive. I am to give myself to no one apart from my spouse. My relationship with Christ is the same. I am to have "no other gods before me" (Deut. 5:7; Exodus 20:3).

The mystery is not of marriage - the mystery is that of Christ and the Church. Marriage is to be the demonstration of the unity of Christ and His Bride. Every time we come together as husband and wife, we experience different emotions, the same way we do in our relationship with Christ: joy, exhilaration, rest, refreshment, relaxation, release from stress and tension.

Physical intimacy is grace personified. Grace is freely given to us by God. It is not something we deserve, nor work for, nor are good enough to receive. No, grace is given simply because God gives it. It is unmerited favor. In the same way, physical intimacy is given as a gift to please the heart of the beloved. Physical intimacy delivers us from our natural selfish bent and allows us to give unreservedly to our mate. This truly glorifies God.

Intimacy with God takes time. But, it is worth every day spent. Intimacy with our spouse takes time and effort. But it's worth the time spent. We must never mistake physical intimacy as an act between two bodies. It is far more than that. It is to be a picture of the union, Christ has with His Bride.

Truth 4: Physical Love Demands a Time Priority

In 1 Corinthians 7 and in the Song of Solomon, God implies that successful lovemaking requires a time priority. Solomon created a special bedroom and took his bride away from the activities of life. The preparation and time taken imply that God ordained special emphasis in sexual matters. Is your bedroom a special place?

In Deuteronomy 24:5, young men were instructed: "When a man takes a new wife, he shall not go out with the army nor be charged with any duty; he shall be free at home one year and shall give happiness to his wife whom he has taken." The words "give happiness" refer to sexual pleasure. Since older men of God knew how vital the sexual relationship was to marriage, they placed sex above other very important matters to allow the couple to initially establish their sexual relationship. Any couple who expects to be sexually satisfied must spend time developing their relationship. Not only is the honeymoon important; the years that follow require time and effort to maintain mutual satisfaction.

Truth 5: Physical Love Requires a Transfer of Body Ownership

Sexual love is so important to Christian marriage that the Scripture suggests that couples exchange rights to their own bodies for the sake of their sexual oneness. "The husband must fulfill his duty to his wife, and likewise also the wife to her husband. The wife does not have authority over her own body, but the husband does; and likewise also the husband does not have authority over his own body, but the wife does" (1 Corinthians 7:3–4).

This command clearly establishes God's commitment to physical oneness in marriage. Gracious sacrifice is part of every sexual union from God's perspective. Your body is not yours, but your mate's. God wants you to trust Him and give your body for your mate's pleasure. God intends this to be for mutual pleasure and not for selfish purposes. God makes sex a sacrificial act that is redemptive in that it gets your eyes off your needs and onto the needs of your mate.

Truth 6: Physical Love Is Passionate and Creative

The Song of Solomon describes Solomon and his wife expressing their sexual union in creative and passionate terms. Through this divinely inspired "Song of Songs" (1:1), God implies that mutual sexual communication is needed. Both the wife and the husband must creatively communicate their sexual thoughts and desires. In several passages, Solomon excitedly describes his wife's body. The Shulammite bride responds with an equally passionate description of Solomon's body (4:1–7; 5:10–16; 7:1–9). Study the two passages and feel free to smile at the language used.

> How beautiful are your feet in sandals, O prince's daughter! The curves of your hips are like jewels, the work of the hands of an artist. Your navel is like a round goblet which never lacks mixed wine; your belly is like a heap of wheat fenced about with lilies. Your two breasts are like two fawns, twins of a gazelle. Your neck is like a tower of ivory, your eyes like the pools in Heshbon by the gate of Bath-rabbim; your nose is like the

tower of Lebanon, which faces toward Damascus. Your head crowns you like Carmel, and the flowing locks of your head are like purple threads; the king is captivated by your tresses (Song of Solomon 7:1–5).

Notice that Solomon's eyes start at her feet, progress to the midsection, on to her head, then back to the midsection (verses 6–8). His primary interest is her midsection. He is physical.

In contrast, the wife's interest is different:

My beloved is dazzling and ruddy, outstanding among ten thousand. His head is like gold, pure gold; his locks are like clusters of dates and black as a raven. His eyes are like doves beside streams of water, bathed in milk, and reposed in their setting. His cheeks are like a bed of balsam, banks of sweet-scented herbs; his lips are lilies, dripping with liquid myrrh. His hands are rods of gold set with beryl; his abdomen is carved ivory inlaid with sapphires. His legs are pillars of alabaster set on pedestals of pure gold; his appearance is like Lebanon, choice as the cedars. His mouth is full of sweetness. And he is wholly desirable. This is my beloved and this is my friend, O daughters of Jerusalem (Song of Solomon 5:10–16).

She starts with his head, proceeds to his abdomen, legs, and then back to his head. Clearly, the Shulammite is primarily interested in Solomon's face. She is relational. His face reflects his person—the compelling aspect of her relationship with him.

In 6:13, Solomon describes a dance the Shulammite does to excite him sexually. Mutual pleasure can be explored this way with God's blessing. Creative and passionate marital love is good in the sight of God. Hebrews 13:4 says, "Marriage is to be held in honor among all, and the marriage bed is to be undefiled."

Truth 7: Scripture Advocates Sexual Verbalization

In Song of Solomon 2:6, the Shulammite gives specific instructions during the act of making love: "Let his left hand be under my head and his right hand embrace me." In 4:16, she adds, "Awake . . . make my garden breathe out fragrance . . . May my beloved come into his garden and eat its choice fruits!"

God demonstrates how significant verbalizing one's desires is to sexual love. Yet sexual communication is difficult for most people when first married. Learning to verbalize in marriage becomes more comfortable as time passes. Expressing your thoughts and feelings concerning sexuality pays great dividends as you mature together. Avoid being negative during the sexual act. Instead, it's helpful to communicate briefly sexual preferences. The day after your sexual encounter, inquire what you can do to improve your partner's satisfaction. (We will revisit this truth in chapter 13 under "Sexual Verbalization.")

Truth 8: Physical Love Should Occur Regularly

God specifically instructs married couples to have sexual relations regularly. He warns that disobeying this command leaves the partners open to a loss of self-control, that is, lust problems, which could include sexual fantasies about other women, pornographic materials, masturbation, or even affairs. "Stop depriving one another, except by agreement for a time, so that you may devote yourselves to prayer, and come together again so that Satan will not tempt you because of your lack of self-control," Paul warned (1 Corinthians 7:5).

The issue here is not to establish a standard for the number of times to have intercourse per week. Instead, the focus is to have regular, mutually satisfying sexual contact. Notice that there is no age limit mentioned. The Bible gives accounts of sexual love for the elderly. Abraham and Sarah enjoyed sexual relations in their nineties as Sarah conceived and gave birth to Isaac (Genesis 21:2–6). Regularity may change, but there are biblical, medical, and psychological reasons why the sexual relationship is as important at age sixty as it is at age twenty-five.

Song of Solomon 5:1 says "Eat, O friends, and drink; drink your fill, O lovers" (NIV). Your fill may be different from that of other couples. God wants you as a couple to determine what is mutually satisfying in your unique relationship, both in regularity and in creativity.

Truth 9: Physical Love Is More Than Physical

Don't focus on the physical aspects of sexuality to the neglect of the emotional, spiritual, and intellectual needs. Scripture never makes this mistake. When God said Adam and Eve were naked and unashamed, He was plainly speaking of more than physical transparency. When studying the Song of Solomon, notice that this couple's communication incorporates one another's total needs. The Shulammite rejects Solomon momentarily (5:2–8). He responds to her with love and blessing (6:4–10). The importance of the total person in lovemaking is evident. God compares the union of husband and wife with the union of Christ and His church (Ephesians 5:32).

We highly recommend chapters 2 and 3 of Tim LaHaye's book, *The Act of Marriage*, because they communicate the wholeness of the individual man and woman.

Truth 10: Physical Love Gives Comfort and Healing

David and Bathsheba were utterly distraught following the death of their baby.

"Then David comforted his wife Bathsheba, and he went to her and lay with her. She gave birth to a son, and they named him Solomon" (2 Samuel 12:24 niv). Often when one or both partners have experienced a loss of some kind, the sexual union presents an opportunity to comfort and relax one another. It is a time for the couple to pull together and experience the unity that they so desperately need. Losing a job, feeling stress from work, moving, having problems with children, and losing a loved one are times when comfort is desperately needed. And physical comfort, including holding, kissing, and even sexual union, can give care and warmth.

A wise couple will come together in physical and emotional unity during times of trial because such times naturally pull them apart. In His wisdom, God knows this is a danger point and therefore takes care to draw the couple back together tenderly and patiently.

Truth 11: Sexual Attitudes of Parents Are Transferred to Children

Children should learn that sex was created for the marriage relationship alone. This training should not start in the teenage years, but as early as nine or ten years old. Sexual intimacy was created as a gift from God to allow two people to express marital unity.

It is no accident that a whole book is devoted to the sexual and romantic life of a married couple in the Word of God. The very last chapter of the Song of Solomon ends with an admonition concerning sex and children. The Shulammite's brothers greet her and Solomon as they return home for a visit. The brothers ask about their younger sister who has yet to reach puberty, and discuss her character development in the area of sexual values. "If she is a wall, we shall build on her a battlement of silver; but if she is a door, we shall barricade her with planks of cedar" (Song of Solomon 8:9). "A wall" indicates strength, suggesting strong convictions and determination in abstaining from sexual relationship. "A door" indicates easy entry, or being sexually promiscuous. Significantly the bride responds by saying "I was a wall" (verse 10); she remained a virgin until her wedding day.

If you observe your teens to be walls, firmly resisting sexual temptations, reward them with more freedom. However, if they appear to be doors, open to pressures from friends, you are to lovingly put more fences around them to insure their protection from early experimentation. It is important that the older children assist the parents by being examples in the protection of the siblings. Some children need more boundaries than others. Observant parents will communicate readily with each child concerning sexuality values.

Throughout the Song of Solomon the phrase appears, "Do not arouse or awaken love until it pleases" (Song of Solomon 2:7; 8:4; see also 3:5). According to these verses, no one should open himself or herself to arousal before the time of marriage fulfillment. Early teens should be taught the importance of avoiding tempting situations that can lead to such arousal. Constant communication as they grow to adulthood is not optional, but crucial. Pray continually for the Lord's protection for each child. Pray that each child will be a "wall" and not a "door". Pray especially for the older children to be examples for the younger ones to follow.

The sex talks we had with our children started when they were about eight or nine years old. Dating was not allowed until age sixteen and that was group dating. We communicated very thoroughly with our children all the way through junior high school, high school, and college. Open communication and asking the right questions along the way encouraged them to wait for marriage to have sex.

To a large degree, children learn from the attitudes of their parents. Deuteronomy 6 states that parents teach by what they do and say. Your convictions and actions play a major role in raising children. What you model to them becomes their strongest impression of sexual love.

Attitudes are also communicated by the parents' behavior. Research indicates that children learn very little from what you say and a great deal more from what you do. If Mom and Dad are not excited about each other, the children will miss the most important illustration of what love and marriage are all about. Couples may think they can subtly hide their attitudes from their children. Not so. If a father doesn't have a loving relationship with his wife, it could affect his daughter's concepts of femininity, and her future role in marriage. If the father doesn't have a good relationship with his daughter, it could affect her relationship with her future husband. This is also true of the father-son relationship, and the son's concepts of being a godly father and husband.

In summary, all these ten truths from God's Word teach one thing: *Physical intimacy was created by God and He wants His married children to enjoy His good gift!* Sex in marriage should be a pleasurable expression of a faith relationship. It is altogether good for us.

CHAPTER THIRTEEN

Naked and Unashamed

⬡ "TWO CHAPTERS ON THE SEXUAL RELATIONSHIP! Isn't that a bit too much in a Christian book about unity in marriage?" If those are your thoughts, we can understand. But the physical union in marriage, and the physical pleasures that precede it, are a vital part to the emotional and spiritual unity that God ordained in marriage.

The first couple "were not ashamed," even though "they were both naked" (Genesis 2:25 KJV). Yet many Christian couples are uncomfortable or unsure about their sexual expression in marriage. Part of that is due to the curse of sin and the distortion of sex by our media. But some of the awkwardness comes from not learning about God's plan for marriage sexuality from the pulpit. That's understandable. Many pastors don't deal with the topic as openly as they would like because they have mixed audiences, including children.

Another reason for the awkwardness about sex arises from not knowing about differing sexual needs between women and men. This chapter will look at those differences and encourage wives and husbands to focus on meeting their spouse's needs.

God purposefully made women's sexual needs and motivations different than men's. Over a period of time, these differences reveal a great deal about the total relationship of the couple. The couple who is experiencing an agape marriage relationship will begin to see these differences as opportunities to serve and broaden the sexual experience.

As we look at the different motivations, remember that knowing your spouse's motivation for romance and responding to his or her sexual needs can benefit your whole relationship.

DIFFERING MOTIVATIONS FOR ROMANCE

Sexual Motivation for Women

Women are motivated greatly by the emotional dimension of their sexual relationships. Romantic love and feminine needs cannot be separated. Tender moments that communicate admiration and respect help to prepare wives for an exciting sexual experience. In fact, in the absence of romantic tenderness and emotional appreciation, wives sometimes enter the sexual union with feelings of "being used."

Women also are motivated by thoughts of a deep intimacy, of which the physical union is but one expression. Therefore, wives appreciate tender expressions, both verbally and physically. Women enjoy tenderness before, during, and after the sexual experience. Men, holding your wife after a sexual encounter is probably the most vital gift you can give to her. Sensitive communication about matters other than sex for twenty minutes before or after sex does a great deal to demonstrate your love. Doing so shows that you care about her, not just sex.

Many women tend to be cyclical in their sexual desire. That is, their desire tends to rise, then drop for several days after a sexual experience, only to rise again later. Women tend to be excited gradually and respond to tender touches and caresses. Privacy and a non-threatening environment are important to helping her release her emotions. Sensitive verbalization can soothe and motivate her.

Sexual Motivation for Men

In contrast, *men are motivated much more by the physical dimension* of their relationship. Normally, a man can struggle with a problem all evening and still be tremendously attracted to his wife's body. His sex drive is not cyclical, but continual. Tim LaHaye mentions several related issues in his book, *The Act of Marriage.* A man's sex drive is connected to his ability "to be the aggressor, provider, and leader of his family. The woman who resents her husband's sex drive while enjoying his aggressive leadership had better face the fact that she cannot have one without the other."[1]

Few things in life give a man more a sense of having finished a task well than satisfying his wife sexually.

Men usually respond spontaneously and instantaneously to physical stimuli. They are as likely to be stimulated through the eye as much as the touch. A man normally likes to caress his wife in the light, so he can see her clearly. Men are excited much more quickly than women, and distractions usually don't bother them. They experience immediate release in their sexual orgasm and may fall asleep immediately thereafter. With some effort on their part, however, they too can greatly enjoy those moments after intercourse, which are extremely important to their wives.

Few things in life give a man more a sense of having finished a task well than satisfying his wife sexually. To him, it is like wrapping up a package and tying a ribbon around it. The sexual dimension of marriage is so exhilarating, relaxing, and fulfilling.

Couples should never allow resentment to build toward one another in regard to these differences. Understand them, anticipate them, and work with them. A creative plan can turn these differences into real enjoyment. The woman who understands a man's natural, God-given sexual drive is overwhelmed when he tenderly meets her needs in spite of his own natural desires.

HELPING YOUR MATE TOWARD SEXUAL ONENESS

Expressing sexual love changes all through marriage, including early experimentation in marriage, hormonal and physical changes during pregnancy and nursing, years with small children with little time for privacy, the middle years, and finally the older years—each stage of life presents different sexual expressions. Yet, lovemaking during all these seasons can be extremely satisfying. All the changes that take place can be beautiful tests of your mutual and enduring love. Because life is always changing, so will your sexual experiences. Enjoy the changes, experiment, and communicate. Remember, through sexual oneness a husband and wife sometimes best express their spiritual and emotional commitments to each other.

Most sexual problems develop because of ignorance in the early years of marriage. Couples will ask advice on buying a house or car, or perhaps the discipline of their children. Few will seek help on the sexual relationship. Yet helping your spouse to desire and enjoy sexual oneness is important to having a healthy marriage. We encourage couples to read together Christian books on sex[2] and to seek counsel when problems persist over several months.

Here is some advice to married men and women from thirty years of our counseling experience.

Advice to Men
Men, your responsibility is to love your wife sacrificially as your own body. (See Ephesians 5:25, 28.) If you relate to her in a godly manner, you will enjoy a rewarding sexual relationship. Sacrificial love will pay great dividends for the

rest of your life. Here are some simple guidelines.

ACCEPTANCE AND COMMUNICATION. In the Scriptures, God instructs you to be excited and satisfied with your wife's body. Make it a point to tell her how you are drawn to her body. Fall in love with her so completely that you will not be affected by the inevitable changes produced by having children and aging. Convince your wife of your love and appreciation of her body. The man who fails to explicitly do this will eventually discover that she begins to hide her body from him. The result will be devastating. A husband has the power to make or break his wife's self-image concerning her body. The mirrors in your house and the young bodies pictured in advertisements all remind your wife that her looks are fading. Only you can convince her she still is pleasing to you physically and emotionally.

Good communication includes knowing your wife's fears and frustrations. A husband must take responsibility for helping his wife understand her sexual frustrations. Wives who develop sexual anxiety may not be initially aware of it. Insecurities about her appearance, the size of her breasts, her thighs, her stomach, or whatever, can cause a wife to lose her desire for sexual intimacy.

Husbands are to "live with [their] wives in an understanding way," according to 1 Peter 3:7. Your communication and reassurance are vital if you hope to keep your wife from labeling herself as unattractive. Never communicate, either through words or innuendo, that she needs to lose a few pounds or that she should have surgery in any given area of her body. She will be devastated by such insensitive comments and may never get over them.

LOVING ACTIONS. Since so much of a woman's sexual enjoyment is tied to her emotional preparation, the husband must be prepared to take charge of easing his wife's burdens. A messy house, unattended children, uncertainty of personal attractiveness, criticism from her husband, and social pressures are typical problems that keep wives from releasing themselves emotionally. For example, an effective husband may get up on Saturday morning and let his wife sleep in. He dresses and feeds the children and helps clean the house. He may also take the children for several hours that afternoon so she can have her hair done or go shopping, enabling his wife to relax.

Such loving actions unburden a wife emotionally, which in turn allow her to become more aware of the husband's need.

When we first married, I used to blame Sally when she was not "up" sexually. Now I blame myself. I usually have not been romantically creative, or have not been sensitive to her needs. Sometimes such love will need to be sacrificial, inconvenient, or even difficult for the man. But the husband will do it because in his love he wants to please his wife and ease her burden.

A RELAXING, PLEASANT ENVIRONMENT. Men, protect your wife

from sexual anxiety. This may seem obvious, but never take your cleanliness for granted! Brush your teeth and take a shower. Do things that take the pressure off the sexual union. Hot baths, rubdowns, and walks together just prior to intimate involvement foster communication and associate pleasure with sexual experiences. Candlelight and soft music reduce anxiety and help your wife to be uninhibited. Holding her and taking time to talk to her before sex add definite pleasurable associations with the act itself.

No man can guarantee a woman's sexual response every time, but he can create a satisfying experience for both of them most of the time.

Don't allow your wife to endure sexual pain! Occasional momentary pain upon entry is not abnormal, but if pain persists, seek medical help together. Rashes, infections, or more severe problems such as endometriosis can cause pain. Manual stimulation for both the man and woman gives pleasure and may alleviate tension or rejection brought on by painful intercourse. If these problems persist for an extended time in spite of proper medical help, seek counsel immediately.

NATURAL MOTIVATION. When a marriage is functioning according to God's perspective, women can be as sexually responsive as men. Unfortunately, outside pressures may frequently inhibit emotional responsiveness of women. On the other hand, men may not be as affected sexually by outside pressures. The following discussion, though addressed to men, can also help women, as husbands and wives learn to balance each other's sexual needs.

In most men and women, the level of sexual aggressiveness is natural, somewhat predictable. The following line represents the total spectrum of all natural sexual drives.

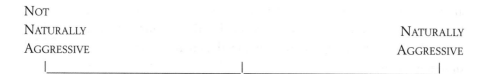

NOT
NATURALLY
AGGRESSIVE

NATURALLY
AGGRESSIVE

Most women tend to be to the *left* of center (not naturally aggressive), while most men tend to be *right* of center (naturally aggressive). In other words, most women don't initiate sexual activity as often as men. These women may not be against sex, or even uninterested. They simply may not naturally think aggressively about sex. However, apart from being properly approached, they may not develop an internal need for sexual fulfillment but every five to fifteen days. If properly motivated and stimulated by their husbands, they would be open to more frequent sexual advances.

Tragically, many husbands interpret this lack of natural aggression by their wives as failure or lack of interest. That's a big mistake. It simply may be a symptom of needed communication and support. The level of her natural aggressiveness should not be a measure of a husband's sexual failure or success. This natural aggressiveness has nothing to do with the couple's ultimate fulfillment.

Men must realize that God created their natural aggressiveness for obvious procreation purposes. It's OK for you to be the aggressor most of the time. It doesn't mean there is anything wrong with your wife. However, if a husband desires sex far too often for the wife, there may be a problem with communication, or feelings of rejection. These feelings can stem from his past. If a wife's sexual aggressiveness is lower than desired, the couple simply needs a mutually satisfying plan to change the balance. Counsel and openness can accomplish the solution to either of these problems.

In our culture, it is not unusual to find men who are less aggressive than their wives. Do not attach one another with labels that destroy emotional security. This will only worsen the problem. For husbands and wives, the solution is the same: Seek godly counsel.

Advice to Women

ENJOYING SEX. When we first married, I (Don) thought if I could just have my sexual needs met I would be happy. Before long I realized that the greatest need I had was not my own enjoyment, but my wife's. Sexually speaking, the greatest gift a woman can give to her husband is enjoying her own sexual experience. This is very motivating to a husband.

Too many wives look at sex merely as their duty to satisfy their husband's needs. Every woman should know that God wants her to feel good and to enjoy sex. If a wife has the freedom to look at her physical union as an enjoyable experience, her attitude will change tremendously. In order to enjoy the sexual union and to reach orgasm, most women need to concentrate on their own bodies, while the man enjoys concentrating and thinking about her body.

For maximum enjoyment, a wife needs a positive attitude concerning sex and marriage based on the Scriptures. She also needs to sense personal freedom in several areas, including (1) good communication with her mate, (2) satisfaction with her mate, (3) respect from and for her husband, (4) freedom to discover what feels good, (5) freedom to verbalize enjoyment, feelings, instructions, and (6) assurance that her husband will sensitively approach her, with her needs being his first priority. In addition, as we noted earlier, the woman will need to feel relaxed from her daily responsibilities, secure in her sexual setting, and secure that her body is attractive to her mate. She will also want personal cleanliness for herself and her husband.

BEING FEMININE. God gave men a tremendous desire to pursue and serve their wives. In the natural sense, this drive manifests itself through sexual attraction. Wives should take advantage of this God-created desire instead of resenting it. Rather than condemn him, learn to motivate him and enjoy his instinctive desire.

How you dress is very important to him. Most men like their wives to wear feminine clothing as much as possible. Nice feminine undergarments are extremely motivating to husbands. Makeup and perfume can also affect his natural desire. Ask your husband what he enjoys about your clothing, or what he would like you to change.

Most men do not want their wives to be alluring to other men, so watch how short or tight fitting your skirts are. He may want you to wear particular outfits for him on occasion, but take care to be very modest in public.

FULL SEXUAL EXPRESSION

Again, because of the influences of our culture, wives and husbands often focus on sexual intercourse as the sole goal of sexual expression. Yet full sexual expression consists of much more than the physical union of husband and wife. Here are four aspects of the sexual relationship that contribute to a fulfilling sexual encounter between husband and wife.

A Focus on Your Mate's Total Person

Each couple should place the focus of their sexual relationship on being naked and unashamed instead of just having an orgasm in intercourse. While orgasm is a very important icing on the cake, it is not the cake. No couple can be assured of a successful orgasm experience every time, but every couple can be assured of a successful intimate experience. Characterize your physical love-making by focusing on each mate's total person.

Our caution is: Do not limit your sexual experiences to just intercourse. Many couples confine their sexual expression to fifteen quick minutes of intercourse. Couples who allow their sexual experience to dwindle to this point have, many times, guaranteed that the wife will have lower enjoyment for several reasons. Research shows that there is a large possibility that intercourse alone will not produce an orgasm for the wife. Second, fifteen-minute "quickies" foster servitude feelings in wives, not encouragement. They are very likely to feel used. Third, fifteen minutes does not allow wives to experience a total-person encounter. A naked and unashamed experience can take up to an hour. A woman needs time to be reassured, to be listened to, to have her hurts mended, as well as to give her body time to prepare.

What are we saying? Husbands, you need to level the playing field! You can normally have an orgasm over 90 percent of the time. But quick lovemaking may limit her ability to have an orgasm to, at best, 40 percent of the time. You may be angry with God for not giving you a more sexually aggressive wife, but you may have failed repeatedly in the sensitivity and creativity department.

A woman needs time to be reassured, to be listened to, to have her hurts mended, as well as to give her body time to prepare.

Guys, wake up! If you take time to deeply engage your wife's emotions, she will enjoy the sexual encounter even if she cannot have an orgasm. Cake is good, even without the icing. Do not allow your wife just to serve your needs. If she is at all frustrated, both of you must seek counsel. If this applies to you, don't expect a four-or five-day recovery. It may take months to repair as her trust in you grows.

Body Freedom

Since the sexual relationship involves a physical act, it is very important for partners to be excited about their mate's body as well as their own. Research indicates that sexual feelings intensify when couples are open and creative with each other's bodies. The woman who can uninhibitedly open her mind, body, and body movements to her husband's rhythm and motion will certainly experience increased enjoyment and success.

Today, it is common for a man to be attracted to his wife's body and even to express that verbally. It's not so common for a wife to express her appreciation for her husband's body. It is helpful for wives to reprogram their minds through Scripture by reading the Song of Solomon. For instance, consider Solomon's Shulammite wife, who said, "He is wholly desirable. This is my beloved and this is my friend" (Song of Solomon 5:16).

It is generally much easier for a husband to develop freedom with his body and with his mate's body. Generally, women are not so free. They tend to compare themselves with the youthful, unblemished bodies of models on TV, which can result in insecurity. Christian teaching has not helped women to be free with their husbands. Some women believe that the lower parts of their bodies are extremely unattractive and even unsanitary. This sets them up for sexual anxiety. Yet men, when polled on what part of their wife's body is most attractive, overwhelmingly said the lower parts. This is a shocking revelation to wives!

Because of these natural differences, husbands need to slow down and allow their wives time to adjust. With patience and sensitivity, after several months, the couple can learn to be open and free with one another's bodies.

Once a wife experiences her husband's tenderness and patience, sex will become a more enjoyable experience for her.

Sexual Verbalization

As with all communication in marriage, sexual communication is a nonnegotiable. Talking about sexual excitement, instructions, hurts, fears, disappointments, joys, and anticipation are very important. The couple's ability to verbalize these to each other is imperative.

Several problems occur in sexual verbalization. It is not natural for men or women to verbalize during lovemaking for fear of losing their focus. Communicating criticism is easier than encouragement. "Don't do that," or "I don't like that," are said all too often instead of encouraging things like, "That feels good," or "One thing I love for you to do is . . ."

Because of the personal aspect of the sexual relationship, egos are easily injured. A mate who tries hard to please his partner, only to be criticized for his effort, may eventually stop trying. Hurt can turn a beautiful sexual experience into a bitter exchange of insults. Don't criticize *during* the physical act of lovemaking. If you have concerns, wait till the following day to discuss those issues. Approach the subject with humility and sensitivity and with much prayer.

Learning to verbalize can involve creating a sexual vocabulary. Sally and I conscripted terms from the Song of Solomon and developed words that we personally felt comfortable with. We laughed a lot and had a good time developing our intimate vocabulary. After years of marriage, it is amazing how comfortable we are with our terminology. Read the Song of Solomon out loud to each other. Have the wife take the part of the Shulammite and the husband, Solomon. You will laugh at some of the terminology, but you will begin to feel natural using sexual terms from this book. It is a beautiful poetic book and needs to be read often by couples.

Time Priority

Sexual freedom and blessing should increase the longer you're married. Moderate your past disappointments by considering the following fail-safe plan that changes your time priorities.

First, have a two-hour sexual experience weekly for the rest of your marriage. Schedule it if you have to, but make it happen. Plan an evening with no TV and without the children (or wait till they have gone to bed). You will be surprised at how creative you will become with your two-hour encounter.

The second commitment is very important as children come along. We suggest to couples that they take a twenty-four-hour time period alone together once a month. You can takes turns watching children with another couple who are doing the same thing. It's fun to sometimes have breakfast in bed, or sleep late, or have an early morning love-in. Be creative!

Begin now to establish a habit of making time for just the two of you. If a couple takes a night each week and a day every month to concentrate on their physical and emotional needs, most problems can be conquered together. Obviously, accomplishing this faithfully in the real world is hard. Yet, if you only take half of these days during the year, you will still characterize your sex life as being very satisfying. Begin now to establish a habit of making time for just the two of you. Your children will grow up and characterize your marriage as great. They will sense that you enjoy spending time together and that you love each other. That is the greatest gift you can give one another and your children.

What About Sex If You're Engaged?

Many counselors and well-meaning friends contend that premarital sex releases people from their inhibitions, strict morals, and religious hang-ups. If you are engaged and planning for a wedding, the commitment is there, and it's helpful to get to know each other, they say. Although we agree that certain hang-ups need emotional understanding, premarital sex is not the answer. Rather than freeing couples, premarital sex does just the opposite. It adds emotional pressure and puts you in bondage. It can rob you of the ability to clearly see God's will for marriage.

God's will is for sexual expression to occur only in the committed bonds of marriage. To God, sexual love expresses the more important spiritual commitment and unity between two married people. Sexual love, apart from marriage, reduces sex to a purely physical experience.

Some readers who are engaged have had premarital sex—perhaps you are involved in it right now. Recognize that it is sin. God didn't tell you to avoid premarital sex because He wanted to take away your fun. He has said no because He loves you and has a better way. If you have had premarital sex, I strongly encourage you to see a Christian counselor to help you seek God's forgiving perspective and to provide accountability.

Recognize that sin is forgivable regardless of the form it takes and that you need to ask God's forgiveness. If you are presently involved in premarital sex, you must now make a decision of your will to refrain. This will ensure a much better transition into marriage.

Because of our human makeup and the cultural fantasy that is perpetrated on couples today, sexual involvement before marriage causes an unnatural emotional response. An air of false excitement and expectancy alters the normal marital sexual response. Therefore, a couple involved prior to marriage may have problems adjusting when this false expectancy is removed after the wedding. Stopping now will allow God to begin to give you an anticipation of a sexual relationship in marriage that is free from guilt and open to godly expression.

Here are some practical ideas that will help with this struggle. First, make a spiritual and verbal commitment together to stop your premarital sexual activities. Men, take the leadership in this decision. Women are as responsible before the Lord as men, but God expects you to exhibit leadership. Your future wife will respect you even more for being strong here.

Here is an alternative to sexual involvement that has worked for many couples. Although actual sexual involvement frustrates a relationship, the real need is not sexual contact, but sexual recognition and communication. I suggest to couples that after making their commitment to stop all sexual involvement, they try the following. When you spend time together, just before you part, excuse yourselves from family or friends and privately kiss affectionately. Then both of you should express your excitement for future marital love. The statement should be brief and stated as unto the Lord. Yet it should be a complete expression of what you feel and need in general terms.

Express your excitement for future marital love. . . . A brief statement, communicated sincerely, can meet the need of being recognized and appreciated sexually.

Either the man or the woman might say, "Darling, I want you to know that I am excited about giving myself to you after the wedding. You are so attractive to me. I am going to pray specifically tonight that God will cause me to be a great lover to you after we marry." I have found that a brief statement, communicated sincerely, can meet the need of being recognized and appreciated sexually. Creativity by both will aid the development of sexual verbalization.

The key to this project is to *attempt this communication just as the couple is parting.* The sexual battle is usually lost not at the point of contact but at the point of putting yourself in a tempting situation. A couple who plans a day at the apartment watching television is in trouble from the start. Be verbally creative in meeting the other's need for physical attention.

We do not recommend a long engagement period for obvious reasons. If the wedding is a year away, consider moving up the date a few months. Usually it does not take more than four to six months to plan a wedding. This may not be possible, but it is easier to refrain sexually for six months than a year. If you still struggle with sexual involvement after these suggestions, the next step is to make yourselves accountable to someone else. Go together to a godly person in your church whom you can trust. Communicate your frustrations and make a commitment to do what is asked of you. Usually this type of accountability will do the job. Premarital counseling is a must if you desire for your marriage to have a good beginning.

Most importantly, remember that God created sex to be a very vital, fulfilling aspect of married life. Trust Him that He wants you to be more fulfilled than you even desire for yourself.

Notes

1. Tim and Beverly LaHaye, *The Act of Marriage* (Grand Rapids: Zondervan, 1976), 22.
2. We recommend the following four books on the sexual relationship, each written from a Christian perspective: Ed and Gaye Wheat, *Intended for Pleasure* (Grand Rapids: Baker, 1981); Linda Dillow and Lorraine Pintus, *Intimate Issues* (Colorado Springs, Waterbrook, 1999); Tim and Beverly La Haye, *The Act of Marriage* (Grand Rapids, Zondervan, 1976); and Clifford and Joyce Penner, *The Gift of Sex* (Waco, Tex.: Word 1981).

CHAPTER FOURTEEN

Financial Freedom

■ YEARS AGO, SUSAN, RECOGNIZED AS A SPIRITUAL
leader in our community, gave us an unexpected call. She had had major financial problems, and as her story unfolded, I (Sally) was surprised by how much financial stress she lived with. Through bitter tears, Susan revealed the disappointment and resentment that had built up over the years regarding her husband's financial habits. She had prayed and prayed, but she could not resist resentment in this area.

Her husband habitually let bills become past due before paying them. When they arrived in the mail, he would pay them—months later! All of this came to a head one day when she was shopping, unfortunately with three friends. She attempted to charge a dress and was refused because of their payment record. She was extremely embarrassed and humiliated, and decided to seek counsel immediately.

Susan was a godly wife, yet her story taught us the dangers to a marriage of poor or absent financial planning. Financial stress is a major problem in most marriages. Frequently couples spend restless nights over financial fears. Howard Dayton, president and founder of Crown Ministries, and Larry Burkett, president and founder of Christian Financial Concepts, agree that money-related issues are the number one cause instigating divorce. Indeed, 50 percent of couples who divorce cite finances as a major cause of disagreement. Few things generate more bitterness and resentment than money management.

Paul was certainly correct when he said to Timothy: "For the love of money is a root of all sorts of evil, and some by longing for it have wandered away from the faith and pierced themselves with many griefs" (1 Timothy 6:10).

The key phrase is "*some by longing for it.*" The first financial problem to be solved in marriage is attitude. Jesus taught, "For where your treasure is, there your heart will be also"(Matthew 6:21). What role does money play in your marriage? Is it a blessing from God or a source of strife and division? Can you trust God even if you have little money? Every couple needs to agree on some financial absolutes to minimize attitude problems. Mature, solid marriages exhibit a balance of both biblical attitudes and financial discipline. Some couples have great attitudes, but still become financially strapped because they fail to anticipate, record, and control their budget.

Financial responsibility requires proper attitudes and faithful control. Problems occur when our worldly desires conflict with God's perspective. The following chart illustrates how our culture subtly says one thing about financial responsibility, while God's Word says another.

A CONTRAST IN PERSPECTIVES

OUR CULTURE'S VIEW	GOD'S PERSPECTIVE
1. Fix your attention on money and possessions.	"But seek first His kingdom and His righteousness, and all these things will be added to you" (Matthew 6:33).
2. Wealth and possessions determine happiness in life.	"Beware, and be on your guard against every form of greed; for not even when one has an abundance does his life consist of his possessions" (Luke 12:15).
3. I'll be satisfied when I have more _____.	"He who loves money will not be satisfied with money, nor he who loves abundance with its income." (Ecclesiastes 5:10).
4. A man's wealth is his security.	"God is our refuge and strength, a very present help in trouble. Therefore we will not fear, though the earth should change, and though the mountains slip into the heart of the sea" (Psalm 46:1–2).
5. Financial success is the first priority.	Matthew 6:33 (above); also, "Not addicted to wine or pugnacious, but gentle, peaceable, free from the love of money" (1 Timothy 3:3).

You might be tempted to read quickly over these conflicting statements without a lot of personal conviction, but don't! Any person who has grown up in America cannot help but be influenced by our culture's thought patterns. The resulting pressures and conflicts are painful. The more couples follow God's thought patterns, the more freedom and blessing they will experience.

FINANCIAL FAITHFULNESS

To develop God's perspective on finances, first look at the example of Christ Himself. Jesus indicated that financial faithfulness is a thermometer of our relationship with God.

> *He who is faithful in a very little thing is faithful also in much; and he who is unrighteous in a very little thing is unrighteous also in much. Therefore, if you have not been faithful in the use of unrighteous wealth, who will entrust the true riches to you? And if you have not been faithful in the use of that which is another's, who will give you that which is your own? No servant can serve two masters; for either he will hate the one, and love the other, or else he will be devoted to one, and despise the other. You cannot serve God and wealth (Luke 16:10–13).*

Jesus compared money to a "little thing." He made it clear that in comparison to the important things in life, money is a small item. But this little thing is a big indicator of a man's faithfulness in serving God. The way a man handles his finances is a strong indicator of his trustworthiness as a person. Jesus asked (verse 11) how God could give His servants true riches if they could not be trusted financially. "The true riches" refers to the grace, hope, and peace that God gives to a person or couple who adheres to His perspective. Today, men crave money to find peace, but God says money does not bring peace or contentment.

Jesus said that every person is either trusting God or trusting in the security of money. Which do you trust as a person or couple? Couples who apply faith in finances experience blessing and peace. Couples who put their hope in money and possessions, however slightly, will struggle greatly. Often the struggle results in questioning God or feeling depressed. There is seldom any middle ground. We are convinced that God uses finances as few other things to teach dependence upon Him.

To find God's perspective on money, consider the following truths. Accepting these four perspectives will do more to insure financial peace of mind than anything the world can provide.

FOUR PILLARS OF FINANCIAL MATURITY

1. Ownership

Interestingly, I (Don) began to feel a compulsion to own things *the minute* I bought my first car. This compulsion forced me to compare myself with others who owned more, and I became discontent. Indeed, the advertising industry attempts to accomplish one thing: to make us dissatisfied with what we have. Advertisers tell us that their products will make us happier, whether the item is a house, car, stereo, or simply toothpaste. If their claims were true, there would be a lot of satisfied people in this country; but just the opposite is true. We always seem to want more. The Scriptures challenge that desire. King David, a man after God's own heart (1 Samuel 13:14; Acts 13:22), knew that true riches are found in knowing and giving to the mighty God.

> *Yours, O Lord, is the greatness and the power and the glory and the victory and the majesty, indeed everything that is in the heavens and the earth; Yours is the dominion, O Lord, and You exalt Yourself as head over all. Both riches and honor come from You, and You rule over all, and in Your hand is power and might; and it lies in Your hand to make great and to strengthen everyone. Now therefore, our God, we thank You, and praise Your glorious name. But who am I and who are my people that we should be able to offer as generously as this? For all things come from You, and from Your hand we have given You. For we are sojourners before You, and tenants, as all our fathers were; our days on the earth are like a shadow, and there is no hope. O Lord our God, all this abundance that we have provided to build You a house for Your holy name, it is from Your hand, and all is Yours (1 Chronicles 29:11–16).*

The Scriptures declare that God is head over all and that all things come from Him. We are simply stewards of God's possessions for a short time, and we are to worship and glorify Him with what He has given us. When others are in need, God desires that we should be free to give from our abundance. Sally and I often discuss how God uses the possessions He has given us to test us. God just wants to know if we see ourselves as *owners* or only *stewards* of His possessions.

Our first test came early in our marriage following the purchase of a brand-new washing machine. At the time, we were close friends with a couple in seminary who had very little money, and we told them they could wash their clothes in our machine. Every Saturday they came over to do laundry. Sally began to feel uneasy about this, thinking that the machine might break because of overuse, leaving us stuck with the repair bill. But we reminded ourselves that the machine was the Lord's and not ours. By faith, we had given all our possessions to Him to be used however He chose. As a result, we changed our attitude from one of possessiveness to gratefulness, believing that God had blessed us with a machine that others could use. That machine lasted more than ten years. It was never repaired, and we later sold it in a garage sale. God faithfully takes care of all His possessions!

Sally and I don't struggle very long anymore with possessiveness. It seems the Lord always reminds us who gave it, who plans to use it, and who is going to pay the bills. And He reminds us who may even take it away! We continually give Him our lives, our possessions, our money, our children and families, and so on. He has repeatedly tested our hearts in giving. However, in return, He has given us peace and contentment, along with more material blessings than we could have ever dreamt. Being a steward is very freeing indeed. However, when we occasionally take ownership back, peace becomes elusive, our struggle returns, and God graciously reminds us of who owns it all.

According to Deuteronomy, these struggles help us to recognize our motives and test our obedience: "Remember how the Lord your God led you all the way . . . to humble you and to test you in order to know what was in your heart, whether or not you would keep his commands" (8:2 NIV).

2. God's Providence

Another constant struggle for Christians is that of comparing their financial resources to others. Feeling superior over those with less, or hating and resenting those with more can destroy God's perspective in your life. There is even a great tendency among some today to feel proud about their simple lifestyles. God clearly speaks about differences in financial situations.

> But you, why do you judge your brother? Or you again, why do you regard your brother with contempt? For we will all stand before the judgment seat of God. For it is written, "As I live," says the Lord, "Every knee shall bow to Me, and every tongue shall give praise to God." So then each one of us will give an account of himself to God. Therefore let us not judge one another anymore (Romans 14:10–13).

> The Lord makes poor and rich; He brings low, He also exalts. He raises the poor from the dust, He lifts the needy from the ash heap to make them sit with nobles, and inherit a seat of honor; for the pillars of the earth are the Lord's, and He set the world on them (1 Samuel 2:7–8).

God leaves no doubt on this issue: He makes both rich and poor. There are no accidents in business. Whatever your state, God put you there, not luck or breaks. We have all seen sure deals collapse and totally hopeless deals pay tremendous financial dividends. Don't waste your time blaming or watching others, because the one to look to is Christ Himself. It is not man, but God, who causes all things to happen.

The issue is not what you have . . . but what you do with what you have.

The issue is not what you have or don't have, but what you do with what you have. You are accountable to God for what He has given you. God's ultimate purpose is to conform us to the image of His Son, Jesus Christ, and He uses finances to shape us. Can you thank Him at all times for what you have or don't have? Everything we have is a gift from Him, and is a part of His plan for our lives.

3. Contentment

So, if we do not really own anything, and God is the one who makes rich or poor, what should be our attitude? Apart from basic food and clothing, we must recognize that there is no real hope in things—there is only the *appearance* of hope. So be content with food and clothing if that's all you have.

As Paul wrote, "For we have brought nothing into the world, so we cannot take anything out of it either. If we have food and covering, with these we shall be content." He then warned, "But those who want to get rich fall into temptation and a snare and many foolish and harmful desires which plunge men into ruin and destruction"

God is the only one who can give you genuine contentment.

(1 Timothy 6:7–9). The writer of Hebrews also wrote, "Make sure that your character is free from the love of money, being content with what you have; for He Himself has said, 'I will never desert you, nor will I ever forsake you'" (13:5).

If you have wealth, or desire it, then you must be very cautious. Remember that God is still responsible for meeting your needs. "He Himself has said, 'I will never desert you, nor will I forsake you.'" Trust Him to meet your needs. He has promised to do so; and in many cases He has given us many of our wants as well. And consider this insight from wise King Solomon. "Give me neither poverty nor riches; feed me with the food that is my portion, that I not be full and deny You and say, 'Who is the Lord?' or that I not be in want and steal, and profane the name of my God" (Proverbs 30:8–9).

It is human nature to always want more. God is the only one who can give us genuine contentment. As hard as it is to grasp, you must realize the difference between needs, wants, and desires, and claim God's promises to meet your needs. The ability to be content in these promises is a major ingredient in God's recipe for financial maturity. Throughout your married life, you will experience times of real financial need. Such times offer wonderful opportunities to acknowledge your needs to God, ask Him to meet those needs, and then watch Him answer.

There is such contentment and joy in answered prayer! Over many years Sally has kept a careful journal of prayers and answers to prayer. Our faith has grown tremendously as we read of God's past faithfulness. This gives us faith as we face the future. Our children also learned the faithfulness of God because we often recounted ways in which He met the family's needs. Now, as adults, they do not doubt His care for us.

Paul wrote that Christians should let God know needs and wants. "Be anxious for nothing, but in everything by prayer and supplication with thanksgiving let your requests be known to God. And the peace of God, which surpasses all comprehension, will guard your hearts and your minds in Christ Jesus" (Philippians 4:6–7). These verses don't mean that God will give you your wants; but if He doesn't, He will give you His peace. And what more could you want than the peace of God, which surpasses your ability to comprehend?

4. Security

The last pillar of God's perspective on finances is security. Real security is not found in the uncertainty of riches. Instead, security is found by fixing your hope on God, who gives you everything you need. Scripture abounds with this concept, both in finances and in human relationships. Paul wrote to Timothy: "Instruct those who are rich in this present world not to be conceited or to fix their hope on the uncertainty of riches, but on God, who richly supplies us with all things to enjoy. Instruct them to do good, to be rich in good works, to be generous and ready to share, storing up for themselves the treasure of a good foundation for the future, so that they may take hold of that which is life indeed" (1 Timothy 6:17–19).

If you place your hope and security in God to the point that you actually share with others, then God promises "life indeed." Faith is acting on a statement from God, even when it goes against human reason. Financial freedom and security are in God, not in earthly possessions.

These four pillars of financial freedom—ownership, God's providence, contentment, and security—give you the foundation to use money properly in your life. When you understand that His gracious hand has given all of your material goods, you will be more careful how you give, save, invest, and spend. Prayerfully, you will become faithful stewards of God's money and possessions.

UNDERSTANDING AND APPLYING:
GIVING, SAVING, INVESTING, AND SPENDING

The four financial pillars are tested and proved in the practical financial activities of giving, saving, investing, and spending. Scripture instructs us in each of these important activities. Develop a careful strategy for each one.

Giving

The importance of giving financially to the church (or Temple in Old Testament times) and to others is a theme throughout Scripture. The Old and New Testaments give very specific direction on amounts to give, when to give, and to whom to give.

Paul instructed each believer to put aside money in order to give regularly, based on how much God has given you. (See 1 Corinthians 16:1–2.) We Christians are to set aside the money *before* we spend, or we won't have it to give. In the Old Testament, men gave 20 percent as required by the Law. If you lived in Israel, the 20 percent was divided between the government (under the rule of God) and the Temple (also under the rule of God). Thus, 10 percent went to the Lord's work, and 10 percent went to keep the government operating.

In the New Testament, we are to ask the Spirit of God to direct our giving. "Each one must do just as he has purposed in his heart" (2 Corinthians 9:7). For some, it will be 10 percent, some 20 percent, and some more. Give with a gracious spirit and not one of "compulsion, for God loves a cheerful giver" (verse 7). Curiously, surveys show that *the more* a couple earns, the more possessive and materialistic they become. Each couple should take seriously God's command to give liberally.

Why does God desire that we give generously? Giving is a redemptive act—God graciously and tenderly lets you help to meet the needs of others. Doing so forces your eyes off your needs and yourself. It allows you to keep the right perspective on who really owns your money, and who gives it. You will receive a blessing from God if you give sacrificially to others. I challenge you to let the Holy Spirit tell you what to give and to whom.

The Scripture instructs us to give to those who minister to us (Galatians 6:6). The ability of God's full-time servants to be available depends on our faithfulness to support them financially, be that in our local churches, Christian organizations, or missionary agencies. Above all, we are to be visionary in our giving. Trust the One who has given so much to you. God wants to use you as a reservoir to meet needs! Allow God to use you greatly so He can enlist you as a supplier for His work.

Giving triggers a blessing cycle: The more you give, the more God gives. Jesus expressed it this way: "Give, and it will be given to you. They will pour into your lap a good measure—pressed down, shaken together, and running over. For by your standard of measure it will be measured to you in return" (Luke 6:38).

Even when you loan money to others, consider giving the money instead. Giving releases you from always wondering if the recipient will repay the loan. Loaning money can cause you to become resentful and bitter toward the person.

I am not saying that a loan should not be repaid, but God says your contentment should not depend on another person's lack of responsibility. Always keep an open and giving spirit toward others. God does amazing work in our lives when we give unselfishly. (See the command to give generously in Deuteronomy 15:10–11.)

Beyond your regular tithing to the church and your offerings to the church and Christian organizations, here are some creative ways to give out of your abundance:

- Food: when someone is out of a job, has a baby, or has a death in the family
- Clothing: for others less fortunate or to mission organizations
- Furniture: for church people or young couples in need
- Cars: for a missionary or pastor who is in need
- Stock: given as a benefit to the recipient and you

Rather than selling your items, ask God to whom you should give it. Your part is to give and God's part is to bless.

Saving

Saving is vital to financial peace and joy. We often deal with couples struggling with debt, or those who have no money at the end of the month. A poor family with a little money in savings is much freer financially than a rich family who is overextended.

Scripture says there is wisdom in saving for future needs. According to Proverbs 21:20, "There is precious treasure and oil in the dwelling of the wise, but a foolish man swallows it up." Similarly, Proverbs says concerning a father's savings, "A good man leaves an inheritance to his children's children, and the wealth of the sinner is stored up for the righteous" (13:22).

We encourage couples to begin a habit of saving, no matter how small the amount, even if it's only $50 a month. If you run out of money at the end of the month, the pressure is much less if you have an additional $500 in savings. A good rule of thumb is to save 10 percent of your salary each month. Saving, like giving, needs to come *before* and not after spending. If you begin saving when first married, you will be amazed how much you will accumulate for a home, college education, and emergencies. Money in savings can tide you over if a job is lost. Most Americans are one paycheck away from bankruptcy. Are you?

Investing

God's Word teaches key principles for making wise investments and saving. First, avoid get-rich-quick schemes. Build security slowly, Proverbs warns us (21:5; 28:22). We believe the best strategy is to put a little aside each pay period.

Second, do not have a strong desire to get rich, remembering Paul's warning, "But those who want to get rich fall into temptation and a snare and many foolish and harmful desires which plunge men into ruin and destruction" (1 Timothy 6:9). Obtain money by hard work, for "Wealth obtained by fraud dwindles, but the one who gathers by labor increases it" (Proverbs 13:11).

Third, always seek counsel from someone with successful experience. (See Proverbs 20:18.) Those who are older and more mature often have more wisdom. Don't be afraid to ask questions when it comes to investing. Find someone who will take the time to listen and help you create a plan. It is not wise to borrow against projected future income to make investments, or to cover expenditures in the present. Also, be careful about seeking counsel from someone who is selling an investment product or service. Their advice might be biased toward making the sale.

Finally, remember that security is not in wealth but in the gracious hand of God, who has ultimate control of our lives.

> Come now, you who say, "Today or tomorrow we will go to such and such a city, and spend a year there and engage in business and make a profit." Yet you do not know what your life will be like tomorrow. You are just a vapor that appears for a little while and then vanishes away. Instead, you ought to say, "If the Lord wills, we will live and also do this or that." But as it is, you boast in your arrogance; all such boasting is evil. Therefore, to one who knows the right thing to do, and does not do it, to him it is sin (James 4:13–17).

Uncontrolled Spending (Debt)

Debt has literally destroyed many marriages, and the national debt may lead our country to financial collapse. (See *The Coming Economic Earthquake* by Larry Burkett.) Though an improving economy at the end of the 1990s has lessened the debt somewhat, it remains a staggering $5.7 trillion. Debt is considered normal today, both on the national and personal level. Personal debt is at an all-time high, and personal bankruptcy filings "are expected to exceed two million by the year 2001."[1] According to the American Bankruptcy Institute, more than 90 percent of those bankruptcies will be the result of out-of-control credit card spending.[2]

Credit card debt is extremely stressful in marriage. Most financial problems occur in the spending area. "Americans spend on average $1.10 for every $1.00 they earn."[3] You should know at all times how much you owe so you won't go deeper into debt. And then begin to escape your credit card debt by paying off high interest cards first. Then commit to make purchases with cash. If you have credit cards, pay the balance each month so you don't accumulate debt. Limit yourself to two or three credit cards at the most.

Paul exhorts the Romans to "owe nothing to anyone except to love one another" (Romans 13:8). Although he was not speaking directly of finances, the application is valid.

Establish a budget to govern your purchases. If you don't do this, you will have problems in your marriage. Often two people come together in marriage with totally different ways of looking at spending. Pay off high monthly payments (car and house) as quickly as possible. When your car is paid off, resist the urge to buy a new car. Instead, put the same money in the bank for the purchase of a newer car when needed. Buying a newer car with limited mileage may be a better investment than a brand-new car. If you have a thirty-year loan on your house, begin paying an extra $100–150 a month toward the principle. You will be amazed at how fast the house gets paid off. Taking out a fifteen-year loan is better than a thirty-year loan because of the thousands of dollars of interest saved.

The following chart, "Questions to Ask Before Spending," is an example of the type of questions you might ask yourself to determine if your expenditures are in line with God's perspective. Study this with your spouse.

Questions to Ask Before Spending

QUESTION	SCRIPTURE
1. Is my spending motivated by the love of money?	1 Timothy 6:9; 1 John 2:15
2. Has God already led me to meet a need with this money?	2 Corinthians 8:14
3. Do I have a doubt about it?	Romans 14:23
4. Have I given God an opportunity to use it?	Psalm 37:5; Proverbs 10:3
5. Will this spending hinder my spiritual growth?	1 Corinthians 6:12; Hebrews 12:1; 2 Corinthians 11:3
6. Is this spending a good investment?	Proverbs 20:14
7. Does it put me into debt?	Proverbs 22:7
8. Will it be meaningful to my family?	1 Timothy 3:4; 5:8

Each of these factors should be considered when making a financial decision. Wise counsel from another person helps. Couples who keep tight control over their purchases will have little trouble keeping God's perspective on money management. Peace and contentment will be their reward.

ABOUT A BUDGET

Any family that desires to get control of their finances should start by setting up a monthly budget. A budget is simply a projection of future income and expenses. A simple budget really does not take much time but, over a period of five to six months, can help a couple manage their finances. Typically the budget won't be absolutely accurate at first, but it should be reviewed and adjusted faithfully each month. The couple can then evaluate any problem areas together, find solutions, and adjust their spending patterns. Several good financial management books and computer programs are available. We highly recommend the resources of Christian Financial Concepts in Gainesville, Georgia.[4] Also, a twelve-week course on managing finances God's way has been produced by Crown Ministries in Longwood, Florida, and has changed the lives of thousands of couples.[5]

Couples are never more aware of their lack of oneness than when they are dealing with finances.

It is very important to compare your actual expenses each month with your budget. Then you can see exactly what you are spending and where you tend to overspend. A budget's value is realized as you continuously review and update it. Couples who plan usually tend to make do, and their money goes farther.

Couples are never more aware of their lack of oneness than when they are dealing with finances. Since each of you will have different ways of handling money, it is essential to discuss how you are going to approach financial problems. You must agree on your priorities for purchasing and establish your financial values. Apply the faith commitments of Genesis 1 and 2 to your finances. Agree together to transfer to the Lord all of your possessions. Conflict results when there is no mutual commitment or when one spouse acts independently from the other.

INDIVIDUAL RESPONSIBILITIES FOR FINANCES

Men have the primary responsibility for the financial integrity of the home. God has instructed husbands to provide for their families (1 Timothy 5:8), and He has never changed that mandate. The man is responsible to provide for the family's welfare through working, though the wife also may work. (A layoff or poor health may at times shift the responsibility to the woman.) The husband also has the chief responsibility to control the expenditures, pay the bills, initiate giving, and save for a rainy day. That does not mean he is smarter, more gifted, or even more successful at these things, but he is *primarily* responsible. With humility, take your leadership very seriously.

If your wife is more gifted than you are in the area of managing finances and desires to help, give her major responsibility. The husband still must bear the financial pressure, being sure there is enough to pay the bills and grow the savings, even as the wife does the bookkeeping. If the husband begins to hedge on his responsibility, however, or if the wife struggles, she should give the financial record keeping back to him.

Wives, you must be careful when you take such responsibility not to "put your husbands down" in their areas of weakness. Neither of you should belittle the other when it comes to money. Remember, you are "joint heirs" of the grace of life. If a couple communicates well in the area of finances, their marriage will exhibit peace.

The husband . . . should always seek his wife's input and advice and include her in financial decisions.

Although the husband should take leadership with the family finances, he should always seek his wife's input and advice and include her in financial decisions. If the wife works outside the home, try not to become dependent on her income. It would be wise to invest her salary. This will allow you to set money aside for the future and it will also give your wife the potential to stop working if she so desires. It can give her more flexibility to respond to the needs of any children at home. Becoming too dependent on her salary will eventually affect how a mother cares for her children. Don't allow a desire for material things to compete with the needs of the children. After the children leave home, she may want to return to work. However, she should always be free to work or not to work.

Both the husband and wife should maintain a spirit of joy, freedom, and creativity in the household. Some people become extremely creative when they are low on money. They have joy in giving and yet have a tight budget. Refinishing furniture, selling crafts, having garage sales, and performing do-it-yourself repairs on the home are among the creative money savers that low-budget families adopt. When their circumstances are approached by faith, low-budget families can often be happier than couples who have more financial resources.

Most couples will struggle financially, especially early in marriage. It seems that God uses money more than anything else to teach dependence on Him. When you struggle, reread this chapter to review God's perspective, and the Holy Spirit will encourage and direct you.

NOTES

1. March 1998 study by the WEFA Group; the projected figure of 2.2 million bankruptcies by 2001 comes from Visa U. S. A., the credit card company, based on the WEFA report. See "2 Million Bankruptcies by 2001," 14 July 1998, at http://www.visa.com.

2. Elif Sinanoglu, "I Chucked My Credit Cards and Saved More Than $150 a Month," Money, August 1996, 64.

3. Larry Burkett, Money Matters Newsletter, April 1997, Christian Financial Concepts, Gainesville, Ga.

4. Contact Christian Financial Concepts at 1-800-722-1976.

5. Contact Crown Ministries at 1-407-331-6000.

CHAPTER FIFTEEN

Loving Those In-laws

■ ALTHOUGH IN-LAW JOKES ARE COMMON, MOST couples fail to find this relationship amusing. Few fully realize the potential stress, anxiety, and hurt that can come if they are unprepared for potential in-law problems. To be forewarned is to be forearmed!

About the time wedding invitations are sent, wedding showers begin, and plans for the ceremony are under way, couples realize that parents usually have strong opinions about the wedding. By the time the wedding arrives, simple parent-child relationships may have turned into a complex minefield of disagreement and hurt. The bride cries, "Oh, why can't Mom understand?" and the groom wonders, "How did I upset them so much?" Caught off guard, the couple has unintentionally created a source of conflict that cuts deeply into the emotional needs of both the couple and their parents. Before they realize it, their in-laws have already developed opinions about their future son- or daughter-in-law.

The toughest aspect of preparing for a positive in-law relationship is you don't get a practice run! Your introduction to them can be either tremendously personal and meaningful, or negative and hurtful. After all, the future of their son or daughter is at stake. Only after having children of our own have we understood this pressure. When our oldest daughter was only eight, Don began to realize that one day some guy would tell us he deserved our little girl. And sure enough, eighteen years later, he did! Fortunately, God was gracious in giving us a fine son-in-law. We know parents desire close relationships with their future sons- or daughters-in-law, but their initial introduction can sometimes be emotionally stressful on them.

Sometimes these introductions take place while planning the wedding. Other times couples have known each other a long time. In our transient society, it is common for a son or daughter to bring his or her future mate home just weeks or months before the wedding. Forcing two families who are usually complete strangers to come together amiably is not a natural thing. In fact, it is a miracle if it goes well.

DON'S IN-LAW BEGINNING

I can still remember meeting Sally's parents for the first time, *only one week before the wedding.* The reason was that we met and dated in a different state than Sally's home, and we were engaged within three months. Mom and Pop Hill are extremely likable people, and the slight problems we encountered were due to the awkward situation, and not them.

I arrived in Boulder, Sally's hometown, about 2 p.m. I had stopped earlier to clean up and put a suit on before meeting Sally's family. Since they lived in the mountains above Boulder, I decided to drop in on Sally's dad at work to get directions to their house. Pop was a well-known auto mechanic in Boulder. When I entered his shop, the supervisor told me Mr. Hill was working under a car, several cars down the line.

I was spotlessly dressed, overly aggressive, and somewhat nervous. I walked up to the car and said to his feet, which were sticking out, "Mr. Hill, I am Don Meredith." Stunned, Mr. Hill got about halfway out from under the car before I grabbed his greasy hand and said "Hello!" He was embarrassed about the grease, and we both felt rather awkward. He gave me directions to their house, and I left with my clean suit and greasy hand.

That night the pressure escalated. I quickly discovered that Sally's house had only one bathroom, and you had to go through her parents' bedroom to get there! After going to bed, my worst fears came true. I had to use the bathroom. I'm a very modest person. I waited as long as I could, and then I walked through their bedroom. I flushed the toilet and it sounded like Niagara Falls. I was so embarrassed! I felt emotional pressure from that point forward.

Later in the week we had a serious problem concerning the phone expenses. Sally and I had made some long-distance calls related to our wedding plans. However, we forgot to tell the Hills that we intended to pay for the calls. All the calls were long, full of questions, congratulations, and general catch-up, and they were all expensive. Finally, Sally mentioned her parents' concern over all the calls. This was perfectly understandable, but in light of the tension, I reacted strongly against Sally. I took pride in my financial responsibility and felt my integrity being questioned.

These problems sound foolish as I retell them, but at the time they were very serious. Four people, who under normal circumstances would have hit it off perfectly, started out on the wrong foot. Since then, things have smoothed out, and, by God's grace, our in-law problems have been minor. Our family greatly enjoys our times at Sally's parents' home, and we all look forward to our visits. This is true of my family as well.

Many couples start off wrong and are then burdened with poor in-law relationships for years. Once again, it will take faith to develop positive in-law relationships. For this reason, couples need to know what God says concerning in-laws.

LEAVING ONE'S FATHER AND MOTHER

God established His foundational thoughts concerning in-laws at the time He created marriage: "For this cause a man shall leave his father and his mother, and be joined to his wife; and they shall become one flesh" (Genesis 2:24). In this passage the man is commanded to leave upon marriage, yet throughout the Old Testament numerous examples are given of women leaving. The Hebrew word used in Genesis 2:24 for "leave" means to abandon or break off completely. God is saying that before a significant new relationship can begin, the old parent-child relationship must cease. By this, God means that in issues of authority the parents no longer have responsibility.

After twenty or so years of responding to parental authority, there [is] a tendency to continue the dependence even after marriage.

God does not mean that the parental relationship should end altogether. Obviously, *children should never stop honoring their parents.* God is not against parents. His strong command to men and women is to put their full trust in God and their mates. Total mate satisfaction and respect can occur only when a couple has established a new primary allegiance.

God knew that after twenty or so years of responding to parental authority, there would be a tendency to continue the dependence even after marriage. Therefore, God indicates that one dependent relationship should end so that another can begin.

Although the parents' authority ends with the creation of the new relationship, the couple's responsibility to honor their parents continues. Deuteronomy 5:16 tells us that the duty of a child is to honor his parents. This word "honor" speaks primarily of valuing at a high price, showing deep respect or reverential awe. In marriage, parental experience and advice are very important. Still, decisions must be made by the couple apart from parental control. Even though parental advice may be necessary at times, it is better for the couple to go to the parents and not vice versa.

WAYS THAT COUPLES DON'T LEAVE

During our counseling, we have observed four common ways couples fail to leave their parents. These examples of failure to leave can be so subtle that couples may feel frustration without even understanding why.

1. Parental Wealth and Social Benefits.

This problem reveals a conscious or subconscious dependence on parents for financial or social benefits to the point that the couple fails to acknowledge their own independence. For instance, a husband may allow his mother to criticize his wife so that the financial relationship with his parents won't be endangered. Other couples tend to spend too much time at the home of parents because of social or financial advantages. This dependence may hinder the development of the new relationship. This can be a two-way problem when some parents spend too much time with their children, often resulting in the in-law child resenting the new parents.

2. Parental Model.

Some couples, again consciously or subconsciously, compare some area of their mate's performance to that of their parents. This comparison can ultimately cause dissatisfaction. I have seen men become completely disillusioned with their wives because they do not develop a particular housekeeping habit or cooking ability that the husbands' mother may have had. On the other hand, I have seen women lose respect for their husbands because they did not project the same financial stability as their fathers. These expectations are especially true in early marriage. Unfair comparisons like these can destroy marital oneness and commitment.

3. Parental Approval.

Some mates remain dependent on their parents' approval after marriage due to an extremely strong or domineering parent. The need for parental approval may block trust in their new mate. Women have told me that they love their husbands, yet they perform to please their own mothers because they need Mom's approval. These new wives may be frustrated if their mothers disapprove of their husbands. They clean house the way Mom would want, discipline the children with Mom in mind, all the while hoping for her recognition or approval. Women who need approval in this way will jeopardize their husbands' sense of security and leadership. Similarly, men who are overly dependent on their father's approval can lower their wives' respect for them.

4. Parental Relationship Substitute.

Nothing deflates a spouse more than for the mate to continue looking to their parents to meet primary emotional needs, especially when the spouse's own emotional needs go unmet as a result. We have counseled men and women who continue to call or go see their parents about most key issues in their lives, sometimes before they consult their mate. They give affection, receive most of their security, share their criticism, and even express most of their creative abilities with their parents. This behavior not only excludes their mates, but deeply hurts and divides them. It also creates confusion and a lack of dependence on the spouse.

HOW TO TRULY CLEAVE TO YOUR MATE

Failing to leave your parents hurts them in the long run as well as your mate and yourself. Agree together on a mutual plan to leave the authority of your parents. Here are several suggestions for truly leaving your parents' authority and cleaving to your spouse for help, comfort, and advice in decision making.

First, evaluate everyone's needs.

Parents are not your enemy; they just do what comes naturally. If misunderstandings arise between you and your parents or parents-in-law, don't strike out at them for loving you, even if their method is wrong. Since both mates have an innate need to be at peace with their parents, don't be disrespectful to your in-laws.

Instead, when frustrations occur, analyze the situation with your mate and agree together about the cause. Evaluate everyone's real need, what went wrong, and most importantly, look for a *creative solution.* If either mate has wronged a parent, ask forgiveness. If a decision is needed to protect the integrity of the marriage, make it together. Then look for a creative way to communicate this to the parents.

Second, maintain privacy.

Commit together never to share any intimate needs or decisions with either set of parents without your mate's permission. A husband may be dreaming of a new car, and his wife simply mentions it to her dad. The father then voices his disapproval to her husband, and the husband feels betrayed. Couples must build their lives together, and everything should remain private unless agreed otherwise.

Third, handle critical statements with care.

Never be critical about your mate to your parents or allow them to make critical statements about your mate. Sharing something critical about your mate is damaging, not only to your mate, but also to your parents. Why? Because parents never forget the problems shared, and rarely allow your mate to change (in their minds). Your parents naturally become overly protective of their own children. We know one wife who revealed a financial irresponsibility by her mate in the first year of their marriage, and her parents are still bringing it up after twenty years. Parents don't have the opportunity to see your mate change and improve as you do. They only have your comments to go on.

If in-laws tend to visit too much, agree on a plan; then the child of that in-law should talk to the parent

Do yourself and your parents another favor. The next time they make a critical statement about your mate, respond with a strong but loving rebuff. I know of one man whose mother was just leading up to a critical remark about his wife. He interrupted with, "Mom, I love you a lot, but please don't be critical of my wife. I want you to know she is God's gift to me, and I don't want to hear those criticisms."

His mother hastily replied, "Don't be silly; I wasn't going to be critical of her."

The wise son responded with, "Forgive me, Mom. I just so want you two to be friends, because I love you both so much." He was strong but kind to his mother.

Fourth, develop a plan for visiting in-laws.

Before visiting your parents, especially early in marriage, agree on the *length* of time that you plan to stay. One idea is to allow your wife to go home to her parents a few days earlier than you in order to give her parents the attention they need before you arrive. Men, occasionally go home to see your parents alone. Sometimes parents need time alone with their children after they are married. If you live close to either parent, this will not be a problem.

Most importantly, when visiting as a couple, let your mate have the freedom to love his own parents. If you feel somewhat ignored while at your spouse's parents' home, anticipate and discuss it before your next visit.

For example, you might want to go somewhere with your wife while at her home. Since she is the one who is naturally accepted in her home, take her aside and tell her your plan. That way she can announce the need for you both to go somewhere at the appropriate time. She takes total responsibility for the decision. You are free from the possibility of hurting her parents, and they better understand and accept the decision. If in-laws tend to visit too much, agree on a plan; then the child of that in-law should talk to the parent. Don't put your mate in a position that might offend or hurt your parents. It's easier to deal with your parent yourself so your spouse is still approved and not involved in tough discussions.

Fifth, be considerate toward your in-laws.

Ask your mother-in-law and father-in-law what they would prefer that you call them. Let them know you will be glad to call them Mom and Dad if they prefer. You may be more comfortable calling them by their first names, especially if you have known them for a long time. Asking gives them the freedom to say, "It's up to you."

Another thing that demonstrates consideration is dropping your parents-in-law an occasional card, thanking them for their role in your mate's life or for allowing you to visit. Courtesy with parents not only brings joy to them and to you, but increases the possibility of an exciting grandparent-child relationship in the future.

MONEY MATTERS WITH PARENTS OR IN-LAWS

A key area that can bring either gratitude or resentment is receiving financial assistance. The husband should work out a definite plan for receiving money offered by parents on either side, and then communicate that plan to both sets of parents. If a husband communicates with his father-in-law the first time that parent attempts to give the couple a gift, her father will always respect his son-in-law. We discourage parental loans in almost every situation, but parents should have the freedom to give gifts to their children. However, a husband needs to set boundaries that ensure his authority as well as the parents' respect.

By nature, most parents are givers and children are takers. This tendency doesn't necessarily end when the child marries. Take the example of going out to dinner. Parents have always bought dinners for their children. How does a child begin to be an adult around the parent? These are the questions that need to be addressed. Who pays? When do you pay? Who invited whom?

As with most problems, communication is the key. A good rule of thumb is to address the issues before they ever come up. Every once in awhile, take your parents out to dinner. If you offer to pay, and your parents reject the offer, then you have done your part. If your parents ask you to go somewhere that is clearly beyond your means (i.e., a trip, expensive restaurant, etc.), make sure to discuss what they think is appropriate to contribute.

Because moms and dads handle money differently, they also have different expectations of their adult children. Make sure that you talk to *both* of your parents about money issues so that resentment does not develop. Remember that resentment over money issues can cause great bitterness.

Parents and parents-in-law can be a source of joy or a source of irritation.

Wise is the couple who has a plan, communicates that plan (to all parents), and is flexible in meeting the needs of all parties. Be sure to keep your own marriage healthy. This will communicate to the parents, more than anything else, that you and your mate are one.

A WORD TO PARENTS AND PARENTS-IN-LAW

This chapter is for couples, of course, but we have included a final section that you may want to let your parents read. Explain that the chapter on relationships with parents and in-laws has been helpful and it includes a chapter they would enjoy reading (by a couple who have been parents for thirty years and in-laws for a shorter time).

Regarding her married children, one mother said, "Lord, give me the wisdom to bite my tongue." Our hope for parents is that you trust the Lord with your children so that you won't need to bite your tongue. Let them make some mistakes (by your standards). Parents tend to give advice on how they would run things, how they would spend money, how they would raise kids, and so on. If your children don't do what they know you expect them to do, they may feel guilt.

Realize that times have changed, not scriptural values. Your children may live in nicer housing than you did at the same age. Your children may leave their children with childcare far more often than you did. Avoid developing a critical attitude. Criticism will wound your children. No one enjoys being with a critical person. Over time your children may begin to distance themselves from you, and you may destroy your opportunity to watch them grow to maturity and to enjoy them as friends.

It is wise to say to your children, "Listen to what I say, and then do as you please." This assures you of always having the freedom to offer advice and suggestions based on your experience, yet it assures your children that they can make their own decisions. This leaves the door of communication open for all of you. Allow them to then do as they please without further unsolicited advice or an "I-told-you-so" attitude.

Remember this: Criticizing your children or their spouses will only drive them away from you. If it continues, they will avoid you and will dread their times with you. Think before using the statements, "You never . . ." and "You always. . . ." Also, don't do something nice for your children, and then remind them of it. Sometimes it is best to just drop a subject than to cause conflict.

Don't forget to be sensitive to their need for privacy. If you live in close proximity, call before you visit and *don't overstay your welcome or visit too often*. Instead, establish a visiting pattern that fits everyone. Exchange visits at appropriate times. When grandchildren come, more communication will be required. Exchanged visits then become even more important. Never assume your children won't mind if you just drop over, especially early in marriage. When both husband and wife work, their time in the evenings and on weekends may be their only time for privacy. Be as considerate of them as you would your other friends.

Make sure your daughter-in-law or son-in-law feels welcome in your home and with your family. Balance your gifts equally to your married children and their spouses. Treat them as part of the family and they will be. If you do, God will use you in their lives in ways you would never dream. This may be their first opportunity to observe mature Christian parents. Fathers, initiate time with your son-in-law so the daughter can spend time with her mom.

Finally, many couples today have several sets of in-laws if their parents have been divorced. This obviously can cause problems, especially around the holidays. If this is the case with you, allow your children and spouses to visit all the parents involved.

With sensitivity and love, you can become a source of joy to your children all the days of your lives.

CHAPTER SIXTEEN

God's Testing Times

◈ I REMEMBER WHEN I (DON) FIRST BEGAN TO understand the biblical importance of trials as a new Christian. My initial assumption was that successful Christians missed the most trials, similar to running through a minefield and dodging the mines. Years of study, counseling, and personal experience have changed my perspective. I've hit a few of those mines, and you probably have also. Indeed, many of the trials we face in marriage are universal. Therefore, we should identify them and be prepared to deal with them.

Here is God's perspective on trials: "For you have been called for this purpose, since Christ also suffered for you, leaving you an example for you to follow in His steps" (1 Peter 2:21).

At first, I could not imagine that it was actually part of God's plan for me to experience trials. But the more I thought about the above verse and its message, the more it made sense. If I had been called to salvation by Jesus Christ and given His inheritance, it seemed reasonable that I would be called to share in His suffering also.

The same is true with our marriages. Without trials we probably would not depend on the Lord very often. As husbands and wives, our human natures are bent toward lustful desires and self-centeredness. In His grace, God reminds us through trials of our need for Him in the marriage. Trials humble us and cause us to depend on God. When a husband is humbled, he tends to notice his spouse instead of himself. Similarly, a wife facing trials, tough as they are, finds they are redemptive in her life. Often the only anchor a husband and wife have during a trial is the reality of Christ and His Word.

GOD'S PURPOSE IN TRIALS

God's purpose for allowing trials in your life and marriage is revealed in James

1:2–4: "Consider it all joy, my brethren, when you encounter various trials, knowing that the testing of your faith produces endurance. And let endurance have its perfect result, so that you may be perfect and complete, lacking in nothing." Several things stand out in this passage. First, James says *when*, not if, you encounter trials. As a Christian, you will definitely encounter trials. They are not an option. Further, these trials will result from a variety of sources. The word various comes from a Greek word that means "multicolored." Trials come in many hues and from different sources.

In a world where unfulfilled marriages are robbing people of their best hope in relationships, having endurance is no small thing. God promises that the result of endurance will be that you may be "perfect and complete, lacking in nothing." Trials not only develop endurance but maturity. The phrase "lacking in nothing" means equipped with every resource. Endurance, complete maturity, and being equipped with every resource—that's quite a promise!

Trials . . . develop endurance, . . . complete maturity, and [equip us] with every resource—that's quite a promise!

Maintaining a joyful spirit when either you or your mate is experiencing a trial is not a natural human response, but a faith-oriented response. Christ suffered because He knew that by going to the Cross you and I would someday be with Him in eternity. "For the 'joy' set before Him [He] endured the cross, despising the shame" (Hebrews 12:2). He looked beyond the suffering of the Cross to those of us who would spend eternity with Him. When it comes to trials, we must do the same thing—look beyond the suffering.

James also indicates that God will approve the person who perseveres. "Blessed is a man who perseveres under trial; for once he has been approved, he will receive the crown of life which the Lord has promised to those who love Him" (James 1:12). The word *blessed* refers to the very highest experience; in this case, God's approval. "Approved" was the word stamped on cookware after it came out of the potter's fire with no cracks. God may sometimes turn up the heat to remove the cracks in your life. After being tested, each person is promised a stamp of approval.

With a thought of joy and expectation, look at some of the trials you may suffer in marriage. Don't be caught off guard by trials when they come. When shocked by trials, you may have a tendency to blame others. Often couples go through trials and blame their mates for what God is allowing to happen in their lives.

OUR PERSONAL "THORNS IN THE FLESH"

Almost every person has one or two areas in his or her life that are just plain tough. Paul mentioned one such problem in 2 Corinthians 12. In order to limit his pride, God gave him a "thorn in the flesh" (verse 7) to keep him from exalting himself. We cannot be sure what Paul's problem was, but he clearly called it a weakness.

> Concerning this I implored the Lord three times that it might leave me. And He has said to me, "My grace is sufficient for you, for power is perfected in weakness." Most gladly, therefore, I will rather boast about my weaknesses, so that the power of Christ may dwell in me. Therefore, I am well content with weaknesses, with insults, with distresses, with persecutions, with difficulties, for Christ's sake; for when I am weak, then I am strong (verses 8–10).

Many people have burdens to bear. Your acceptance of the thorns you have is vital to maturing in your Christian life. You can prepare yourself for the possibility that you and your mate will have at least one area that will probably never change and you will have to view it as Paul did his thorn.

For some people it might be stubbornness, a weight problem, temper, sloppiness, or low self-image. I have seen some great men with pride problems and some with insecurities. In my own life, my insecurity related to public speaking is definitely a problem, my "thorn in the flesh." I am convinced that it is there for my good and that it will become a source of strength in my life. Public speaking is an area I have fought, questioned, and agonized with God about; it has caused my family some trauma, and me some heartache, yet it is still there.

In working through my thorn, I have been able to recognize other peoples' thorns. I know there are millions of marriages where mates are paralyzed because of some unchangeable weakness in themselves or their mates that has robbed them of all hope and joy.

If you or your mate have a problem that seems impossible to work with, approach it as Paul did. If it never changes, then thank God for it and ask Him to use it in your life to develop endurance, patience, maturity, and compassion.

VARIOUS TRIALS:
OUR JOBS, CHILDREN, AND RELATIONSHIPS

We will face many trials as married adults. Many of the tensions, arguments, and heartaches are caused by the transgression or misunderstanding of others.

But often the trial comes through our own personal sins or irresponsible behavior. In this section, we will consider how to respond to our own sins and those of others.

If you determine that you brought the trial into your life through sin or a bad decision, confess it to God. After confessing, begin to take the appropriate steps to resolve it. Be sure to seek forgiveness from others when appropriate.

The following three areas are examples of trials people create—problems resulting from unresolved broken relationships with friends, family, and children, financial irresponsibility, jealousy, gossip, and uncontrolled anger.

Concerning trials on our jobs:

Let's recognize first that as career men and women move through life, they go through many cycles in their working relationships. Everyone needs to work hard and feel both productive and appreciated. There are a number of factors that affect a person's happiness at work, such as knowing he or she is in the right job, being excited about going to work, enjoying his or her work, and being proud of the job done.

Men and women—including wives and mothers, who as homemakers have tasks that can give both satisfaction and benefit others—need to prepare for trials in their work. You may be happy one day and dissatisfied the next. Wives need to trust and support their husbands during periods of dissatisfaction, which can last for extended lengths of time. Husbands, likewise, need to understand and encourage their wives who work in the home or in an outside job.

Job frustration is a normal and predictable problem in life. One of the main sources of stress while working outside the home is fellow workers. Jealous supervisors, insensitive owners, coworkers who gossip, and those with irritating personalities are not unusual. Their negative actions, like ours, are caused by sinful, selfish natures, yet we cannot ignore them. At times, going to work is painful.

Here are some suggestions to deal with trials in the workplace. First, identify these incidents as trials. Then talk to your mate about them. An understanding and supportive mate will strengthen you at such times. Pull together! Support each other while developing a plan to correct the problems (where it's in your power to do so). Seek counsel if you need to.

Working men and women can become accountable to several older adults of the same sex, preferably in their church, to help them evaluate and keep perspective during trials. For women working as homemakers, both husbands and older, mature Christian women can provide support for the daily tensions of maintaining the home.

Continually evaluate if you are doing what you enjoy and do well. If not, consider contacting an agency for counsel and a career assessment. We recommend Life Pathways, a division of Christian Financial Concepts. Life Pathways can help you to develop a conservative strategy and to move slowly toward what you enjoy and do well.

Concerning the rearing of children:

We believe that children are a major blessing in life, yet realize they can also be a source of major trials along the way. They, like us, are sinners, and we are rearing them to become independent adults. That means they will make mistakes and disappoint us. We need to be patient and forgiving of them. It also means we will make mistakes as we correct and help them. During the child-rearing years, the trials will come regularly.

Men, if you support your wife in these trials, you will make these times much easier and a greater blessing for your family. A woman's major mission field is often her children. She will tend to evaluate her worth in life in terms of her children's success. It is not a surprise, then, that God would use children to teach women dependence. If husbands share this responsibility properly, wives will feel less stress.

The initial trials with children can develop as early as during pregnancy and the first year of a child's life, for the newborn and unborn are indeed needy. An understanding and patient husband will help with meals and housework both during pregnancy and the first months of the baby's life. Though some trials are momentary and passing, babies can disrupt a mother with their sickness, sleeping problems, and scheduling. The husband must be able to help his wife during these times, and not allow her to take all of the responsibility.

When children reach school age, parents begin to observe potential emotional, intellectual, and spiritual needs. Anticipate these trials and support one another. Fathers, stay involved in your children's accomplishments, failures, and disappointments. Don't let those failures and disappointments— including those that are actually based on your own expectations or preferences—make you upset; instead, encourage your children. And don't leave school discipline problems to your wife. Instead, plan to visit your child's teacher with your wife.

The process of disciplining children is a continual trial, especially for mothers. Husbands can save their wives much frustration by taking responsibility for part of the discipline. We recommend that the father take a three-day period every two months to run a discipline check and then fine-tune his children's discipline. Children respond beautifully to fathers who take authority and spend quality time with them. A father who disciplines but fails to spend time loving his children makes a serious mistake. It takes both love and discipline to develop healthy relationships.

Concerning personal relationships:

Realize that as husband and wife, each of you will face challenges and disappointments with friends and acquaintances on the job, in the neighborhood, and at church. How you deal with hurtful relationships as a couple will largely determine your happiness in life. Why? Dealing with hurt quickly can prevent anger and bitterness from developing. Not dealing with such tensions can lead to the bitterness that robs couples of hope and faith.

Long–term bitterness is faith's enemy.

Prepare for trials in working relationships. Realize that people will fail to appreciate you, use you for selfish purposes, blame you for failure, question your abilities, and even cut you out of future plans. These typical hurts can cause bitterness. Gear up for these occasional shocks and protect your spouse when he or she encounters such trials. Losing a job or missing a promotion is a small thing for the Lord to overcome. Remember: Long-term bitterness is faith's enemy. Help one another to maintain hope in the Lord and His Word during these trials. Also remember that *people are not your enemies.* Satan wants you to believe that they are in order to distract and discourage you.

Church relationships, close friends, family, and neighbors are sources of potential trials. Aggressively apply the law of love, but expect occasional hurts. When it happens, renew your mind, and pull together as a couple. Above all, don't be critical of others.

TRIALS OF GREAT PAIN:
DEATH OF FAMILY MEMBER, INFERTILITY, DIVORCE

Many couples face trials that produce great pain, including the death of a family member, infertility, and divorce.

Whether it be a parent, child, or friend, eventually you will lose a family member. Christ removed the sting of death, yet we still suffer the loss here on Earth. *Death* can be very discouraging and depressing. Husbands and wives must stand together in their pain, pray for one another, and seek help when necessary.

Losing a child is one of the most painful and devastating trials in life. The pain often lasts years, and only God can bring you through it with hope and healing. As Christians, our view of death is different than the world's perspective. God also gives us other people to offer comfort, and we can welcome them. Others who have experienced this loss can become valuable allies in time of need. Support groups are very important as well.

And, as you receive comfort, remember God gives you a great opportunity to give back to others: "[God] comforts us in all our troubles, so that we can comfort those in any trouble with the comfort we ourselves have received from God. For just as the sufferings of Christ flow over into our lives, so also through Christ our comfort overflows" (2 Corinthians 1:4–5 NIV).

Infertility may be more common than you think. Even if you never personally face infertility, it is likely you will meet someone who will. The number of couples having difficulties conceiving children has increased significantly in recent years, though the reasons for the dramatic climb have remained unclear. New research seems to point to longer use of the birth control pill and pregnancy in later years as the largest factors causing infertility. Past abortions may also have a negative effect. The latest statistic is that one in six couples has difficulty getting pregnant. Some cannot get pregnant without medical help.

The emotional and financial toll caused by this problem can be hurtful, as well as discouraging. At times the wife may feel like a failure. The husband must convince her that his love is not contingent upon her ability to conceive and bear children. Remind her from Scripture that God not only makes rich and poor, but He also controls the womb. Help turn her perspective to God by reminding her that she is your provision from the Lord, with or without children. A wife needs to emotionally support her husband who may be the reason for the infertility. He can blame himself for the inability of his wife to conceive, also.

A husband . . . must convince her that his love is not contingent upon her ability to conceive and bear children.

There are many doctors today who specialize in fertility. Good support groups exist to help couples confront this potentially painful situation, and they can give much guidance and comfort. Couples who face this trial should seek God's perspective on each possible solution.

His perspective will give comfort. For instance, many infertile couples feel that they are being judged by God for some past sins. Although infertility was a temporal curse under the Mosaic Law (see, for example, Leviticus 26:9, 15; Deuteronomy 28:4, 11, 18), those warnings are part of the Old Covenant God had with the children of Israel. We cannot apply the Old Covenant to God's relationship with us in the New Covenant. To do so is to misuse the Scriptures.

Properly applying the Scriptures can actually give infertile couples hope for one loving remedy: adoption. Adoption is used as one of the most significant descriptions of our relationship with God in the New Covenant. When we trust Christ as our personal Savior, God "adopts" us as His own children forever, according to the Scriptures. (See Romans 8:15, 23; Galatians 4:4–6; and Ephesians 1:5–6.) Since God has adopted us into His forever family, we can consider human adoption as a divine alternative to infertility. What a divine blessing to be able to love and disciple children who would not otherwise come in contact with the things of God. Adoption can be very fulfilling for those who sense in prayer that God is directing them into this joyful adventure. If you choose to adopt, remember that adopted children, like biological children, will bring challenges that require love, patience, and understanding.

Finally, *divorce* represents one of the most painful periods of any person's life, hurting both spouses and any children. If you are considering divorce, we urge you to view that as a last resort. Get counsel, read the Scriptures, and see if the marriage can be healed.

If divorce (or separation) has already occurred, seek God's wisdom in His Word and from godly mentors and counselors. Those who have undergone divorce often feel they're failures and unworthy; sometimes they are unable to trust anyone afterward. The divorced must deal with grief and release anger and bitterness. It's OK to grieve and be angry for a season, but don't stay there and become bitter. The divorced also must learn to forgive and often need to reestablish their faith in God. With forgiveness comes healing of the soul and mind.

During such crisis points, solace comes ultimately in God—seeking His face through Bible study, prayer, and sometimes fasting. If you are contemplating remarriage, be sure you have come to the point of once more trusting God and trusting others. Forgiveness reestablishes faith, and faith causes us to mature, in spite of deep pain in our lives.

When it comes to any trial, if you have not brought the trial into your life, assume it is from God's loving hand for your benefit and His glory. Begin to apply the perspectives taught in Scripture concerning trials. Thank the Lord for each trial and you will be blessed for your faith.

TRIALS OF THE EVERYDAY

Often our trials are not the heartache of death, the absence of children, or the pain of fractured relationships. There are the trials of the everyday living as husband and wife. Two trials you should be alert to as a family are the pressures of moving and busy schedules.

America is such a mobile society that people change residences frequently. Yet few things affect the emotional security of a family more. Selling your home and buying another one, followed by the move, are only the beginning. Many other things change: relationships, church and organizational ties, friends, and security. New frontiers must be forged, new relationships built, a new job begun, and a new church home established. Probably the most difficult part of a move is making new friends. It takes several years to replace good friends.

Your children also experience tremendous loss, especially their close friends. Be very patient and tender with them as they go through their tears and ask "why?"

Since moving is so common, it is important as a couple to support one another in all the changes. Begin by making the decision together; include the whole family when possible, and then work out a total plan that gives everyone hope. God doesn't often move people into a spiritual vacuum. Before you finalize your move, also try to find a church home.

Pray about everything as you plan the move. Years ago, before our move from Dallas to Little Rock, we prayed for specific things. Todd prayed for a creek in the backyard, Carmen prayed for a two-story house, and Sally prayed for red brick with yellow trim. We flew to Little Rock, found a realtor, and told her what we wanted. She said, "I've got just the house." And it was. We also prayed for a neighborhood with children, friends for Sally, and a church like the one in Dallas. We ended up starting a church just like the one in Dallas. God specifically answered all of these requests. We had not prayed specifically for our previous moves, and for the most part, those moves were more anguishing. I am convinced that if we spend time on our knees, God will know our requests! He will glorify Himself by meeting our needs as a family.

You need time for yourself, for romance, for the children, for ministry, for hobbies.

And what about busy family schedules? Managing time usually becomes one of the biggest trials in married life. You need time for yourself, for romance, for the children, for ministry, for hobbies—even time just to read a good book. Many Christians trying to do what is right in their marriages usually lose the battle with their schedules.

You must get tough with establishing priorities. There are so many responsibilities and good things to distract you that only a clear commitment to time priority will suffice.

Men, take responsibility here. A wife cannot do much without her husband's involvement. First, decide on your major priorities, listing what you need to accomplish in each area. After that, you will have to eliminate almost everything else. Sally and I discuss our schedules in order to gain input and suggestions from each other. Just communicating helps us to eliminate unneeded or unwanted things in our schedules. We have learned that trials result from becoming overcommitted. Husbands and wives can help each other say, "No, I can't do that right now." Those are difficult words to say, but it helps if we understand our limitations.

Because of the importance of time control and schedule in relation to a man's priorities, I occasionally will ask two or three close Christian brothers to sit down and go over my schedule. After Sally gives her perspective, I try to schedule a meeting with these men six weeks later to evaluate my schedule and priorities. Sally also makes herself accountable with other women. If they agree with us on our busy schedules, then we know it is momentarily workable and our priorities are in the order the Lord would desire.

For accountability, husbands should consider joining a men's accountability group. Because men usually have difficulty expressing feelings, hurt, frustration, and struggles, a group creates accountability in these areas. For women, small prayer groups or Bible studies are invaluable for friendships, as well as accountability and encouragement. Couples would do well to learn to be leaders of small groups within their churches. These small groups could include marriage studies, parenting issues, the Christian faith, and financial studies.

FINDING VISION
THROUGH OUR TRIALS

Often the very trial you go through may in fact be saving your life and may eventually save someone else's. Our ministry organization, Christian Family Life, and this book were the result of trials we encountered in early marriage. Many organizations and support groups, such as Mothers Against Drunk Driving and Alcoholics Anonymous, started because of painful trials in someone's life. Almost all biblical characters endured various trials. So you are not alone. The very trial that you may be experiencing now may, in fact, lead you to your life's work. Life, at best, brings uncertainty and trials, but these trials are always good for us. They teach us contentment in life and dependence on God. As the apostle Paul wrote:

> Not that I speak from want; for I have learned to be content in whatever circumstances I am. I know how to get along with humble means, and I also know how to live in prosperity; in any and every circumstance I have learned the secret of being filled and going hungry, both of having abundance and suffering need. I can do all things through Him who strengthens me (Philippians 4:11–13).

The better you are at anticipating trials, the more growth you will experience in your faith. The greater your faith, the greater your spiritual maturity. There is a difference in anticipating trials and living in worry and anxiety. Look beyond the trial and ask God how He wants to use it. God is good, and He has a purpose for every trial that we encounter.

Epilogue

IN CHAPTER 1 WE RECOUNTED HOW THE TWO OF US experienced a turbulent beginning to marriage, like many couples. Our struggle provoked this question, "If God designed marriage, can He make it work?" We found the answer to be a resounding yes. We trust this book has led you to the same answer.

Our central message declares that spiritual marriages require faith. When speaking of Scripture's greatest examples of faith, the writer of Hebrews said, "And without faith it is impossible to please Him, for he who comes to God must believe that He is and that He is a rewarder of those who seek Him" (Hebrews 11:6). Faith demonstrates our belief in God and, as a result, pleases Him. It is no surprise that God designed marriage to increase our faith in Him. We cannot please Him without faith.

Faith requires two things. First, it requires that we know and trust Him as God, the creator of heaven and earth. Second, if we truly know Him, we are to trust Him to reward us according to His magnificent promises. No individual can love by faith without believing that God's Word is more powerful than their mate's weaknesses.

True faith always produces good works. As your faith produces good works toward your mate, God will astonish you by fulfilling His magnificent promises to you from His Word. Faith allows us to override our natural selfishness by choosing to act on God's Word. Faith then releases God to do what He said He would do.

To experience a supernatural "faith marriage," your spouse and you must embrace each of the commitments discussed in this book. Let's quickly review these commitments:

1. Each of you must openly confess your selfish tendencies. Commit to change the course of your marriage in the future by seeking a faith relationship.

2. Each of you must accept your responsibility from God to fulfill His purposes of *reflecting* God's image, *reproducing* His image through children and disciples, and *reigning* on earth to His glory. These purposes require oneness between husband and wife.

3. Each of you must accept from God that you were created with a relational need that can be met only by God. Then, by faith, you must receive your mate as God's personal provision for your aloneness need.

4. Loving your mate by faith will require you to individually submit your will to the Holy Spirit's ministry in your life. This means you must allow the Holy Spirit to convict, teach, lead, and empower you. Remember, marital oneness cannot exist apart from the Holy Spirit.

5. Marital oneness requires each of you to understand God's agents for change in marriage. Scripture endorses two forces of change: (1) sacrificial love as demonstrated by Christ and (2) returning a blessing when wronged. You must trust God to change your mate as you faithfully love and bless him or her.

6. The divine order of oneness is love and submission, as illustrated in the Trinity of God (1 Corinthians 11:3 and John 17:20–21). It takes great faith, spiritual insight, and trust to joyfully love and respect each other. Each of you must ask God for wisdom on a daily basis to defeat Satan's worldly deceit.

7. Displaying godly traits toward each other requires your being people of faith. Such traits will bring harmony and peace to your home.

These commitments form the basis of a supernatural faith relationship. Good intentions or natural desires will never result in a faith relationship. A faith relationship results from knowing and applying God's Word. How do you know if you have a faith relationship? The only way to know is for both mates to commit to the above insights by faith. Sally and I, as good as our original intentions were, did not understand these insights when we married. Later we understood and committed to these principles, and our marriage changed dramatically.

Such faith commitments will affect the practical areas of marriage, including sex, finances, and communication. Each of you must discover what God's Word says on each subject and then apply it by faith.

It takes time and effort to fully discover a supernatural faith relationship. But make no mistake—a faith relationship starts by understanding and applying the six insights just summarized. Do not put this book down until you have made these commitments by faith. Then share them with others to deepen and revitalize your understanding over time.

In 1979, when we first wrote this book then titled *Becoming One* (having been married only twelve years), Sally and I experienced firsthand the results of God's principles of marriage in our own lives. Now, thirty-plus years later, we have been more than pleased to still experience joy in each other, to laugh and play together, to work together, to write and create together. But most rewarding is the fact that all four of our children are walking with God. As we have tried to reflect God's image as a couple and reign together as a couple, God has rewarded us with a godly heritage.

All four of our children have married spouses who love and walk with God. We have been blessed also with all of their spouses' godly families. What rich rewards! We say all of this not because our kids have been perfect but because God said if we obey Him, He would bless us. And bless us He has! We say this to give the honor where honor is due: to God the Father, God the Son, and God the Holy Spirit.

Sally and I pray that you too will be able to apply the following verses to your marriage: "For this reason a man shall leave his father and his mother, and be joined to his wife; and they shall become one flesh. And the man and his wife were both naked and were not ashamed" (Genesis 2:24–25). We wish each of you the joy of being totally exposed to each other with no fear or threat. If you miss this joy of being one, you will have missed much of God's blessing on this earth. Only faith can release God's blessing in your marriage.

OTHER RESOURCES
FROM CHRISTIAN FAMILY LIFE

Don and Sally Meredith founded Christian Family Life, Inc., in 1971 to further the training of professional counselors as well as laypeople. In 1976, they helped start the Family Life Ministry of Campus Crusade for Christ. The Merediths, who are marriage counselors, developed a discipleship course designed for married and engaged couples.

The course is contained in the *Two Becoming One Workbook.* The workbook helps couples to implement the principles from *Two Becoming One* into their lives. We encourage you to consider the workbook as a follow-up tool for applying the principles of this book and enriching your marriage. For more information, or to order workbooks and other supplies, visit us at *www.2becoming1.com* or call (800) 264-3876.

You may want to consider promoting or leading a church or at-home class to study the workbook. If you would like more information on organizing or leading such a group study, we invite you to visit us online at *www.2becoming1.com.*

A PUBLICATION OF
CHRISTIAN FAMILY LIFE, INC.

Christian Family Life teaches engaged and married couples God's faith principles for marriage so they may know Christ more intimately and be free to serve Him more effectively. The ministry of Christian Family Life is extended primarily through small groups, publications, Sunday School and the Internet. For more information about Christian Family Life, please visit us on the Internet at www.2becoming1.com.

To order resources please go to www.2becoming1.com or call toll-free (800) 264-3876.

Christian 💕
FamilyLife

Christian Family Life, Inc.
13415 Reese Blvd. West
Huntersville, NC   28078

1-704-987-8270